DISC INCLUDED

Evidence-based Infectious Diseases

Evidence-based Infectious Diseases

Edited by

Mark Loeb
Department of Pathology and Molecular Medicine,
Department of Clinical Epidemiology and Biostatistics,
McMaster University, Hamilton, Ontario, Canada

Marek Smieja
Department of Pathology and Molecular Medicine,
Department of Clinical Epidemiology and Biostatistics,
Department of Medicine,
McMaster University, Hamilton, Ontario, Canada

Fiona Smaill
Department of Pathology and Molecular Medicine,
Department of Medicine,
McMaster University, Hamilton, Ontario, Canada

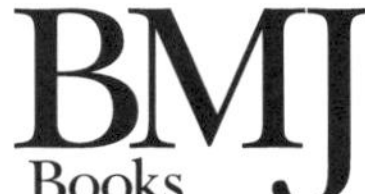

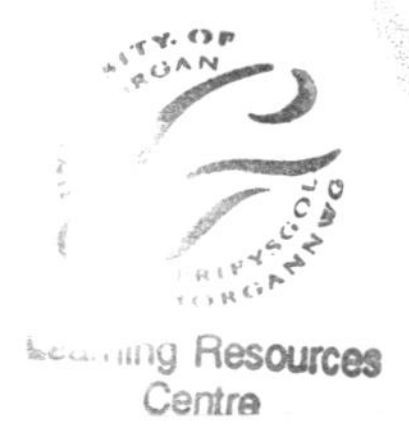

BMJ Books is an imprint of the BMJ Publishing Group Ltd

First published in 2004
by BMJ Books, BMA House, Tavistock Square,
London WC1H 9JR

www.bmjbooks.com

British Library Cataloguing in Publication Data

A catalogue record for this book is available from the British Library

ISBN 0 7279 1691 2

Typeset by SIVA Math Setters, Chennai, India
Printed and bound by MPG Books, Bodmin, Cornwall

Contents

Contributors

Elias Abrutyn
Department of Medicine, MCP Hahnemann School of Medicine, Philadelphia, PA, USA

Brian J Angus
Nuffield Department of Medicine, University of Oxford, John Radcliffe Hospital, Headington, Oxford, UK

Doug Austgarden
Department of Emergency Medicine and Critical Care, York Central Hospital, Richmond Hill, Ontario, Canada

A Bouckenooghe
Regulatory Affairs, Merck Sharp & Dohme (Europe) Inc., Brussels, Belgium

Eric J Bow
Sections of Infectious Diseases and Haematology/Oncology, University of Manitoba, Canada

Guy de Bruyn
Program in Infectious Diseases, Fred Hutchinson Cancer Research Center; Division of Allergy and Infectious Diseases, Department of Medicine, University of Washington, Seattle, USA

Robert Burrell
Chemical and Materials Engineering, University of Alberta, Edmonton, Alberta, Canada

Manjula Datta
Department of Epidemiology, The Tamilnadu Dr M.G.R. Medical University, Chennai, India

Thomas Fekete
Section of Infectious Diseases, Temple University School of Medicine, Philadelphia, USA

David N Fisman
Drexel University School of Public Health and Drexel University College of Medicine, Philadelphia, PA, USA

William Gillespie
The Hull York Medical School, UK

Carolyn V Gould
Department of Medicine, Division of Infectious Diseases, University of Pennsylvania School of Medicine, Philadelphia, PA, USA

Scott D Halpern
Center for Clinical Epidemiology and Biostatistics; Department of Biostatistics and Epidemiology; Center for Education and Research on Therapeutics, University of Pennsylvania School of Medicine, Philadelphia, PA, USA

Anthony Harris
University of Maryland, VA Maryland Health Care System, Baltimore, Maryland, USA

Ebbing L Lautenbach
Department of Medicine, Division of Infectious Diseases; Department of Biostatistics and Epidemiology; Center for Clinical Epidemiology and Biostatistics; Center for Education and Research on Therapeutics, University of Pennsylvania School of Medicine, Philadelphia, PA, USA

Christine H Lee
Department of Pathology and Molecular Medicine; Department of Medicine, McMaster University, Hamilton, Ontario, Canada

Mark Loeb
Department of Pathology and Molecular Medicine; Department of Clinical Epidemiology and Biostatistics, McMaster University, Hamilton, Ontario, Canada

Sarvesh Logsetty
Department of Surgery and Firefighters' Burns Treatment Unit, University of Alberta, Edmonton, Alberta, Canada

Eli Perencevich
University of Maryland, VA Maryland Health Care System, Baltimore, Maryland, USA

Timothy Peto
Nuffield Department of Medicine, University of Oxford, John Radcliffe Hospital, Headington, Oxford, UK

Robert Rennie
Medical Microbiology, University of Alberta Hospital, Edmonton, Alberta, Canada

David C Rhew
Zynx Health Incorporated, Beverly Hills, California, USA

Stuart Rosser
Sections of Infectious Diseases and Critical Care, University of Manitoba, Canada

Fiona Smaill
Department of Pathology and Molecular Medicine; Department of Medicine, McMaster University, Hamilton, Ontario, Canada

Marek Smieja
Department of Pathology & Molecular Medicine; Department of Clinical Epidemiology & Biostatistics; Department of Medicine, McMaster University, Hamilton, Ontario, Canada

Brian L Strom
Center for Clinical Epidemiology and Biostatistics; Department of Biostatistics and Epidemiology; Center for Education and Research on Therapeutics; Division of General Internal Medicine, University of Pennsylvania School of Medicine, Philadelphia, PA, USA

Edward E Tredget
Dept of Surgery, University of Alberta, Edmonton, Alberta, Canada

Preface

As busy academic physicians we are often approached about assuming new roles and responsibilities, and frankly are sometimes hesitant about placing yet another item on the "to do" list. However, when we were first approached about editing this book, our reaction was different. The idea of editing the first book about evidence-based infectious diseases was exciting. Although there are many standard textbooks on infectious diseases, none that we were aware of use an "evidence-based" approach.

We emphasize in this book both the methodological issues in assessing the quality of evidence, as well as the "best evidence" for practicing infectious diseases. We have divided the book into two parts. In Part I, we focus on specific infections, including skin and soft tissue infections, bone and joint infections, infective endocarditis, meningitis and encephalitis, community-acquired pneumonia, tuberculosis, diarrhea, urinary tract infections, sexually transmitted infections, and human immunodeficiency virus (HIV). In Part II, we focus on infections that occur in specific populations and settings. These include infection control, infections in the neutropenic host, surgical infections, the thermally injured patient, and infection in healthcare workers. We have asked chapter authors to begin with a clinical scenario, to help focus on relevant clinical questions, and then to briefly summarize the burden of illness or background epidemiology. The remainder of each chapter summarizes the best evidence with respect to diagnosis, prognosis, treatment, and prevention, with a focus, where possible, on systematic reviews.

As we discuss in the introductory chapter, we believe that important clinical questions that arise should be approached in a systematic fashion. The chapters in this book will never be as up to date as the information that you can derive by searching the most recent literature. This is particularly relevant when we are faced with new emerging infections, such as severe acute respiratory syndrome (SARS). However, browsing through these chapters will give a good context and will provide you with key evidence that you can update by conducting a search to see if there is any useful new information. While evidence from well-designed studies informs the decision-making process, it obviously does not replace it. The outcomes of a clinical trial, for example, may suggest a default antibiotic to use for pneumonia, but does not preclude our individualizing treatment based on patient allergies, the biology of the responsible organism, or the pharmacokinetics and pharmacodynamics of the drugs to be administered in that patient.

We hope that our approach will help to emphasize aspects of diagnosis, prognosis, treatment, or prevention in which there is already excellent evidence, while highlighting areas in which more compelling evidence is needed. In these latter areas in which our confidence is limited, the reader should be particularly careful to look for newer published data when faced with a similar clinical problem.

We are grateful to the chapter authors who made this book possible. We appreciate the guidance (and patience) of Christina Karaviotis and Mary Banks from BMJ Books. We thank our families (Andrea, Julia, and Nathalie Loeb; Cathy Marchetti and Daniel, Nicole, and Benjamin Smieja; Peter Seary) for their patience and support.

We hope you find this book informative and stimulating, and we shall certainly appreciate any feedback.

Mark Loeb
Marek Smieja
Fiona Smaill

Evidence-based Infectious Diseases CD Rom

Features

Evidence-based Infectious Diseases PDF eBook

- Bookmarked and hyperlinked for instant access to all headings and topics
- Fully indexed and searchable text – just click the "Search Text" button

BMJ Books catalogue

- Instant access to BMJ Books full catalogue, including an order form

Also included – a direct link to the Evidence-based Infectious Diseases update website

Instructions for use

The CD Rom should start automatically upon insertion, on all Windows systems. The menu screen will appear and you can then navigate by clicking on the headings. If the CD Rom does not start automatically upon insertion, please browse using "Windows Explorer" and double-click the file "BMJ_Books.exe".

Tips

The viewable are of the PDF ebook can be expanded to fill the full screen width, by hiding the bookmarks. To do this, click and hold on the divider in between the bookmark window and the main window, then drag it to the left as required.

By clicking once on a page in the PDF eBook window, you "activate" the window. You can now scroll through pages using the scroll-wheel on your mouse, or by using the cursor keys on your keyboard.

Note: the Evidence-based Infectious Diseases PDF eBook is for search and reference only and cannot be printed.

Troubleshooting

If any problems are experienced with use of the CD Rom, please send an email to the following address stating the problem you have encountered:

cdsupport@bmjbooks.com

Evidence-based Infectious Diseases update website

Further information and updates can be found at:
http://www.evidbasedinfectiousdisease.com

Abbreviations

AFB	acid fast bacilli
ACE	angiotensin-converting enzyme
ADC	AIDS dementia complex
ALC	absolute lymphocyte count
ALP	alkaline phosphatase
ALT	alanine aminotransferase
AMC	absolute monocyte count
AML	acute myeloid leukemia
ANC	absolute neutrophil count
ARDS	adult respiratory distress syndrome
ARR	absolute risk reduction
ASCUS	atypical squamous cells of undetermined significance
AST	aspartate aminotransferase
BAL	bronchoalveolar lavage
CABG	coronary artery bypass graft
CAP	community-acquired pneumonia
CE	contrast enema
CI	confidence interval
CG	control group
CMV	cytomegalovirus
COPD	chronic obstructive pulmonary disease
CS	corticosteroid
CSF	cerebrospinal fluid
CT	computed tomography
CXR	chest *x* ray film
DFA	direct immunofluorescent antibody
DILD	diffuse infiltrative lung disease
DOT	directly observed therapy
DQ	Diff-Quik
EBID	evidence-based infectious diseases
EG	experimental group
EIA	enzyme immunoassay
ELISA	enzyme-linked immunosorbent assay
FNE	febrile neutropenic episode
FTA-Abs	fluorescent treponemal antibody absorbed assay
GGT	gamma glutamyl transferase
GM-CSF	granulocyte-macrophage colony-stimulating factor
HAART	highly active antiretroviral therapy
HBO	hyperbaric oxygen therapy
HBsAg	hepatitis B surface antigen
HEPA	high efficiency particulate air

HICPAC	Hospital Infection Control Practices Advisory Committee
HPV	human papillomavirus
HSV-1	Herpes simplex virus type 1 infection
HSV-2	Herpes simplex virus type 2 infection
ICU	intensive care unit
IE	infective endocarditis
IFA	indirect immunofluorescent antibody
IG	immunoglobulin
ITT	intent-to-treat
IVIG	intravenous immunoglobulin
IVU	intravenous urography
LCR	ligase chain reaction
LDH	lactate dehydrogenase
LEE	liver enzyme elevation
LOS	length of hospital stay
LR	likelihood ratio
LTBI	latent TB infection
MAC	*Mycobacterium avium* complex
MBS	microbiologic study
MCV	mean corpuscular volume
MDR-TB	multidrug resistant tuberculosis
MEMS	Medication Event Monitoring System
MODS	multiple organ dysfunction syndrome
MRSA	methicillin-resistant *Staphylococcus aureus*
MVP	mitral-valve prolapse
NNH	number needed to harm
NNIS	National Nosocomial Infections Surveillance
NNT	number needed to treat
OI	opportunistic infection
OR	odds ratio
PCP	*Pneumocystis carinii* pneumonia
PCR	polymerase chain reaction
PHI	primary HIV infection
PI	protease inhibitor
PID	pelvic inflammatory disease
PM	printed materials
PML	progressive multifocal leukoencephalopathy
PORT	Patient Outcomes Research Team
PPM	polypropylene mesh
PSI	Pneumonia Severity Index
PTFE	polytetrafluoroethylene
RCT	randomized controlled trial
ROC	receiver operating characteristic
RR	relative risk
RR	respiratory rates

RRR	relative risk reduction
SARS	severe acute respiratory syndrome
SIRS	systemic inflammatory response syndrome
SMX	sulfamethoxazole
SOC	suboptimal concentration
SSI	surgical site infections
STI	sexually transmitted infections
STI	structured treatment interruption
STSS	streptococcal toxic shock syndrome
TB	tuberculosis
TBSA	total body surface area
TCAA	trichloroacetic acid
TEE	transesophageal echocardiography
TMP	trimethoprim
TMP-SMX	trimethoprim-sulfamethoxazole
TTE	transthoracic echocardiography
UTI	urinary tract infection
VRE	vancomycin-resistant enterococcus
ZN	Ziehl–Neelsen

1

Introduction to evidence-based infectious diseases

Mark Loeb, Marek Smieja, Fiona Smaill

Our purpose in this chapter is to provide a brief overview of evidence-based infectious diseases practice and to set the context for the chapters which follow. We highlight evidence-based guidelines for assessing diagnosis, treatment, and prognosis, and discuss the application of evidence-based practice to infectious diseases, as well as identifying areas in which such application must be made with caution.

What is evidence-based medicine?

Evidence-based medicine was born in the writings of clinical epidemiologists at McMaster University, Yale, and elsewhere. Two series of guidelines for assessing the clinical literature articulated these, then revolutionary, ideas and found a wide audience of students, academics, and practitioners alike.[1,2] These guidelines emphasized the randomized clinical trial (RCT) for assessing treatment, now a standard requirement for the licensing of new drugs or other therapies. David Sackett, the founding chair of the Department of Clinical Epidemiology and Biostatistics at McMaster University, defined "evidence-based medicine" as "the conscientious, explicit and judicious use of current best evidence in making decisions about the care of patients".[3]

These guidelines, which we summarize later in the chapter, were developed primarily to help medical students and practicing doctors find answers to clinical problems. The reader was guided in assessing the published literature in response to a given clinical scenario, to find relevant clinical articles, to assess the validity and understand the results of the identified papers, and to improve their clinical practice. Aided by computers, massive databases, and powerful search engines, these guidelines and the evidence-based movement empowered a new generation of practitioner and have had a profound impact on how studies are conducted, reported, and summarized. The massive proliferation of randomized clinical trials, the increasing numbers of systematic reviews and evidence-based guidelines, and the emphasis on appropriate methods of assessing diagnosis and prognosis, have affected how we practice medicine.

Evidence-based infectious diseases

The field of infectious diseases, or more accurately the importance of illness due to infections, played a major role in the development of epidemiological research in the 19th and early 20th centuries. Classical observational epidemiology was derived from studies of epidemics – infectious diseases such as cholera, smallpox, and tuberculosis. Classical epidemiology was nevertheless action-oriented. For example, John Snow's observations regarding cholera led to his removal of the Broad Street pump handle in an attempt to reduce the incidence of cholera. Pasteur, on developing an animal vaccine for anthrax, vaccinated a number of animals with members of the media in attendance.[4] When unvaccinated animals subsequently died, while vaccinated animals did not, the results were immediately reported throughout Europe's newspapers.

In the era of clinical epidemiology, it is notable that the first true randomized controlled trial is widely attributed to Sir Austin Bradford Hill's 1947 study of streptomycin for tuberculosis.[5] In subsequent years, and long before the "large simple trial" was rediscovered by the cardiology community, large-scale trials were carried out for polio prevention, and tuberculosis prevention and treatment.

Having led the developments in both classical and clinical epidemiology, is current infectious diseases practice evidence-based? We believe the answer is "somewhat". We have excellent evidence for the efficacy and side effects of many modern vaccines, while the acceptance of before-after data to prove the efficacy of antibiotics for treating bacterial meningitis is ethically appropriate. In the field of HIV medicine we have very strong data to support our methods of diagnosis, assessing prognosis and treatment, as well as very persuasive evidence supporting causation. However, in treating many common infectious syndromes – from sinusitis and cellulitis to pneumonia – we have many very basic diagnostic and therapeutic questions that have not been optimally answered. How do we reliably diagnose pneumonia? Which antibiotic is most effective and cost-effective? Can we improve on the impaired quality of life that often follows such infections as pneumonia?

While virtually any patient presenting with a myocardial infarction will benefit from aspirin and thrombolytic therapy, there may not be a single "best" antibiotic for pneumonia. Much of the "evidence" that guides therapy in the infectious diseases, particularly for bacterial diseases, may not be clinical, but exists in the form of a sound biologic rationale, the activity of the antimicrobial against the offending pathogen and the penetration at the site of infection (pharmacodynamics and pharmacokinetics). Still, despite having a sound biologic basis for choice of therapy, there are many situations where better randomized controlled trials need to be conducted and where clinically important outcomes, such as symptom improvement and health-related quality, are measured.

How, then, can we define "evidence-based infectious diseases" (EBID)? Paraphrasing David Sackett, EBID may be defined as "the explicit, judicious and conscientious use of current best evidence from infection diseases research in making decisions about the prevention and treatment of infection of individuals and populations". It is an attempt to bridge the gap between research evidence and the clinical practice of infectious diseases. Such an "evidence-based approach" may include critically appraising evidence for the efficacy of a vaccine or a particular antimicrobial treatment regimen. However, it may also involve finding the best evidence to support (or refute) use of a diagnostic test to detect a potential pathogen. Additionally, EBID refers to the use of the best evidence to estimate prognosis of an infection or risk factors for the development of infection. EBID therefore represents the application of research findings to help answer a specific clinical question. In so doing, it is a form of knowledge transfer, from the researcher to the clinician. It is important to remember that use of research evidence is only one component of good clinical decision-making. Experience and clinical skills are essential components. EBID serves to inform the decision-making process. For the field of infectious diseases, a sound knowledge of antimicrobials and microbiologic principles are also needed.

Posing a clinical question and finding an answer

The first step in practicing EBID is posing a clinically driven and clinically relevant question. To answer a question about diagnosis, therapy, prognosis, or causation, one can begin by framing the question.[2] The question usually includes a brief description of the patients, the intervention, the comparison, and the outcome (a useful acronym is "PICO"). For example, if asking about the efficacy of antimicrobial-impregnated catheters in intensive care units,[6] the question can be framed as follows: "In critically ill patients, does use of antibiotic-impregnated catheters reduce central line infections?" After framing the question, the second step is to search the literature. There are increasingly a number of options for finding the best evidence. The first step might be to assess evidence-based synopses such as Evidence-Based Medicine or ACP Journal Club (we admit to bias – two of the editors [ML, FS] are associate editors for these journals). These journals regularly report on high quality studies that can impact practice. The essential components of the studies are abstracted and the papers are reviewed in an accompanying commentary by knowledgeable clinicians. However, since these journals are geared to a general internal medicine audience, many questions faced by clinicians practicing infectious diseases may not be addressed.

The next approach that we would recommend is to search for systematic reviews. Systematic reviews can be considered as concise summaries of the best available evidence that address sharply defined clinical questions.[7] Increasingly, the Cochrane Collaboration is publishing high quality infectious diseases systematic reviews (http://www.cochranelibrary.com). Another source of systematic reviews is the *Data Base of Abstracts of Reviews of Effects (DARE)* (http://nhscrd.york.ac.uk/darehp.htm). To help find systematic reviews, MEDLINE can be searched using the systematic review clinical query option in PUBMED (http://www.ncbi.nlm.nih.gov/PubMed/). If there are no synopses or systematic reviews that can answer the clinical question, the next step is search the literature yourself by accessing MEDLINE through PUBMED. After finding the evidence the next step is to critically appraise it.

Evidence-based diagnosis

Let us consider the use of a rapid antigen detection test for group A streptococcal infection in throat swabs. The first question to ask is whether there was a blinded comparison against an accepted reference standard. By blinded, we mean that the measurements with the new test were done without knowledge of the results of the reference standard.

Next, we would assess the results. Traditionally, we are interested in the sensitivity (proportion of reference-standard positives correctly identified as positive by the new test) and specificity (the proportion of reference-standard negatives correctly identified as negative by the new test). Ideally, we would also like to have a measure of the precision of this estimate, such as a 95% confidence interval on the sensitivity and specificity, although such measures are rarely reported in the infectious diseases literature.

Note, however, that while the sensitivity and specificity may help a laboratory to choose the best test to offer for routine testing, they do not necessarily help the clinician. Thus, faced with a positive test with known 95% sensitivity and specificity, we cannot infer that our patient with a positive test for group A streptococcal infection has a 95% likelihood of being infected. For this, we need a positive predictive value, which is calculated as the percentage of true positives among all those who test positive. If the positive predictive value is 90%, then a positive test would suggest a 90% likelihood that the person is truly infected. Similarly, the negative predictive value is the percentage of true negatives among all those who test negative. Both positive and negative predictive value change with the underlying prevalence of the disease, hence such numbers cannot be generalized to other settings.

A more sophisticated way to summarize diagnostic accuracy, which combines the advantages of positive and negative predictive values while solving the problem of varying prevalence, is to quantify the results using likelihood ratios. Like sensitivity and specificity, likelihood ratios are a constant characteristic of a diagnostic test, and independent of prevalence. However, to estimate the probability of a disease using likelihood ratios, we additionally need to estimate the probability of the target condition (based on prevalence or clinical signs). Diagnostic tests then help us to shift our suspicion (pretest probability) about a condition depending on the result. Likelihood ratios tell us how much we should increase the probability of a condition for a positive test (positive likelihood ratio) or reduce the probability for a negative test (negative likelihood ratio). More formally, likelihood ratio positive (LR+) and negative (LR–) are defined as:

$$\text{LR+} = \frac{\text{odds of a positive test in an individual } \textbf{with} \text{ the condition}}{\text{odds of a positive test in an individual } \textbf{without} \text{ the condition}}$$

$$\text{LR}- = \frac{\text{odds of a negative test in an individual } \textbf{with} \text{ the condition}}{\text{odds of a negative test in an individual } \textbf{without} \text{ the condition}}$$

A positive likelihood ratio is also defined as follows: sensitivity/(1-specificity). Let us assume, hypothetically, that the sensitivity of the rapid antigen test is 80% and the specificity 90%. The positive likelihood ratio for the antigen test is (0·8/0·1) or 8. This would mean that a patient with a positive antigen test would have 8 times the odds of being positive compared with a patient without group A streptococcal infection. The tricky part in using likelihood ratios is to convert the pretest probability (say 20% based on our expected prevalence among patients with pharyngitis in our clinic) to odds: these represent 1:4 odds. After multiplying by 8, we have odds of 8:4, or a 67% post-test probability of disease. Thus, our patient probably has group A streptococcus, and it would be reasonable to treat with antibiotics.

The negative likelihood ratio, defined as (1–sensitivity)/specificity, tells us how much we should reduce the probability for disease given a negative test. In this case, the negative likelihood ratio is 0·22, which can be interpreted as follows: a patient with pharyngitis and a negative antigen test would have their odds of disease multiplied by 0·22. In this case, a pretest probability of 20% (odds 1:4) would fall to an odds of 0·22 to 4, or about 5%, following a negative test. Nomograms have been published to aid in the calculation of post-test probabilities for various likelihood ratios.[8]

Having found that the results of the diagnostic test appear favorable for both diagnosing or ruling out disease, we ask whether the results of a study can be generalized to the type of patients we would be seeing. We might also call this "external validity" of the study. Here we are asking the question: "Am I likely to get the same good results as in this study in my own patients." This includes such factors as the severity and spectrum of patients studied versus those we will encounter in our own practice, and technical issues in how the test is performed outside of the research setting.

To summarize, to assess a study of a new diagnostic test, we identify a study in which the new test is compared with an independent reference standard; we examine its sensitivity, specificity, and positive and negative likelihood ratios; and we determine whether the spectrum of patients and technical details of the test can be generalized to our own setting.

In applying these guidelines in infectious diseases, there are some important caveats.

- There may be no appropriate reference standard.
- The spectrum of illness may dramatically change the test characteristics, as may other co-interventions such as antibiotics.

For example, let us assume that we are interested in estimating the diagnostic accuracy of a new commercially available polymerase chain reaction (PCR) test for the rapid detection of *Neisseria meningitidis* in spinal fluid. The reference standard of culture may not be completely sensitive. Therefore, use of an expanded reference ("gold") standard might be used. For example, the reference standard may be growth of *N. meningitidis* from the spinal fluid, demonstration of an elevated white blood cell count in the spinal fluid along with Gram negative bacilli with typical morphology on Gram stain, or elevated white blood cell count along with isolation of *N. meningitidis* in the blood.

It is also important to know in what type of patients the test was evaluated, such as the inclusion and exclusion criteria as well as the spectrum of illness. Given that growth of micro-organisms is usually progressive, test characteristics in infectious diseases can change depending when the tests are conducted. For example, PCR conducted in patients who are early in their course of meningitis may not be sensitive as compared to patients that presented with late stage disease. This addresses the issue of spectrum in test evaluation.

Evidence-based treatment

The term "evidence-based medicine" has become largely synonymous with the dictum that only randomized, double-blinded clinical trials give reliable estimates of the true efficacy of a treatment. For the purposes of guidelines, "levels of evidence" have been proposed, with a hierarchy from large to small RCTs, prospective cohort studies, case–control studies, and case series. In newer iterations of these "levels of evidence", a meta-analysis of RCTs (without statistical heterogeneity, indicating that the trials appear to be estimating the same treatment effect), are touted as the highest level of evidence for a therapy.

In general, clinical questions about therapy or prevention are best addressed through randomized controlled trials. In observational studies, since the choice of treatment may have been influenced by extraneous factors which influence prognosis (so-called "confounding factors"), statistical methods are used to "adjust" for identified potentially confounding variables. However, not all such factors are known or accurately measured. An RCT, if large enough, deals with such extraneous prognostic variables by equally apportioning them to the two or more study arms by randomization. Thus, both known and unknown confounders are distributed roughly evenly between the study arms.

For example, a randomized controlled trial would be the appropriate design to assess whether dexamethasone administered prior to antibiotics reduces mortality in adults who have bacterial meningitis.[9] We would evaluate the following characteristics of such a study: who was studied; was there true random assignment; were interventions and assessments blinded; what was the outcome; and can we generalize to our own patients?

When evaluating clinical trials it is important to ensure that assignment of treatment was truly randomized. Studies should describe exactly how the patients were randomized (for example, random numbers table, computer generating). It is also important to assess whether allocation of the intervention was truly concealed. It is especially important here to distinguish allocation concealment from blinding. Allocation of an intervention can always be concealed even though blinding of investigators, participants or outcome assessors may be impossible. Consider an RCT of antibiotics versus surgery for appendicitis (improbable as this is). Blinding participants and investigators after patients have been randomized would be difficult (sham operations are not considered ethical). However, allocation concealment occurs before randomization. It is an attempt to prevent selection bias by making certain that the investigator has no idea to what arm (antibiotics versus surgery) the next patient enrolled will be randomized. In many trials this is done through a centralized randomized process whereby the study investigator is faxed the assignment after the patient has been enrolled. In some trials, the assignment is kept in envelopes. The problem with this is that, if the site investigator (or another clinician) has a preference for one particular intervention over another, the possibility for tampering exists. For example, if a surgeon who is a site investigator is convinced that the patient he has just enrolled would benefit most from surgery, the surgeon might be tempted to hold the envelope up to a strong light, determine the allocation, and then select another if the contents of the envelope do not indicate surgery as the allocation. This would lead to selection bias and distort the result of the clinical trial. This type of tampering has been documented.[10]

The degree of blinding in a study should also be considered. It is important to recognize that blinding can occur at six levels: the investigators, the patients, the outcome assessors, adjudication committee, the data monitoring committee, the data analysts, and even the manuscript writers (although in practice few manuscripts are written blinded of the results).[11] Describing a clinical trial as "double-blinded" is vague if in fact blinding can occur at so many different levels. It is better to describe who was blinded than using generic terms.

Similarity of groups at baseline should also be considered when evaluating randomized controlled trials to assess whether differences in prognostic factors at baseline may have had an impact on the result. A careful consideration of the intervention is also important. One can ask what actually constitutes the intervention – was there a co-intervention that really may have been the "active ingredient"?

Follow up is another important issue. It is important to assess whether all participants who were actually randomized are accounted for in the results. A rule of thumb is that the potential for the results to be misleading occurs if fewer than 80% of individuals randomized are not accounted for at the end (i.e. loss to follow up of over 20% of participants). More rigorous randomized controlled trials are analyzed on an intention to treat basis. That is, all patients randomized are accounted for and are analyzed with respect to the group to which they were originally allocated. For example, an individual in our hypothetical appendicitis trial who was initially randomized to antibiotics but later received surgery would be considered in the analysis to have received antibiotics.

Having assured ourselves that the study is randomized, the randomization allocation was not prone to manipulation, and the randomized groups have ended up as comparable on major prognostic factors, we next examine the actual results. Consider a randomized controlled trial of two antibiotics A and B for community-acquired pneumonia. If the mortality rate with antibiotic A is 2% and that with B is 4%, the absolute risk reduction is the difference between the two rates

(2%), the relative risk of A versus B is 0·5, and the relative risk reduction is 50%, that is the difference between the control and intervention rate (2%) divided by the control rate (4%). In studies with time-to-event data, the hazard ratio is measured rather than the relative risk, and can be thought of as an averaged relative risk over the duration of the study. Absolute risk reduction, relative risk, and hazard ratios are all commonly reported with a 95% confidence interval (CI) as a measure of precision. A 95% CI that does not cross 1·0 (for a relative risk or hazard ratio) or 0 (for the absolute risk reduction) has the same interpretation as a *P* value of $< 0{\cdot}05$: we declare these results as "statistically significant". Unlike the *P* value, the 95% CI gives us more information regarding the size of the treatment effect. Note that statistical significance simply tells us whether the results were likely due to chance, the CI also tells us the precision of the estimate (helpful especially for underpowered studies, in which the wide CI warns us that a larger study may be required to more precisely determine the effect). It is important to be aware that statistical significance and clinical importance are not synonymous. A small study may miss an important clinical effect, whereas a very large study may reveal a small but statistically significant difference of no clinical importance. In well-designed studies, researchers prespecify the size of a postulated "minimum clinically important difference" rather than solely relying on statistical significance.

Measures of relative risk, hazard ratios, or absolute risk reduction may be difficult to apply in clinical practice. A more practical way of determining the size of a treatment effect is to translate the absolute risk reduction into its reciprocal, the number needed to treat (NNT). In this example, the number needed to treat is the number of patients who need to be treated to present one death. It is the inverse of the absolute risk reduction (1/0·02), which is 50. Therefore, if 50 patients are treated with antibiotic B instead of A, one death would be prevented. A 95% CI can be calculated on the NNT, although we would only recommend such calculations for statistically significant treatment effects. This recommendation is based on the curious mathematical property that, as the absolute risk reduction crosses 0, the NNT becomes infinite, and thereafter crosses over into the bounds of a "number needed to harm".

It is important to determine if all important outcomes were considered in the randomized controlled trial. For example, a clinical trial of a novel immunomodulating agent for patients with severe West Nile virus disease would need not only to consider neurological signs and symptoms but also to assess functional status and health-related quality of life. When deciding whether the results of a randomized trial can be applied to your patients, the similarity in the setting and patient population needs to be considered. Finally, you must consider whether the potential benefits of the therapy outweigh the potential risks.

Rather than relying on individual RCTs, it is generally preferable to try to identify systematic reviews on the topic. Systematic reviews, however, also need to be critically evaluated. First, one must ensure that the stated question of the review addresses the clinical question that you are asking. The methods section should describe how all relevant studies were found: that is, including the specific search strategy as well as the inclusion and exclusion criteria. Study validity should be assessed, although there is no universally accepted method for scoring validity in systematic reviews. Both size and precision of treatment effects need to be considered. Similar to evaluating randomized controlled trials, whether all important outcomes were assessed in the review is important. Asking whether the findings are generalizable to your patients and whether the likely benefits are worth the potential harms and benefits is also important.

In summary, to assess a treatment we would find a systematic review or clinical trial; assess whether patients were properly randomized; whether various components of the study were blinded; whether there was a high proportion followed up for all clinically relevant outcomes. We then consider the actual results, and express these ideally as a "number needed to treat" to appreciate the importance (or lack thereof) for individual patients. Finally, we consider whether these results are applicable to the type and severity of disease that we may see in our clinics.

In examining a treatment in infectious diseases, a few caveats to these guidelines are in order.

- For many infections there may be a very strong historic and biologic rationale to treat; in such cases an RCT using placebo will be unethical.
- Many infections may be too rare to study in RCTs, and some infected populations (such as injection drug users) may be difficult to enrol into treatment studies. Observational methods, such as case–control or cohorts to examine therapies or durations associated with cure or relapse, may be the most appropriate methods in these circumstances.
- While the individually randomized clinical trial is held up as an ideal, it may be more sensible to study many infections through so-called "cluster randomization" in which the unit of randomization may be the hospital, a school, neighbourhood, or family. Such studies may detect a treatment effect where herd immunity is important, and may be more feasible to run. However, the confidence intervals for a cluster-randomized study are somewhat wider than if individuals are randomized.
- Even when individually randomized, the infection itself may represent a "cluster". Thus, a highly effective therapy for one strain of multidrug resistant (MDR) *M. tuberculosis* may be useless against another MDR strain. Hence, biological knowledge of the pathogen and therapy need to be considered when the results of an RCT are generalized to a particular clinical setting.

Evidence-based assessment of prognosis

Many studies about risk factors and outcomes for infectious diseases are published but the quality is variable. The best designs for assessing these are cohort studies in which a representative sample of patients is followed, either prior to developing the infection (to determine risk) or after being infected (to determine outcome). Patients should be assembled at a similar point in their illness (the so-called "inception cohort"), and follow up should be sufficiently long and complete. Important prognostic factors should be measured, and adjusted for in the analysis. As with clinical trials, the outcome measures are a relative risk, absolute risk, or hazard ratio associated with a particular infection or prognostic factor. For example, to assess the outcome of patients with severe acute respiratory syndrome (SARS), one would optimally want an inception cohort of individuals who meet the case definition within several days of onset of symptoms. These individuals would then be followed prospectively. One of the challenges with SARS was the lack of a "real-time" diagnostic test with high sensitivity and specificity. In general, as diagnostic tests improve, our ability to detect early disease will improve. If SARS re-emerges and therapeutic agents are developed, this will change the natural history, hence the importance of noting whether therapy was administered in the cohort study. If strains of SARS coronavirus mutate as immunity to the virus builds, this may reduce the virulence of the agent. Therefore, it is important to keep in mind that estimates of risk and outcome may change with changes in the infectious agent.

Summary

We hope that the approaches described in this chapter will prove useful for evaluating articles about diagnosis, prognosis, treatment, or prevention in the infectious diseases literature. Using the principles described in this chapter, the chapters that follow attempt to summarize the best evidence for key clinical issues about infectious diseases.

References

1. Department of Clinical Epidemiology and Biostatistics. How to read clinical journals: I. why to read them and how to start reading them critically. *CMAJ* 1981;**124**:555–8.
2. Oxman A, Sackett, DL, Guyatt GH. Users' guides to the medical literature. I. How to get started. *JAMA* 1993;**270**: 2093–5.
3. Sackett DL, Rosenberg WM, Gray JA, Haynes RB, Richardson WS. Evidence-based medicine: what it is and what it isn't. *BMJ* 1996;**312**:71–2.
4. Dubos R. *Pasteur and Modern Science*. Washington: ASM Press 1998.
5. Daniels M, Hill AB. Chemotherapy of pulmonary tuberculosis in young adults: an analysis of the combined results of three medical research council trials. *BMJ* 1952;**1**:1162–8.
6. Darouriche RO, Raad II, Heard SO *et al.* A comparison of two antimicrobial-impregnated central venous catheters. *N Engl J Med* 1999;**340**:1–8.
7. Cook DJ, Mulrow CD, Haynes RB. Systematic reviews: synthesis of best evidence for clinical decisions. *Ann Intern Med* 1997;**126**:376–80.
8. Detsky AS, Abrams HB, Forbath N, Scott JG, Hilliard JR. Cardiac assessment for patients undergoing noncardiac surgery. A multifactorial clinical risk index. *Arch Intern Med* 1986;**146**:2131–4.
9. de Gans J, van de Beek D. Dexamethasone in adults with bacterial meningitis. *N Engl J Med* 2002;**347**:1549–56.
10. Schulz KF, Grimes DA. Allocation concealment in randomized trials: defending against deciphering. *Lancet* 2002;**359**:614–18.
11. Devereau PJ, Manns BJ, Ghali WA *et al.* Physician interpretations and textbook definitions of blinding terminology in randomized controlled trials. *JAMA* 2001;**285**:2000–3.

Part 1
Specific diseases

2
Skin and soft-tissue infections

Doug Austgarden

Cellulitis

Case presentation 1

A healthy 45-year-old man hit his forearm while doing some house renovations, causing a minor abrasion, 3 days prior to his presentation to the Emergency Department. He noted some minor swelling, pain, and erythema yesterday, but this morning he noted much more pain. His right forearm was swollen and erythema covered most of the dorsal surface from wrist to elbow. The emergency physician refers him for consideration of parenteral therapy and inpatient treatment with concerns about the area of involvement and rate of spread. His health is otherwise excellent.

On examining the patient, he is afebrile, pulse rate of 78 per minute and blood pressure of 134/75 mmHg. He has a small abrasion on his dorsal wrist with erythema extending to the elbow. The erythema is not raised, has indistinct borders, with no vesicles or bullae. The lesion is warm, tender to palpation, but there is no increase in pain on movement.

Cellulitis is a common problem in primary care but only a minority are referred to consultants or admitted for inpatient treatment. A review of a patient database in five urban hospitals showed 3929 diagnoses of cellulitis representing 1·3% of Emergency Department visits; 7% required inpatient treatment.[1]

Cellulitis usually presents with pain, erythema with typically indistinct borders and swelling. Fever and regional lymphadenitis are occasionally seen. In a predominately outpatient population, pain, erythema, and swelling were described in 69%, 78%, and 69% of cases, respectively, while fever and lymphadenitis occurred in only 7% and 10% of patients.[1] For an inpatient population, pain, erythema, and swelling were seen in 87%, 79%, and 90%, respectively, and fever occurred in 63% of patients.[2] Unfortunately, these signs and symptoms are not specific and many other processes can present with similar clinical findings, for example superficial or deep vein thrombophlebitis, fasciitis, hematoma, dermatitis, and local reaction to a bite or sting.

Most commonly *Staphylococcus aureus* and *Streptococcus pyogenes* are the pathogens. Less often and usually associated with underlying chronic disease, immunosuppression, or infection at a particular site, for example periorbital cellulitis with sinusitis, pathogens can include *Haemophilus influenzae*, *Pseudomonas aeruginosa*, other *Streptococci* spp., gram-negative bacilli, *Clostridia* spp., and other anaerobes.[3,4] In a data registry of hospitalized patients in Canada and the USA, 1562 bacterial isolates were identified over 1 year in a wide variety of patients with skin and soft-tissue infections: *S. aureus* accounted for 42·6% of isolates, with 24% being MRSA, *P. aeruginosa* (11·3%), *Enterococcus* spp. (8·1%), *Escherichia coli* (7·2%), *Enterobacter* spp. (5·2%), and β-hemolytic streptococci (5·1%).[5] Essentially the same rank was seen in both countries with the exception of *Enterococcus* spp. which was third in the USA and seventh in Canada.[5] If there is a concern with exposure to water, certain specific organisms should be considered. In salt water, *Vibrio vulnificus* can cause a cellulitis and a potentially life-threatening infection in patients with liver disease. In fresh water, *Aeromonas hydrophilia* is a possible pathogen.

Erysipelas is a distinctive form of cellulitis. The lesion is typically bright red, warm, painful (which differentiates it from more superficial infections) with a raised, clearly demarcated border (usually not seen in other forms of cellulitis.) Facial erysipelas with the often described malar "butterfly" rash actually represents only 15–20% of cases and most infections involve the lower extremity.[3,4] Systemic symptoms, for example fever, chills, sweats and rigors are common. Infants, young children, and older adults are most commonly affected. Erysipelas has a predisposition for areas of impaired lymphatic drainage and in these patients recurrent episodes can occur.[4] Group A streptococcus is primarily responsible for erysipelas but groups B, C, and G, as well as *S. aureus* have been described.[5] Only 5% of blood cultures are positive.[3]

Surface cultures, aspiration, and blood cultures all have low diagnostic yield in identifying the infecting organism causing cellulitis. Surface cultures are not recommended because of low yield and contamination with skin flora. Some advocate culturing an intact pustule if present.[3] Several studies have described varying techniques to aspirate from the lesion, resulting in positive cultures from 10% to 100% of the time.[7–10] In a large retrospective study of over 750 patients with cellulitis and 553 blood cultures, only 2% of blood cultures yielded a pathogen, and 73% of these were β-hemolytic streptococci.[11] In the healthy patient without an unusual exposure, microbiological testing is neither necessary or cost-effective.

Routine laboratory investigations have little diagnostic role in managing the healthy patient with cellulitis but may be required in the management of patients with chronic diseases, such as diabetes, liver disease, or renal failure, where an infection may lead to acute deterioration of the underlying disease, influencing the choice and dose of antibiotics and the decision whether to admit.

Plain radiographs to rule out a foreign body are sometimes needed. Often *x* ray films are obtained to screen for tissue air if necrotizing fasciitis is a concern, or for osteomyelitis in an infected diabetic foot ulcer.

Case presentation 1 (continued)

After careful review you decide this patient has cellulitis and unlikely has a fasciitis. Since he is otherwise healthy and no history of unusual exposure you feel no extra tests are required. You are, however, concerned about the size and the rapidity of spread and decide this patient needs parenteral antibiotics, but which one(s) and does he need to be admitted?

In mild and localized cellulitis in otherwise healthy patients presenting to the Emergency Department, an oral agent covering *S. aureus* and *Streptococcus* spp. is sufficient, and there is no advantage to agents with broader spectrum antimicrobial activity.[12] A penicillinase-resistant penicillin, first- or second-generation cephalosporin, or macrolide have appropriate activity, although no studies demonstrating superiority of one agent over another have been done. Seven to ten days of therapy with the agent at its higher dose range is recommended, but no study has addressed the duration needed nor the optimal dose. Prophylactic penicillin is recommended for patients with recurrent episodes, although one study showed that this approach was only effective in patients without predisposing factors.[13,14]

In patients with more severe cellulitis, it is generally accepted that parenteral antibiotics are required. What is not well defined is in which patients cellulitis should be deemed moderate or severe. Studies of moderate or severe cellulitis have included patients with cellulitis and one or more of the following: extensive area, ulceration, abscess, signs of toxicity or sepsis, associated with surgical site, bite, foreign body, trauma, intravenous drug injection site, diabetic foot or pressure ulcer, immunosuppression (for example, HIV), diabetes, or chronic corticosteroid use or failure of previous therapy.[15,16,18,21–24]

Many antibiotic regimens evaluated in methodologically sound studies have demonstrated similar efficacy with inpatient populations and complicated skin infections: pipercillin-tazobactam.[15] ticarcillin-clavulanate,[15,16] levofloxacin,[16,19] teicoplanin,[17,20] meropenem,[18] imipenem/cilastin,[18] ceftriaxone,[20,24–27] ciprofloxacin,[22] ofloxacin,[22] cefotaxime,[21,22] linezolid,[23] oxacillin,[23] and cefazolin.[26,27] Clinical cure rates ranged from 84% to 98·4% and microbiological cure rates from 71% to 94%. Owing to differences in patient populations, no one agent should be considered superior. Any subsequent changes or additions should be based on clinical response and any positive cultures of presumed pathogens.

Many patients may choose to be treated with parenteral therapy on an outpatient basis. Although there have been no randomized controlled trials comparing inpatient versus outpatient therapy for skin and soft-tissue infections, prospective evaluations of outpatient antibiotic programs have shown that they are safe and effective.[20,24–28]

Intravenous ceftriaxone has been widely recommended for outpatient therapy owing to its once daily dosing.[24,25] Two studies have demonstrated that cefazolin and probenecid have equivalent efficacy to ceftriaxone in an outpatient setting.[26,27] Brown *et al.* randomized 194 patients with moderate-to-severe cellulitis to 2 g intravenous cefazolin daily or 2 g intravenous ceftriaxone daily, while both groups received probenecid 1 g orally.[26] Outcomes were similar, 91·8% versus 92·7% clinical cure, with cost savings associated with the cefazolin group. However, the majority of patients were intravenous drug users with injection site infections, follow up was not complete and patients were given a prescription for penicillin and cloxacillin upon enrolment.[26] Grayson *et al.* randomized 116 patients who presented with moderate to severe cellulitis to 2 g intravenous cefazolin and 1 g probenecid orally or 1 g intravenous ceftriaxone and placebo.[27] Clinical cure rates were similar: 86% in the cefazolin arm versus 96% in the ceftriaxone arm ($P = 0{\cdot}11$) and remained equivalent up to 1 month follow up, 96% versus 91% ($P = 0{\cdot}55$).[27] Both studies excluded patients with penicillin allergies, septic patients requiring hospitalization, patients with evidence of osteomyelitis, and significant renal failure.

Oral antibiotics with a broad spectrum of antimicrobial activity and equivalent bioavailability to intravenous regimens offer another alternative for the outpatient management of patients with complicated skin and soft-tissue infections. In a randomized trial comparing intravenous or oral levofloxacin and intravenous ticarcillin/clavulanate alone or followed by oral amoxicillin/clavulanate, 44 of 200 patients in the levofloxacin group had oral therapy only.[16] Forty patients (90·9%) in this subset had clinical cure, which was a similar rate to either group: 84·1% in the levofloxacin group and 80·4% in the ticarcillin/clavulanate group.[16] Although this subset was not specifically analyzed, the authors caution that it may have had less severe disease.[16] The other fluoroquinolones, for example moxifloxacin and gatifloxacin, with improved gram-positive activity, could be expected to be similarly effective.

There are many options for patients with more complicated cellulitis, and choice of antibiotic should be individualized based on the patient's history and any extenuating circumstances. For most patients, outpatient therapy is safe and effective. Once daily regimens such as cefazolin and probenecid provide an easy, effective, and low-cost alternative. Follow up and clinical response should dictate changes of antibiotic therapy.

Necrotizing fasciitis

Case presentation 2

A previously healthy carpenter presents to the Emergency Department with fever and a painful arm. Yesterday at work he began to notice a sore right shoulder, was assessed in the Emergency Department later that evening, and diagnosed with a soft-tissue injury. Today he has pain in his shoulder and upper arm as well as fever and lethargy. On examination he is in moderate to severe distress from the pain, his temperature is 38·9°C, heart rate 122 per minute, and blood pressure of 90/60 mmHg. There is no obvious trauma or rash on his arm, but it is generally swollen and exquisitely tender to palpation and on movement of the shoulder or elbow. You begin to wonder if this man has a life-threatening infection.

Necrotizing fasciitis involves infection of the subcutaneous tissue with rapid spread and destruction of skin, subcutaneous fat, and fascia. Fortunately, it is a relatively uncommon life-and limb-threatening infection, but requires early recognition, prompt surgical intervention, and broad-spectrum antibiotics. Many names have been used based upon clinical circumstances and pathogen, for example classic (clostridial) gas gangrene, clostridial cellulitis, non-clostridial gas gangrene, Fournier's gangrene, Meleney's synergistic gangrene, necrotizing cellulitis, crepitant cellulitis, streptococcal gangrene, and, in the lay press, the term "flesh-eating bacteria" has been coined. Classification systems have also been developed based on pathogen[3] but are unhelpful clinically.

The literature on necrotizing fasciitis is predominately empiric, based on retrospective reviews and small case series. With the emergence of group A streptococcal fasciitis and associated toxic shock syndrome, more knowledge and understanding has been gained, but because of the relative rarity of cases and the complexity of the illness, randomized trials of management will be difficult to undertake.

The incidence of necrotizing fasciitis has been estimated at four cases per million.[29] A prospective cohort study monitoring the incidence of group A streptococcus in Ontario, Canada between 1991 and 1995 showed an increasing incidence from 0·85 per million to 3·5 per million during the study.[30] The CDC has estimated 500 to 1500 cases of group A streptococcus worldwide annually.[31]

The presentation of necrotizing fasciitis can vary from the appearances of a simple cellulitis or soft-tissue injury to the classic hemorrhagic bullae, presence of soft-tissue gas, septic shock, and multiorgan failure. Toxic shock syndrome and multiorgan failure were also present in 47% of patients with group A streptococcus necrotizing fasciitis.[30] Most cases of necrotizing fasciitis initially present with a cellulitis but progress over hours to days with spreading erythema and edema. Hemorrhagic bullae can form as a result of skin necrosis secondary to vessel thrombosis. Pain out of proportion to clinical findings is commonly reported as an important early sign. Anesthetic skin due to destruction of nerves can be a late sign. Soft-tissue gas is a classic finding especially with clostridial infection. Estimates of the frequency of these signs and symptoms are not available.

Necrotizing fasciitis should be considered in any patient with "cellulitis" and systemic symptoms of fever and tachycardia, or rapidly spreading infection. Commonly necrotizing fasciitis starts at a pre-existing skin lesion, such as a surgical site, trauma, chronic skin problems (for example, pressure ulcer, diabetic foot, ischemic ulcer, or psoriasis), and, in children, varicella infection predisposes for necrotizing fasciitis.[3,29,30,32–35] In Kaul *et al.* a predisposing skin lesion was present in 74% of cases of group A streptococcus necrotizing fasciitis.[30] Any underlying medical condition, such as diabetes, alcohol abuse, immunosuppressive illness or treatment, cardiac disease, peripheral vascular disease, chronic lung disease or chronic renal failure, should increase the suspicion for necrotizing fasciitis.[3,29,30,32,33,35] In Kaul *et al.* one or more of these conditions were present in 71% of cases.[30] Any area of the body can be involved, but the lower extremity accounted for 53% of cases, while the upper extremity was involved 29% of the time.[30]

Necrotizing fasciitis can be caused by many organisms and usually is polymicrobial with a mixture of aerobic and anaerobic bacteria. One review showed that 85% of confirmed cases of necrotizing fasciitis were polymicrobial, while *S. aureus*, *S. pyogenes*, and *Clostridia* spp. were the most commonly isolated single pathogen.[36] Usual aerobic pathogens are *S. aureus*, *S. pyogenes*, and *E. coli*, while *Clostridia* spp., *Bacteroides fragilis* and *Peptostreptococcus* spp. are predominate anaerobes. Rarely, and usually as a copathogen, other gram-positive organisms such as *Streptococcus pneumoniae*, gram-negatives such as *Pseudomonas aeruginosa*, *Serratia*, *Vibrio*, *Proteus*, *Enterobacter*, *Pasteurella*, *Eikenella*, *Neisseria*, and anaerobes *Fusobacterium* and *Prevotella* spp. can cause necrotizing fasciitis.

The gold standard for diagnosis is surgical exploration to determine fascial involvement and to provide material for culture and microscopic examination.[3,29,32–35,37] Surgical exploration will also indicate the need for surgical debridement. In a small retrospective study, a frozen-section biopsy with urgent histopathologic analysis reduced mortality.[38] Fine-needle aspirate is positive for bacteria or pus 80% of the time.[39] Soft-tissue gas observed clinically or with plain films is diagnostic, but not always present. Ultrasound, CT, and MRI have all been used to aid in the diagnosis of necrotizing fasciitis[39–45] but performance indicators (sensitivity and specificity) of ultrasound and CT in diagnosing necrotizing fasciitis have not been published. In two studies, totalling 25 patients, MRI had a 100% sensitivity but a specificity of 100% and 75%, respectively.[43,44] Other conditions (i.e. cellulitis and abscesses) can be indistinguishable from necrotizing fasciitis.[45] Imaging should not delay definitive surgical treatment in the unstable patient. Laboratory investigations such as creatine kinase, C-reactive protein, serum sodium, WBC count, serum calcium, creatinine, urea, and coagulation profiles have all been proposed to aid diagnosis, but lack sensitivity to reliably rule out necrotizing fasciitis.[3,29,30,46,47]

Case presentation 2 (continued)

As you page the surgeon and begin resuscitating this young man, you wonder which antibiotics you could give immediately to cover the potential pathogens and whether there are other therapies that might save his life.

Immediate resuscitation, including ventilatory and inotropic support, prompt surgical debridement or amputation and broad-spectrum parenteral antibiotics are the mainstay of management.[3,4,29,30,32–35,37] Owing to the diversity of potential pathogens and because the majority of cases of necrotizing fasciitis are associated with polymicrobial infection, the most commonly recommended initial antibiotic is a β-lactam/β-lactamase inhibitor plus clindamycin.[3,4,29,32–35,37,48] Acceptable alternative regimens include single agents such as carbapenems, second-generation cephalosporins or fluoroquinolones with anaerobic activity and combinations with ampicillin and metronidazole or clindamycin, with either a third-generation cephalosporin, an aminoglycoside, fluoroquinolone, or aztreonam.[3,4,29,32–35,48] With animal models of group A streptococcus necrotizing fasciitis, clindamycin has been shown to have more effective killing power than penicillin, because bacteria reach the stationary growth phase rapidly while penicillin loses effectiveness in this phase.[3] Clinical data seem to support this with improved survival in patients treated with clindamycin.[30,48] Also owing to its effect on protein synthesis inhibition and toxin production, clindamycin may improve survival in patients with group A streptococcus necrotizing fasciitis.[3,30,32] Once a pathogen(s) has been identified, antibiotics should be tailored to the pathogen(s). For group A streptococcus necrotizing fasciitis, penicillin and clindamycin is recommended.[3,30,32] In penicillin-allergic patients, a second- or third-generation (if *Pseudomonas* is a consideration) cephalosporin can usually be safely substituted.[49,50] If a patient has a true penicillin/cephalosporin allergy a fluoroquinolone, macrolide, or vancomycin may be alternatives.

In a case–control study intravenous immunoglobulin (IG) dosed at 2 g/kg appears to decrease mortality in patients with group A streptococcus necrotizing fasciitis, but there are, however, no data from randomized trials to support this.[51] All patients in these studies had toxic shock syndrome. Intravenous IG appears to modulate the superantigen response in group A streptococcus necrotizing fasciitis.[30,51] The Ontario Group A Streptococcal Study Group have proposed a conservative non-surgical approach to group A streptococcus necrotizing fasciitis, using penicillin (4 million units every 6 hours), clindamycin (900 mg every 6 hours) and intravenous IG (2 g/kg). They report six successful cases (three with TSS) treated with this regimen.[52] One patient had exploratory surgery without debridement and one patient had repeated drainage of an olecranon bursitis at the bedside; the others had no surgery.[52] With the significant morbidity of large area debridement, this regimen potentially offers an alternative approach to group A streptococcus necrotizing fasciitis, but these preliminary data need further study, and currently an aggressive surgical approach remains an important component of management. Intravenous IG use in other forms of necrotizing fasciitis has not been studied, and there is no evidence to support its use apart from in invasive group A streptococcal infections.

Hyperbaric oxygen therapy (HBO) has been used as an adjunct for necrotizing fasciitis. Multiple small, retrospective studies have been done on both clostridial and non-clostridial necrotizing fasciitis with variable results. A meta-analysis showed a significant reduction in mortality in both groups: 19% versus 45% in clostridial necrotizing fasciitis and 20·7% versus 43·5% in non-clostridial necrotizing fasciitis.[53] HBO should not delay surgical debridement and unstable patients should not be transferred, but this treatment modality should be used if available.

Mortality for necrotizing fasciitis is estimated to be around 40%.[32] Specifically, group A streptococcus necrotizing fasciitis had an observed mortality of 34 to 43%.[30,33] Hypotension on presentation is associated with an 18-fold increase in death.[30] Age >65, bacteremia, chronic illness, and multiorgan failure also was associated with increased mortality.[30]

Diabetic foot infections

Case presentation 3

A 63-year-old man with a long-standing history of type 2 diabetes, complicated by peripheral neuropathy and chronic renal insufficiency, presents with a 2-day history of increasing drainage from an ulcer on his right foot. Today redness and swelling in his foot was noted. On examination he is afebrile, with a normal heart rate and blood pressure. On his right foot, he has a 2 cm ulcer on the sole between the 1st and 2nd metatarsal heads, with swelling and erythema to the mid-foot dorsally. His blood sugar is 18 mmol/liter and his WBC count is normal. Knowing the difficult nature of diabetic foot infections, you wonder which antibiotic, oral or parenteral, outpatient or inpatient, and other therapies might help in treating this man.

Due to the triad of vascular insufficiency, peripheral neuropathy, and impaired immune function, foot ulceration and infection are common among diabetics. Foot infections are among the most common cause for hospital admission in diabetics.[54,55] Osteomyelitis is present in an estimated 20% of complicated infections[56] and diabetic foot infection accounts for 50% of lower extremity amputations.[57–59] In 1996, 86 000 lower extremity amputations were performed on diabetic patients in the United States.[59] Thus, diabetic foot infections need a multidisciplinary team approach involving endocrinologist, podiatrist, wound care specialist, diabetic educators, plastic, orthopedic, and vascular surgeons, and infectious disease specialist for their care.

Usually diabetic foot infections occur in a pre-existing ulcer. Peripheral neuropathy is the greatest risk factor for foot ulcers and infection,[60] and patients often have no complaints of pain. Patients will usually have discharge from the ulcer, erythema, swelling, and unexplained hyperglycemia. If there is no draining ulcer but the foot is erythematous and swollen, a Charcot foot (diabetic neuroarthropathy) should be considered and it is unlikely that a non-inflamed ulcer is infected.[61]

Diabetic foot infections can be classified into two groups:

- non-limb-threatening, which have <2 cm of surrounding erythema extending from the ulcer, not a full-thickness ulcer and no systemic signs of toxicity
- limb-threatening, which have >2 cm of surrounding erythema, full-thickness ulcer, presence of an abscess or soft-tissue gas, rapid progression, and signs of systemic toxicity.[54,61]

Two-thirds of patients with limb-threatening infections have no fever, chills or elevated WBC count.[62]

Surface cultures from infected ulcers are considered unreliable because of superficial colonization. Curettage of the base following debridement, or aspiration from non-necrotic tissue, may yield more dependable results to identify the infecting pathogen(s).[54,61] In non-limb-threatening infection, *S. aureus* and group B streptococcus are considered the major pathogens.[62–65] *Enterococcus* spp., gram-negatives, and anaerobes are often cultured, but it is unclear if they are colonizers or pathogens.[61,69] In limb-threatening infection, gram-negatives such as *E.coli*, *Proteus* spp., *P. aeruginosa*, *Serratia* spp., and *Enterobacter* spp., and anaerobes, such as *Bacteroides* and *Peptostreptococcus* spp. are considered pathogenic.[54,61–69]

For non-limb threatening infections, initial antimicrobial therapy can be directed towards *S. aureus* and streptococci, and a first generation cephalosporin, for example, cefazolin, is an appropriate choice. In a randomized, prospective trial of non-limb-threatening diabetic foot infections, 56 outpatients received 2 weeks of either oral cefalexin 500 mg four times a day or clindamycin 300 mg four times a day as an outpatient.[62] From curettage specimens, 89% yielded gram-positive organisms (42% as a sole pathogen), 36% gram-negatives and 13% anaerobes. After 2 weeks of therapy, 91% were cured or improved, while of the five failures, three went on to cure with another agent covering gram-positive organisms (clindamycin, ampicillin, or cloxacillin). One of the other treatment failures had polymicrobial growth and, despite parenteral antibiotics for 2 months, ultimately required a forefoot amputation.[62]

For limb-threatening diabetic foot infections, broad-spectrum antibiotics are recommended and many of the trials on complicated or moderate to severe cellulitis included diabetic foot infections. Randomized trials specifically performed on diabetic foot infections included use of ampicillin/sulbactam,[66,68] imipenem/cilastin,[66] cefoxitin,[64] ceftizoxime,[67] and ofloxacin.[68] All the trials had similar results with clinical cure or improvement in the range of 80–90%. In certain circumstances, outpatient therapy would be appropriate depending on diabetic control, extent of infection, and availability of follow up.

There are other interventions that can be used in the management of diabetic foot infections. The type of wound dressing is an underused tool, and new technologies in skin substitutes have shown great promise in chronic ulcers, but have not been studied in infections.[54,70,71] Non-weightbearing and even rigid immobilization is often recommended, although no randomized trials have been performed.[72–74] Hyperbaric oxygenation has been shown to improve healing of chronic ulcers[75] and has been effective in several small studies in diabetic foot infections.[76–78] Urgent vascular bypass surgery can be an option if ischemia is a major contributor to a non-healing ulcer or infection. The risks of such surgery must be balanced with the expected benefit for each patient.[79]

For a further discussion on the management of complicated infections and osteomyelitis in diabetic patients, refer to Chapter 3.

Animal bites

Case presentation 4

A 59-year-old woman, who was trying to intervene in a fight between the family dog and a neighborhood dog, notices a 2 cm laceration over the 5th metacarpophalangeal joint after the squabble was broken up. She has a past history of angina and hypercholesterolemia and is unsure when her last tetanus booster was given. Both pets have been immunized annually. You wonder, should you close the laceration, does she need prophylaxis and, if so, with which antibiotic? Should she receive treatment for rabies?

Animal bites are very common. The vast majority of people never seek medical attention. Dog bites account for 90% of all bites, cats (5%), humans (2%), rodents (2%) and all other animals less than 1%.[80] It is estimated than 4·5 million dog bites occur annually in the USA and 7·3–18 per 10 000 bites seek medical attention.[81–83] An estimated 10 000 hospitalizations and 20 deaths per year occur secondary to dog bites, most being in children.[82,84] Deaths are usually due to the attack itself and only rarely from secondary infectious complications. Most bites are from family pets and a minority from stray animals.

Patients with bites have a bimodal pattern of presentation. If children are bitten, if the injury is significant, or if there are concerns over the potential for infection, or for tetanus and rabies, medical attention is sought immediately. Later, patients will present with signs and symptoms of secondary infection. An estimated 3–18% of dog bites and 28–80% of cat bites become infected.[86] Most bites occur on the hand or arm, children are more likely to be bitten on the face, males are more likely to be bitten by a dog, and females more likely to be bitten by a cat.[85]

Important historical information to focus on include the past medical history of the patient, especially any history of immunosuppression or significant chronic disease, status of tetanus immunization, time of and circumstances surrounding the event (provoked or unprovoked), and details concerning the animal, for example health, ownership, and location. Many patients will be reluctant to divulge information owing to concern over reprisal on the animal by local authorities. Many cities and regions have mandatory reporting of animal bites. The wound should be assessed for site and potential for nerve, tendon, bone, or joint involvement, especially on the hands and feet. Any wound over a metacarpophalangeal joint should be considered a clench fist injury (punch injury). If the patient presents with established infection, systemic signs, site and extent of infection, lymphadenopathy, and possibility of tenosynovitis, osteomyelitis and septic arthritis should be considered.

Copious irrigation, debridement of necrotic tissue and removal of foreign bodies are essential in early management of bite wounds.[84–86] Puncture wounds should be irrigated with a needle or plastic tip catheter inserted into the wound. Infected wounds should be opened if previously sutured, eschar removed and abscesses drained, then irrigated copiously. Closure of bite wounds is controversial, as there are no randomized studies of this intervention. Wounds less than 24 hours old, with no signs of infection, on the face, trunk, or proximal extremities can probably be closed safely.[86] All wounds on hands or feet, should be left open, especially if cat or human.[84–86]

Talan *et al.* have examined the bacteriology of infected dog or cat bites.[87] They examined the pathogens responsible for 50 dog bites and 57 cat bites. There were a mean of five pathogens per wound with a range of 0–16. For dogs, the most common aerobic bacteria were *Pasteurella* spp. (50% of patients) especially *Pasteurella canis*, *Streptococcus* spp. (46%), *Staphylococcus* spp. (46%), *Neisseria* spp. (16%), and *Corynebacterium* spp. (12%), while the most frequent anaerobes were *Fusobacterium* spp. (32%), *Bacteroides* spp. (30%), *Porphyromonas* spp. (28%), and *Prevotella* spp. (28%). Cats had similar bacteria, with the exception that *Pasteurella* spp. grew in 75% of cases with *P. multocida* being the most frequent species. From these data, the authors recommended a β-lactam/β-lactamase inhibitor or a second-generation cephalosporin with anaerobic activity. The combination of clindamycin and a fluoroquinolone was also recommended. There are, however, no prospective trials nor comparative studies of different antibiotic regimens for treating infected animal bites.

In human bites, the usual organisms are *S. aureus*, *Streptococcus* spp., and anaerobes, as well as an organism specific to the oral flora of humans, a fastidious gram-negative rod *Eikenella corrodens*. It has an unusual sensitivity profile in that it is sensitive to penicillin and β-lactam/β-lactamase inhibitors, but relatively resistant to cloxacillin, first-generation cephalosporins, erythromycin, and clindamycin.[84] A β-lactam/β-lactamase inhibitor combination is an appropriate initial choice.

The majority of patients with infected bite wounds can be managed as outpatients with oral antibiotics. Alternatively, parenteral antibiotics could be initiated with step-down to oral therapy when the infection is resolving. This can be accomplished with the patient either an out- or inpatient, depending on clinical circumstances.

Antibiotic prophylaxis of animal bites is controversial. A Cochrane Library systematic review showed a favorable odds ratio for prophylaxis of cat and human bites, but not dogs, and for prophylaxis in hand wounds, but not face/neck or trunk wounds.[88] A randomized, blinded, placebo-controlled trial on 185 patients with animal bites using amoxicillin/clavulanate for prophylaxis, showed no difference in wounds less than 9 hours old, but a significant difference in those 9–24 hours old.[89] Therefore the animal, location of wound, and time to presentation all seem to affect the risk of infection and need for prophylaxis.

Animal bites can potentially transmit rabies and many patients will seek medical attention for fear of rabies infection. This is a rare occurrence in industrialized countries. In Canada, 22 rabies cases have been reported in 56 years.[85] In the USA, 32 cases over 16 years have been reported.[90] Immunized animals who are acting normally over a period of 10 days are not rabid. In certain areas, wild animals such as bats, raccoons, skunks and foxes have been rabid. Local public health authorities can be a valuable resource in ascertaining the risk of rabies transmission in an individual case and the need for postexposure prophylaxis.

Infections of skin and underlying soft tissue are a common problem in primary care. While most infections are managed without complication, those referred to the hospitalist/consultant are often in patients who have failed therapy, have significant comorbidity or have a life- or limb-threatening infection. A thorough understanding of both common and unusual infectious etiologies, and local resistance patterns, are important in guiding antimicrobial choices. As well, other interventions to improve outcome can be employed and should be considered as part of the management of patients.

References

1. Dong SL, Kelly KD, Oland RC, Holroyd BR, Rowe BH. ED management of cellulitis: A review of five urban centers. *Am J Emerg Med* 2001;**19**:535–40.
2. Ginsberg MB. Cellulitis: Analysis of 101 cases and review if the literature. *South Med J* 1981;**74**:530–3.
3. Bisno AL, Stevens DL. Streptococcal infections of skin and soft tissues. *N Engl J Med* 1996;**334**:240–5.
4. Slaven EM, DeBlieux PM. Skin and soft-tissue infections: the common, the rare and the deadly. *Emerg Med Prac* 2001;**3**:1–24.
5. Doern GV, Jones RN, Pfaller MA, Kugler KC, Beach ML. Bacterial pathogens isolated from patients with skin and soft-tissue infections: frequency of occurrence and antimicrobial susceptibility patterns from the SENTRY Antimicrobial Surveillance Program (United States and Canada, 1997). SENTRY Study Group (North America). *Diag Micro Infect Dis* 1999;**34**:65–72.
6. Jorup-Ronstrom C. Epidemiological, bacterial and complicating features of erysipelas. *Scand J Infect Dis* 1986;**18**:519–24.
7. Goldgeiger MH. The microbial evaluation of acute cellulitis. *Cutis* 1983;**31**:649–56.
8. Sachs MK. The optimum use of fine needle aspiration in the bacteriologic diagnosis of cellulitis in adults. *Arch Int Med* 1990;**150**:1907–12.
9. Sigurdsson AF, Sudmundsson S. The etiology of bacterial cellulitis as determined by fine-needle aspiration. *Scand J Infect Dis* 1989;**21**:537–42.
10. Uman SJ, Kunin CM. Needle aspiration in the diagnosis of soft-tissue infections. *Arch Int Med* 1975;**135**:959–61.
11. Perl B, Gottehrer NP, Raveh D *et al.* Cost-effectiveness of blood cultures for adult patients with cellulitis. *Clin Inf Dis* 1999;**29**:1483–88.
12. Powers RD. Soft-tissue infections in the Emergency Department: the case for the use of "simple" antibiotics. *South Med J* 1991;**84**:1313–15.
13. Wang JH, Liu YC, Cheng DL *et al.* Role of benzathine penicillin G in prophylaxis for recurrent streptococcal cellulitis of the lower legs. *Clin Infect Dis* 1997;**25**: 685–9.

14. Kremer M, Zuckerman R, Avraham Z, Raz R. Long-term antimicrobial therapy in the prevention of recurrent soft-tissue infections. *J Infect* 1991;**22**:37–40.
15. Tan JS, Wishnow RM, Talan DA *et al.* Treatment of hospitalized patients with complicated skin and skin structure infections: double-blind, randomized, multicenter study of pipercillin-tazobactam versus ticarcillin-clavulanate. The Pipercillin/Tazobactam Skin and Skin Structure Study Group. *Antimicrob Agents Chemother* 1993;**37**:1580–6.
16. Graham DR, Talan DA, Nichols RL *et al.* Once-daily, high-dose levofloxacin versus ticarcillin-clavulanate alone or followed by amoxicillin-clavulanate for complicated skin and skin-structure infections: a randomized open-label trial. *Clin Inf Dis* 2002;**35**:381–9.
17. Chirugi VA, Edelstein H, Oster SE *et al.* Randomized comparison trial of teicoplanin intravenous, teicoplanin IM and cefazolin therapy for skin and soft-tissue infections caused by gram-positive bacteria. *South Med J* 1994;**87**:875–80.
18. Garau J, Blanquer J, Cobo L *et al.* Prospective, randomized, multicenter study of meropenem versus imipenem/cilastin as empiric monotherapy in severe nosocomial infections. *Eur J Clin Microbiol Infect Dis* 1997;**16**:789–96.
19. Tarshis GA, Miskin BM, Jones TM *et al.* Once-daily oral gatifloxacin versus oral levofloxacin in treatment of uncomplicated skin and soft-tissue infections: double-blind, multicenter, randomized study. *Antimicrob Agents Chemother* 2001;**45**:2358–62.
20. Nathwani D. The management of skin and soft-tissue infections: outpatient parenteral antibiotic therapy in the United Kingdom. *Chemotherapy* 2001;**47**(Suppl. 1): 17–23.
21. Gentry LO, Ramirez-Ronda CH, Rodriguez-Noriega E *et al.* Oral ciprofloxacin vs parenteral cefotaxime in the treatment of difficult skin and skin structure infections. A multicenter trial. *Arch Int Med* 1989;**149**:2579–83.
22. Gentry LO, Rodriguez-Gomez G, Zeluff BJ *et al.* A comparative evaluation of oral ofloxacin versus intravenous cefotaxime therapy for serious skin and skin structure infections. *Am J Med* 1989;**87**:57S–60S.
23. Stevens DL, Smith LG, Bruss JB *et al.* Randomized comparison on linezolid (PNU-100766) versus oxacillin-dicloxacillin for treatment of complicated skin and soft-tissue infections. *Antimicrob Agents Chemother* 2000;**44**:3408–13.
24. Eron LJ, Choong HP, Hixon DL *et al.* Ceftriaxone therapy of bone and soft-tissue infections in hospital and outpatient settings. *Antimicrob Agents Chemother* 1983;**23**:731–7.
25. Tice AD. Once-daily ceftriaxone outpatient therapy in adults with infections. *Chemotherapy* 1991;**37**(Suppl. 3):7–10.
26. Brown G, Chamberlain R, Goulding J, Clarke A. Ceftriaxone versus cefazolin with probenecid for severe skin and soft-tissue infections. *J Emerg Med* 1996;**14**: 547–51.
27. Grayson ML, McDonald M, Gibson K *et al.* Once-daily intravenous cefazolin plus oral probenecid is equivalent to once-daily ceftriaxone plus oral placebo for the treatment of moderate-to-severe cellulitis in adults. *Clin Infect Dis* 2002;**34**:1440–8.
28. Poretz DM. Treatment of skin and soft-tissue infections utilising an outpatient parenteral drug delivery device: a multicenter trial. HIAT Study Group. *Am J Med* 1994; **15**:23–7.
29. File TM, Tan JS, Dipersio JR. Diagnosing and treating the "flesh eating bacteria syndrome." *Clev Clin J Med* 1998; **65**:241–9.
30. Kaul R, McGeer A, Low D, Green K, Schwartz B, Simor AE. Population-based surveillance for group A streptococcal necrotizing fasciitis: clinical features, prognostic indicators, and microbiologic analysis of seventy-seven cases. *Am J Med* 1997;**103**:18–24.
31. Centers for Disease Control and Prevention. Invasive group A streptococcal infections-United Kingdom,1994. *MMWR* 1994;**43**:401.
32. Stevens DL. Streptococcal toxic-shock syndrome: spectrum of disease, pathogenesis, and new concepts in treatment. *Emerg Infect Dis* 1995;**1**:69–78.
33. Ward RG, Walsh MS. Necrotizing fasciitis: 10 years' experience in a district general hospital. *Br J Surg* 1991;**78**:488–9.
34. Bosshardt TL, Henderson VJ, Organ CH. Necrotizing soft-tissue infections. *Arch Surg* 1996;**131**:846–54.
35. Waldhausen JHT, Holterman MJ, Sawin RS. Surgical implications of necrotizing fasciitis in children with chickenpox. *J Ped Surg* 1996;**31**:1138–41.
36. Elliot D, Kufera JA, Myers RA. The microbiology of necrotizing soft-tissue infections. *Am J Surg* 2000;**179**:361–6.

37. File TM, Tan JS. Treatment of skin and soft-tissue infections. *Am J Surg* 1995;**169**(Suppl.5A):27S–33S.
38. Stamenkovic I, Lew D. Early recognition of potentially fatal necrotizing fasciitis: the use of frozen section biopsy. *N Engl J Med* 1984;**310**:1689–93.
39. Lille ST, Sato TT, Engrav LH *et al.* Necrotizing soft-tissue infections: obstacles in diagnosis. *J Am Coll Surg* 1996; **182**:7–11.
40. Kaplan DM, Schulman H, Fliss DM *et al.* Computed tomographic detection of necrotizing soft-tissue infection of dental origin. *Ann Otol Rhinol Laryngol* 1995;**105**: 164–6.
41. Kane CJ, Nash P, McAninch JW. Ultrasonographic appearance of necrotizing gangrene: aid in early diagnosis. *Urology* 1996;**48**:142–3.
42. Struk DW, Munk PL, Lee MJ, Ho SG, Worsley DF. Imaging in soft-tissue infections. *Rad Clin N Am* 2001;**39**:277–303.
43. Schmid MR, Kossman T, Duewell S. Differentiation of necrotizing fasciitis and cellulitis using MR imaging. *Am J Roent* 1998;**170**:615–20.
44. Brothers TE, Tagge DU, Stutley JE *et al.* Magnetic resonance imaging differentiates between necrotizing and non-necrotizing fasciitis of the lower extremity. *J Am Coll Surg* 1998;**187**:416–21.
45. Loh NN, Ch'en IY, Ceung LP, Li KC. Deep fascial hyperintensity in soft-tissue abnormalities as revealed by T2-weighted MR imaging. *Am J Roentgen* 1997;**168**: 1301–4.
46. Wall DB, Klein SR, Black S, de Virgilio C. A simple model to help distinguish necrotizing fasciitis from non-necrotizing soft-tissue infection. *J Am Coll Surg* 2000;**191**: 227–31.
47. Simonart T, Simonart JM, Derdelinckx I *et al.* Value of standard laboratory tests for the recognition of group A beta-hemolytic streptococcal necrotizing fasciitis. *Clin Infect Dis* 2001;**32**:E9–12.
48. Zimbelman J, Palmer A, Todd J. Improved outcome of clindamycin compared with β-lactam antibiotic treatment for invasive streptococcus pyogenes infection. *Ped Infect Dis J* 1999;**18**:1096–100.
49. Levine BB. Antigenicity and cross-reactivity of penicillins and cephalosporins. *J Infect Dis* 1973;**128**:S364–6.
50. Anne S, Reisman RE. Risk of administering cephalosporin antibiotics to patients with histories of penicillin allergy. *Ann Allerg Asthma Immunol* 1995;**74**:167–70.
51. Kaul R, McGeer A, Norrby-Teglund A *et al.* Intravenous immunoglobulin therapy in streptococcal toxic shock syndrome – a comparative observational study. *Clin Infect Dis* 1999;**28**:800–7.
52. Low D, McGeer A. Streptococcal toxic shock and necrotizing fasciitis: new approaches to therapy. *Infect Dis Microbiol Rounds* 2002;**2**:1–6.
53. Clark LA, Moon RE. Hyperbaric oxygen in the treatment of life-threatening soft-tissue infections. *Resp Care Clinics N Amer* 1999;**5**:203–19.
54. Calhoun JH, Overgaard KA, Stevens MC *et al.* Diabetic foot ulcers and infections: current concepts. *Adv Skin Wound Care* 2002;**15**:31–42.
55. Thomson FJ, Veves A, Ashe H *et al.* A team approach to diabetic foot care: the Manchester experience. *Foot* 1995;**2**:75.
56. The Diabetes Control and Complications Trial Research Group. The effect of intensive treatment of diabetes on the development and progression of long-term complications in insulin-dependent diabetes mellitus. *N Engl J Med* 1993;**329**:977–86.
57. Reiber GE, Pecoraro RE, Koepsell TD. Risk factors for amputation in patients with diabetes mellitus. *Ann Intern Med* 1992;**117**:97–105.
58. Armstrong DG, Lavery LA, Quebedeaux TI *et al.* Surgical morbidity and the risk of amputation due to infected puncture wounds in diabetic vs non-diabetic adults. *South Med J* 1997;**90**:321–89.
59. Centers for Disease Control and Prevention. *Diabetes Surveillance Report*, 1999.
60. Rith-Najarian SJ, Stolusky T, Gohdes DM. Identifying diabetic patients at high risk for lower extremity amputation in a primary health care setting. A prospective evaluation of simple screening criteria. *Diab Care* 1992;**15**:1386–9.
61. Caputo GM, Joshi N, Weitekamp MR. Foot infections in patients with diabetes. *Am Family Physician* 1997;**56**:196–202.
62. Gibbons GW, Eliopoulos GM. Infection of the diabetic foot. In: Kozak GP, Hoar CS, Rowbotham JL, Wheelock FC Jr, Gibbons GW, Campbell D, eds. *Management of diabetic foot problems.* Joslin Clinic and New England Deaconess Hospital. Philadelphia: Saunders, 1984.
63. Lipsky BA, Percraro RE, Larson SA *et al.* Outpatient management of uncomplicated lower-extremity infections in diabetic patients. *Arch Intern Med* 1990;**150**:790–7.

64. Sapico FL, Witte JL, Canawati HN *et al.* The infected foot of a diabetic patient: quantitative microbiology and analysis of clinical features. *Rev Infect Dis* 1984;**6**(Suppl. 1):171–6.
65. Jones EW, Edwards R, Finch R, Jeffcoate WJ. A microbiological study of diabetic foot lesions. *Diabetic Med* 1984;**2**:213–15.
66. Grayson ML, Gibbons GW, Habershaw GM *et al.* Use of ampicillin/sulbactam versus imipenem/cilastin in the treatment of limb-threatening foot infections in diabetic patients. *Clin Infect Dis* 1994;**18**:683–93.
67. Hughes CE, Johnson CC, Bamberger DM *et al.* Treatment and long-term follow up of foot infections in patients with diabetes or ischemia: a randomized, prospective, double-blind comparison of cefoxitin and ceftizoxime. *Clin Ther* 1987;**10**(Suppl. A):36–49.
68. Lipsky BA, Baker PD, Landon GC, Fernau R. Antibiotic therapy for diabetic foot infections: comparison of two parenteral-to-oral regimens. *Clin Infect Dis* 1997;**24**: 643–8.
69. Wheat LJ, Allen SD, Henry M *et al.* Diabetic foot infections. Bacteriologic analysis. *Arch Intern Med* 1986;**146**:1935–40.
70. Wieman TJ, Smiell JM, Su Y. Efficacy and safety of a topical gel formulation of recombinant human platelet-derived growth factor-BB (becaplermin) in patients with chronic neuropathic diabetic ulcers. A phase III randomized placebo-controlled double-blind study. *Diab Care* 1998;**21**:822–7.
71. Pham HT, Rosenblum BI, Lyons TE *et al.* Evaluation of Graftskin (Apligraf), a human skin equivalent, for the treatment of diabetic foot ulcers. *Diabetes* 1999;**48** (Suppl. 1):18A.
72. Caputo GM, Ulbrecht JS, Cavanagh PR. The total contact cast: a method for treating neuropathic diabetic ulcers. *Am Family Physician* 1997;**55**:605–15.
73. Helm PA, Walker SC, Pullium G. Total contact casting in diabetic patients with neuropathic foot ulcerations. *Arch Phys Med Rehabil* 1984;**65**:691–3.
74. Sinacore DR. Total contact casting for diabetic neuropathic ulcers. *Phys Ther* 1996;**76**:296–301.
75. Hammalund C, Sundberg T. Hyperbaric oxygen reduced size of chronic leg ulcers: a randomized double-blind study. *Plast Reconstr Surg* 1994;**93**:829–33.
76. Davis JC. The use of adjuvant hyperbaric oxygen in the treatment of diabetic foot. *Clin Podiatr Med Surg* 1987;**4**:429–37.
77. Oriani G, Meazza D, Favales F *et al.* Hyperbaric oxygen therapy in the diabetic gangrene. *J Hyperb Med* 1990;**5**:171–5.
78. Wattel E, Mathieu DM, Fassati P *et al.* Hyperbaric oxygen in the treatment of diabetic foot lesions. *J Hyperb Med* 1991;**6**:263–8.
79. Gibbons GW. Vascular evaluation and long-term results of distal bypass surgery in patients with diabetes. *Clin Podiatr Med Surg* 1995;**12**:129–40.
80. Callaham ML. Human and animal bites. *Top Emerg Med* 1982;**4**:1–15.
81. Thompson PG. The public health impact of dog attacks in a major Australian city. *Med J Austr* 1997;**167**:129–32.
82. Weiss HB, Friedman DI, Coben JH. Incidence of dog bite injuries treated in emergency departments. *JAMA* 1998;**279**:51–3.
83. Sacks JJ, Kresnow M, Houston B. Dog bites: how big a problem? *Injury Prev* 1996;**2**:52–4.
84. Fleisher GR. The management of bite wounds. *N Engl J Med* 1999;**340**;138–40.
85. Tannenbaum DW, Goldstein EJC, Rupprecht CE, Weber DJ. Management of animal bites. *Patient Care* 2002;**13**:54–69.
86. Goldstein EJC. Bite wounds and infection. *Clin Infect Dis* 1992;**14**:633–40.
87. Talan DA, Citron DM, Abrahamian FM *et al.* Bacteriologic analysis of infected dog and cat bites. *N Engl J Med* 1999;**340**:85–92.
88. Medeiros I, Saconato H. Antibiotic prophylaxis for mammalian bites. In Cochrane Collaboration. *Cochrane Library.* Issue 3. Oxford: Update Software, 2002.
89. Brakenbury PH, Muwanga C. A comparative double-blind study of amoxicillin/clavulanate vs placebo in the prevention of infection after animal bites. *Arch Emerg Med* 1989;**6**:251–6.
90. Noah DL, Drenzek CL, Smith JS *et al.* Epidemiology of human rabies in the United States, 1980–1996. *Ann Intern Med* 1998;**128**:922–30.

3

Bone and joint infections

William J Gillespie

Infectious arthritis

Case presentation 1

A 76-year-old woman presents to her family practitioner with a 72-hour history of increasing pain in the left knee associated with fever and malaise. Onset was insidious. She has been unable to walk for 12 hours prior to presentation. She has a 5-year history of osteoarthritis progressively affecting both knees for which she had taken a number of different non-steroidal anti-inflammatory agents, until 4 months ago when her medication was changed to paracetamol 2 g daily on account of medication-associated gastrointestinal discomfort. She has never previously had surgery to the knee. There is no history of other recent illness or of injury.

Physical examination reveals a temperature of 39°C. The left knee is held in 30 degrees of flexion, and any movement from that position is extremely uncomfortable. There is a tense and tender effusion in the knee, which is warm to the touch. The right knee is cool to the touch, without a palpable effusion. Examination of cardiorespiratory, gastrointestinal, and neurological systems is normal. Blood pressure is 140/95 mmHg. Initial laboratory tests have shown hemoglobin of 10·9 mg/dl, WCC of 15 000/mm^3 with 85% neutrophils and an ESR of 86 mm per hour. Urinalysis is negative for sugar and protein. She is admitted to hospital with a working diagnosis of acute inflammatory arthritis of the left knee, probably bacterial.

Burden of illness

Bacterial arthritis may arise by a hematogenous route from a distant infected focus or from invasive procedures at a distant site, or directly from a local bone or soft-tissue infection, following surgery, injection, or penetrating injury.[1] Although in this section we consider infection of native joints, prosthetic joint infections are often included in data collected on the incidence of pyogenic arthritis.

Hematogenous bacterial arthritis of major joints affects predominantly children and the elderly. Most cases of childhood septic arthritis occur in previously healthy children, but concomitant disease, for example disorder of neutrophil function, appears to be a risk factor.[1] In adults, on the other hand, fewer than 20% have no underlying disorder.[1] Risk associations[1] are:

- age over 64
- intravenous drug abuse
- HIV infection
- diabetes mellitus
- immunosuppression
- malignant disease
- underlying joint disorders (rheumatoid arthritis, other inflammatory arthropathies, and osteoarthritis).

Over time and across regional/national boundaries, these associations appear consistent, but actual incidence/prevalence figures have varied.[1–5]

In the past, *Staphylococcus aureus* and streptococci have been the most frequent isolates.[6] While this remains true, their reported frequency of isolation has fallen somewhat[1,7] in recent reports; this appears to be due to the inclusion of prosthetic joint infections in which coagulase negative staphylococci and gram-negative bacilli have become more common.

The natural history of the untreated case is destruction of the infected joint. Theories of pathogenesis proposed from laboratory experiments include both matrix destruction of articular cartilage and bone by inflammatory mediators and proteinases,[8] and apoptosis of chondroblasts and osteoblasts following internalisation of organisms.[9] Systemic outcomes prior to the availability of antimicrobials included death from multiple organ failure: this outcome is still seen occasionally in elderly and immunocompromised individuals.[10]

In evaluating antimicrobial therapy, the benchmark[11] is that, after 5 days of antimicrobial therapy, synovial fluid should be sterile and clinical signs and symptoms should have diminished.

Clinical presentation

In this presentation, the patient's age and history of osteoarthritis taken in conjunction with the history, physical signs, and initial investigations support the working diagnosis, but at this stage one can only be confident that this patient has an inflammatory monoarthritis. The history of effusion and warm joint is compatible with an episode of gout or pseudogout. The fever and the raised WCC are in favor of infection. In this case we estimate the probability of a pyogenic infection, on the grounds of history and clinical examination, at 80%. Laboratory confirmation is required.

Diagnosis

The terms "septic arthritis" and "pyogenic arthritis" are in common use as synonyms for "bacterial arthritis" and it is realistic to expect that to continue. However, bacterial infection can be confidently diagnosed only in cases where bacteria have been seen on microscopy of joint aspirate or synovium, and grown in the laboratory from the aspirate. Thus, these tests alone constitute the true reference standard.

In practice, this reference standard is frequently not met in a clinically characteristic illness. Well-conducted prospective community based surveys of "bacterial" arthritis have reported failure to identify an organism in a proportion of clinically characteristic cases.[1,2,12] The usefulness of bacterial DNA sequencing using the polymerase chain reaction with broad range bacterial primers in the diagnosis of inflammatory monoarthritis is yet to be established. Current evidence[12] suggests that, in the usual diagnostic laboratory setting, bacterial PCR does not represent any advantage over bacterial culture.

Recognizing the inadequacy of the reference standard, attempts to increase the yield of positive cultures by better techniques of sampling and transport have been made. The value of immediate incubation of the aspirate in blood culture bottles is debated; while it appears to increase the rate of successful culture,[13,14] it may increase the risk of false positives from contamination.[15] Trading specificity for sensitivity in a context in which the definitive decision on antimicrobial therapy depends on both is not necessarily helpful.

The diagnostic standard for definitive diagnosis and treatment of an acute inflammatory arthritis is immediate examination of a smear from synovial fluid obtained by percutaneous needle aspiration, biopsy, or arthroscopy, followed by an attempt to culture the etiologic micro-organism to determine its antimicrobial sensitivity. In suspected bacterial arthritis, this intervention is both diagnostic and part of the therapeutic regimen, for reasons discussed below. Cell count in the aspirate is a poor predictor of infection: very high counts may occur in crystal arthropathy and rheumatoid arthritis.[16] Needle biopsy specimens may have greater diagnostic efficiency in bacterial arthritis than simple aspirates. A study of 54 possibly infected knees[17] compared the achievement of a positive bacterial culture from simple aspirate (sensitivity 31%; specificity 97%) and from synovial biopsy (sensitivity 69%; specificity 100%). Likelihood ratios were 11·87 for aspiration and infinite for synovial biopsy.

Treatment

The introduction of antimicrobial therapy revolutionized the outcome of infectious arthritis. Therefore, although there are no recorded placebo-controlled trials examining the use of antimicrobials in septic arthritis, their use is universally accepted. It is evident that therapy should begin as soon as the synovial fluid specimen for laboratory examination has been taken. Definitive choice of antimicrobial agent is ultimately determined by the sensitivity of the etiologic micro-organism. Before the results of culture become available, (and if no culture becomes available) a "best guess" approach based on the history and physical examination, and preliminary findings from aspiration, biopsy, or drainage of the joint is appropriate.

The purpose of aspiration/biopsy/drainage is 2-fold – to obtain material for microbiologic evaluation and to evacuate inflammatory exudates from the joint. Although open-joint drainage, and more recently arthroscopic drainage[18], are widely accepted, evidence for the effectiveness, or for the best method, of joint drainage is not strong. It is based on the belief that reduction of the burden of inflammatory mediators and bacteria will reduce cartilage damage,[8,9] but an experimental study has not confirmed its effectiveness.[19] Nevertheless, joint drainage remains widely accepted. In large joints, particularly the knee, it seems plausible that a more complete evacuation of the inflammatory exudates in the joint can be obtained by arthroscopic lavage than by aspiration. Where quick access to arthroscopy, is available this is plausibly the best approach, but no RCT evidence is available. If not, then aspiration/needle biopsy should be conducted.

Immediately material has been sent for microbiological examination, provisional antimicrobial therapy should be commenced on a "best guess" basis. In this case, the probability that the infection, if confirmed, is caused by *Staphylococcus aureus* or *Streptococus* spp. is > 70%.[1,2] Choice of agent should reflect that probability. Once a definitive microbiological diagnosis becomes available, a change of agent or agents may become necessary. The optimal duration of antimicrobial therapy is not known. A consensus benchmark for RCTs evaluating new antimicrobial agents was 2–3 weeks.[11] Initially in the acutely febrile patient, intravenous therapy has usually been preferred until the temperature has returned to normal in most units, but once again there is no RCT evidence to support practice.

Outcome of treatment

Population-based studies[1,4] indicate that the mortality rate in adult septic arthritis remains above 10%. Residual loss of function is reported as occurring in more than 50% of cases – not surprising in view of the association with pre-existing joint disease.

Discussion

The diagnosis and management of infectious arthritis is largely based on individual experience and reports of accumulated institutional data. The absence of randomized trials evaluating the different strategies for joint drainage, and the optimal route and duration of antimicrobial therapy is disappointing.

A mortality rate of over 10% associated with an infection that presents localized to a joint, in a developed country also raises the question of prevention in high-risk cases. Kaandorp *et al.*[1] noted that, although in theory there is potential in immunocompromized patients to prevent infection, they form a heterogeneous group in whom it would be difficult to establish protocols for prophylaxis against infection of a native joint. Hematogenous infection around joint prostheses, against which prophylactic precautions have been introduced in several countries[20] accounted for only 8% of cases of infectious arthritis in their community-based study. It is hard to argue with their recommendation that good clinical care, including alertness to the possibility of joint infection in the case of bacteremia and rapid treatment are probably the most important factors in achieving a good outcome.

Prosthetic infection

Case presentation 2

A 64-year-old woman with a 10-year history of rheumatoid arthritis, who had undergone an elective right total hip replacement 8 days previously, presents with pyrexia unabated since surgery, a cellulitis extending for approximately 3 cm around the whole length of the wound, and a serosanguinous wound discharge from which a pure culture of *Staphylococcus aureus*, sensitive to oxacillin, rifampin, and ciprofloxacin has been isolated. She is a current smoker (15 pack years), but does not take alcohol.

Surgery had been conducted in an ultraclean air environment, and she had received antimicrobial prophylaxis (three doses of a second generation cephalosporin given over a 12-hour period, the first with the induction of anesthesia). The implant had been stabilized using polymethylmethacrylate bone cement without added antimicrobial agents. Her medication prior to surgery had been methotrexate 7·5 mg weekly (cumulative dose 1050 mg), prednisone 5 mg daily, and paracetamol 2 g daily.

Burden of illness

When replacement of major lower limb joints was first introduced in the 1960s, infection rates were as high as 10%.[20] This led to the development of techniques to reduce the burden of airborne bacteria in the operating room through the use of various ultraclean air systems and improved operating theatre discipline. At the same time, antibiotic prophylaxis was introduced, initially in the face of some scepticism. This raft of measures was successful in reducing the incidence of prosthetic infections. A careful and detailed follow up of over 26 000 prosthetic joint infections from a single institution[21] in North America found a cumulative incidence over the period 1969–1991 of 1·8%; early infections (those becoming apparent within 90 days) accounted for approximately 20% with the remainder being equally divided between 90 days to 2 years, and > 2 years, after implantation. A follow up of 6489 total knee arthroplasties implanted at another institution[22] between 1993 and 1999 reported an infection rate of 1·5%, of which 29% were early.

Both these studies[21,22] evaluated risk factors for infection using a case–control design. Risk factors reported as significant in both studies, using univariate analysis, were prior arthroplasty and diabetes mellitus. Factors reported as significant in only one study were obesity, rheumatoid arthritis, malignant disease, poor nutrition, and steroid therapy. Multivariate analysis[21] indicated that a history of joint arthroplasty, a National Nosocomial Infections Surveillance (NNIS) surgical risk index score[23] of 1 or 2, and the presence of a malignancy were preoperative risk factors for prosthetic infection.

Implant-related infections are hard to eradicate[24,25] owing to formation of surface biofilms on implant materials, not only by *Staphylococcus aureus*, but also by organisms previously uncommon as human pathogens, such as coagulase negative staphylococci. Eventually, the inflammatory mediators produced by infection result in bone resorption and loosening of the prosthesis. Many surgeons have taken the view that the diagnosis of an infected implant therefore requires its removal, and if possible, replacement by another (exchange arthroplasty). Thus, the time until revision (removal of the infected implant, temporarily or permanently) is an outcome measure (survivorship) of the implant.[26,27]

Prosthetic joint infections presenting earlier than 90 days for implantation are usually classified as early.[28] This classification has been widely adopted. It has facilitated comparisons of the outcome of arthroplasty between surgeons and between institutions, but there is no evidence that the 90-day definition of an early infection has any validity in guiding treatment or predicting its outcome. Cure has been defined as lack of clinical signs and symptoms of infection, a C-reactive protein level of < 5mg/mL, and the absence of radiological signs of loosening or dislocation of the arthroplasty, 24 months from the start of treatment.[29]

Clinical presentation

The first type of presentation, which this scenario represents, is a typical, truly acute nosocomial wound infection. This is strongly associated[21] with deep prosthetic infection (OR 35·9;95% CI 8·3, 54·6). In practice, one should assume that this prosthesis is infected.

Diagnosis

The infection has been confirmed. In this acute situation plain radiography of the hip region has little to offer, beyond confirming that the prosthesis is properly situated. If a thorough clinical examination has shown no suspicion of intrapelvic or intra-abdominal spread of the infection, further imaging would be unlikely to facilitate exploration and debridement of the surgical wound.

Treatment and outcomes

Antimicrobial therapy should be commenced as soon as the infecting organism is identified, and altered if necessary once sensitivities are known. The patient, surgeon, and infectious diseases specialist should discuss the options for treatment, which are:

- one-stage exchange arthroplasty, with prolonged antimicrobial therapy
- two-stage exchange arthroplasty, with prolonged antimicrobial therapy
- debridement with retention of the prosthesis and prolonged antimicrobial therapy.

Two-stage exchange arthroplasty, in which the arthroplasty components are removed, and a new arthroplasty implanted at a later date, has been the standard surgical component of the management of the infected hip arthroplasty, eradicating infection in around 80%.[30] One-stage exchange arthroplasty has also been reported to achieve similar results.[31,32] Although both strategies have been strongly advocated, no RCT has been reported. Thus, the choice between the two exchange arthroplasty strategies has a weak evidence base. So also has the choice between exchange arthroplasty and debridement with retention and antimicrobial therapy. The failure to conduct an RCT comparing these options has some justification, since prosthetic retention has, until recently, been associated with very high failure rates, in excess of 60%.[33] However, following successful experimental investigations,[34] a randomized controlled trial[29] involving patients undergoing initial debridement with prosthesis retention was reported in 1998. The intervention group received a 2-week course of intravenous flucloxacillin or vancomycin with rifampin, followed by long-term (3–6 months) ciprofloxacin/

rifampin oral therapy. Controls received a placebo in place of rifampin. The trial was small and was underpowered to confirm the value of rifampin in the intent-to-treat analysis, but the analysis by protocol completion indicated a significantly higher cure rate at 24 months with the addition of rifampin. Were the findings of this study to be replicated, a trial comparing exchange arthroplasty with debridement and retention would probably be ethical.

In the absence of high-quality evidence for choice of treatment, decision analysis modelling has been conducted. Such a comparison,[35] using a Markov model with explicit assumptions, compared two-stage exchange arthroplasty and debridement with retention. Briefly, this model indicated that, if the annual rate of recurrence of infection after debridement was >61%, that particular approach was more expensive and provided lower quality-adjusted life expectancy than two-stage exchange arthroplasty. If the annual rate of relapse after debridement was <19%, debridement and retention became cost-saving. Between these boundaries, debridement and retention was, arguably, associated with a gain in quality-adjusted life expectancy, although the utility value of the health states used in the calculation could be challenged, as they were not derived directly from the preferences of a relevant patient population.

Thus, the decision on treatment in this case is, largely, empirically based. The informed preferences of the patient herself should be pivotal in the decision on whether to choose debridement with retention, or proceed immediately to exchange arthroplasty. There is weak to moderate evidence that the best choice of antimicrobial therapy, whichever surgical strategy is chosen, would be combination therapy with rifampin and a fluoroquinolone. The optimal duration of therapy is not known, but on the available evidence[29] should not be less than 3 months.

Discussion

Was there any point in the management of this case at which a different course of action might have prevented the infection? This patient had a number of relevant risk factors, so strenuous measures were desirable. Surgery was conducted in an appropriate operative environment with antimicrobial prophylaxis. There might have been added benefit from the use of antimicrobial-impregnated bone cement. Although the RCT evidence[36] is inconclusive, evidence from the Norwegian Arthroplasty register[37] indicates a higher rate of revision for infection (failure rate ratio 4·3; 95% CI 1·7, 11) if systemic antimicrobials alone are used than if antimicrobial-containing bone cement is also used in combination. The patient was a current smoker. One RCT[38] has shown significant reduction in wound-related complications from an effective smoking intervention programme 6–8 weeks before surgery. Finally, should administration of methotrexate have been discontinued before surgery? The evidence that this is worthwhile is suggestive, but not strong, being derived from two cohort studies – one retrospective[39] and one prospective.[40]

Diabetic foot

Case presentation 3

A 74-year-old retired schoolteacher presents with an infection in his left forefoot. He gives a history of type 2 diabetes mellitus of 8 years' duration, which has required insulin for control of blood sugar for the last 4 years. He is a non(never)-smoker, with a daily alcohol intake of 4–5 units. His family doctor reports that his blood sugar control has deteriorated over the last year, and that he had an episode a week previously that may have been a transient ischemic attack.

Clinical examination demonstrates ulceration (Wagner stage IV) on the plantar surface of the foot under the 4th and 5th metatarsal heads, and bone and soft tissue on the lateral aspect of the foot on plantar and dorsal aspects over 3rd to 5th metatarsals. Blunt probing of the ulcer contacts bone. Both feet show intrinsic (hammer toe) deformities and are insensitive to the 5·07 Semmes–Weinstein filament test. He has retinopathy and bruits are heard over both carotid regions. No pulses are palpable in either leg below the knee.

Plain radiographs demonstrate soft-tissue swelling and loss of definition of tissue planes, and zonal osteopenia with cortical and medullary destruction in the heads of both 4th and 5th metatarsals.

Burden of illness

Approximately 15% of over 150 million people worldwide with diabetes mellitus will develop foot ulceration at some time in their life.[41] Although rates as high as 11% have been reported in Africa,[41] a community-based study in the Netherlands estimated the mean incidence of active foot ulceration amongst people with type 2 diabetes to be 2·1% per year;[42] 23% of those had an amputation before or after ulceration. The risk of amputation before healing in an established deep foot infection is 44%.[43] As these data are drawn from different sources, extrapolation is risky, but an indicative estimate of the risk of developing a deep infection from an active ulcer appears to be up to 50%.

It is estimated that contiguous soft-tissue infection preceded by skin ulceration accounts for 90% of cases of osteomyelitis in the feet of diabetics.[44] Thus, risk factors for ulceration are, indirectly, risk factors for osteomyelitis. In a prospective cohort study of 749 diabetic veterans,[45] independent risk factors for the occurrence of a full-thickness skin defect on the foot that took more than 14 days to heal were:

- presence of neuropathy measured by insensitivity to the 5·07 Semmes–Weinstein filament
- presence of a neuropathic joint
- past history of amputation or foot ulcer
- insulin use
- increased body mass
- poor vision
- clawing of toes
- reduced skin oxygenation and foot perfusion.

The International Working Group on the Diabetic Foot (IWGDF) has evolved a diabetic foot risk classification, which has been validated[46] as predictive of the risk of both ulceration and of amputation. Patients in Group 0 have diabetes but no evidence of peripheral neuropathy. In Group 1, neuropathy is present, but without foot deformity or peripheral vascular disease. In Group 2, neuropathy is present along with foot deformity and/or peripheral vascular disease. Patients in Group 3 have a history of foot ulceration or a lower-extremity amputation. In the 3-year follow up period in the validation study, foot ulceration occurred in 5·1, 14·3, 18·8, and 55·8% of the patients in Groups 0, 1, 2 and 3, respectively. All amputations occurred in patients classified into Group 2 (3·1%) and group 3 (20·9%).

Clinical presentation 3 (continued)

This patient's foot is at risk of amputation. The clinical history and findings place him in IWGDF Group 3. The changes in the plain radiograph, as is discussed below, indicate either neuropathic bone disease or osteomyelitis. The positive "probe to bone" test,[47] whose sensitivity is 66% and specificity 85%, adds to the clinical suspicion of infection.

Diagnosis

The admission plain radiographs are useful for providing anatomic information, but have poor sensitivity and specificity for infection, as the appearances of neuropathic bone and joint disease are often similar;[44] for the same reason other imaging modalities are also somewhat unreliable. A systematic review of their performance has recently been published.[48] The literature is characterized by small studies of varied design and validity conducted in different environments. Magnetic resonance imaging appears to be the most useful imaging investigation,[44,48] with an average sensitivity in prospective studies of 91% and a specificity of 77%. Three-phase bone scanning has a sensitivity of 96–100%, but specificity of < 35%. Labelled leukocyte scans have a more acceptable performance, with sensitivity of over 80% in most studies, and specificity of over 60%. In this case, at least a limited surgical intervention is likely. The superior anatomical precision of MRI would aid surgical planning.

In identification of the organism or organisms involved in the infection, the reference standard is bone culture, which may be achieved prior to surgery by fine-needle biopsy (sensitivity 87%, specificity 93%).[49] Although the pattern of microbial isolates appears to have changed somewhat over time, the prevalent organisms in contemporary practice are *Staphylococcus aureus*, *Streptococcus* spp., gram-negative species, and anerobes.[50] Mixed infections are common.

Treatment and outcomes

The man whose story is described in this section is at risk of amputation, and of death from septicemia. The clinical and radiological evidence indicates that there is an open ulcer, a cellulitis, and a probable osteomyelitis. Although apparent cure of chronic osteomyelitis in bone infection without operative intervention can sometimes be achieved,[51] the advice to this patient should represent a balanced plan to which diabetologist, infectious disease physician, and surgeon have contributed.[52] As soon as biopsy material from the bone has been sent for histological examination and culture, provisional antimicrobial therapy should be begun on the assumption that while there may be a dominant pathogen, most likely *Staphylococcus aureus* or a *Streptococcus* sp., polymicrobial infection with gram-negatives and anerobes may be present. The results of culture may require a change in therapy.

In the infected foot, tissue levels of most antibiotics, except fluoroquinolones, are often subtherapeutic.[52] Randomized trials of antimicrobial therapy for chronic bone infection are the subject of a recent systematic review.[53] Apart from a trend in two studies[29,54] in favor of improved long-lasting control of infection when rifampin was added in combination with either ciprofloxacin or nafcillin, no clear best choice of antimicrobial therapy or optimal duration has emerged. Specifically in diabetic foot infections, encouraging results from therapy with rifampin/ofloxacin combination therapy have been described in a non-randomized case series.[55] In each case, therefore, therapy will reflect the sensitivities of the pathogens identified, the condition and comorbidities of the patient, and the antimicrobial prescribing policy of the institution.

Recently, one small randomized trial[56] examined the effect of recombinant granulocyte colony-stimulating factor (G-CSF) in limb threatening diabetic foot infection. Forty patients received empiric antimicrobial therapy (ciprofloxacin and clindamycin) and were randomized to receive a 21-day programme of daily injection of G-CSF or placebo. No significant differences were identified between groups in respect of clinical cure or pattern of microbial isolates, but the number of amputations in the 9 weeks following onset of treatment was significantly smaller in the treatment group. G-CSF is promising but its place in managing osteomyelitis is undefined at this stage.

Surgical treatment options follow the principles of surgical management of osteomyelitis – resection of necrotic bone and soft tissue, management of the postresection defect, and wound closure. For each stage, various surgical approaches have been described. One small randomized trial[57] found no difference in outcome between one- and two-stage Syme amputation procedures. No other information from randomized trials is available for surgical options in managing diabetic foot infections.

Discussion

Can limb-threatening infections in the diabetic foot be prevented? At an organizational level,[58] wider access to expert diabetes care may reduce complications of diabetes at various stages. Since a majority of severe infections are associated with active ulceration, more effective methods of healing ulcers might reduce the frequency of infections. The evidence base for best practice in the management of foot ulcers is poor.[59] One small study[60] compared antibiotic treatment with placebo in the management of uncomplicated neuropathic ulcers treated by standard methods of pressure relief and wound care, but found no evidence of benefit. Topical hyperbaric oxygen therapy does not provide any improvement in ulcer healing.[61] The effectiveness of a living skin equivalent, Graftskin, was evaluated in a multicenter randomized trial involving 208 participants.[62] Both groups received standard wound debridement and dressings, with pressure relief. Application of Graftskin for a maximum of 4 weeks resulted in a higher healing rate without adverse effects. The frequencies of osteomyelitis and amputations were lower in the Graftskin group. This intervention is promising but further studies are needed.

Conclusion

The evidence base for treating bone and joint infections is poor.[53,58,59] This may reflect the fact that responsibility for treatment of such infections has lain, since the introduction of antimicrobial agents, at a boundary between internal medicine and surgery. Greater interdisciplinarity, a focus on questions about whose importance there is consensus, collaboration between multiple centers, and good trial design will help in the future.

Acknowledgment

Mrs Lesley Gillespie kindly conducted the literature search, retrieved copies of original papers, and assisted with assembling the bibliography.

References

1. Kaandorp CJE, Dinant HJ, van de Laar MAFJ *et al.* Incidence and sources of native and prosthetic joint infection: a community based prospective survey. *Ann Rheum Dis* 1997;**56**:470–5.
2. Dubost JJ, Soubrier M, Sauvezie B. Pyogenic arthritis in adults. *Joint Bone Spine* 2000;**67**:11–21.
3. Gillespie WJ. The epidemiology of acute haematogenous osteomyelitis of childhood. *Int J Epidemiol* 1985;**14**:600–6.
4. Weston VC, Jones AC, Bradbury N, Fawthrop F, Doherty M. Clinical features and outcome of septic arthritis in a single UK Health District 1982–1991. *Ann Rheum Dis* 1999;**58**:214–19.
5. Morgan DS, Fisher D, Merianos A, Currie BJ. An 18 year clinical review of septic arthritis from tropical Australia. *Epidemiol Infect* 1996;**117**:423–8.
6. David-Chaussé J, Dehais J, Boyer M, Darde ML. Les infections articulaires chez l'adulte; atteintes périphériques et vertébrales à germes banal et à bacilles tuberculeux. *Rev Rhum Mal Ostéoartic* 1981;**48**:69–76.
7. Ryan MJ, Kavanagh R, Wall PG, Hazleman BL. Bacterial joint infections in England and Wales: analysis of bacterial isolates over a 4 year period. *Br J Rheumatol* 1997;**36**:370–3.
8. Murrell GAC, Jang D, Williams RJ. Nitric oxide activates metalloprotease enzymes in articular cartilage. *Biochem Biophys Res Commun* 1995;**206**:15–21.
9. Lee MS, Yen CY, Ueng SW, Shih CH, Chao CC. Signal transduction pathways and apoptosis in bacteria infected chondrocytes. *J Orthop Res* 2001;**19**:696–702.

10. Gupta MN, Sturrock RD, Field M. A prospective 2-year study of 75 patients with adult-onset septic arthritis. *Rheumatology* 2001;**40**:24–30.
11. Norden C, Nelson JD, Mader JT, Calandra GB. Evaluation of new anti-infective drugs for the treatment of infectious arthritis in adults. *Clin Infect Dis* 1992;**15**(Suppl. 1):S167–S171.
12. Jalava J, Skurnik M, Toivanen A, Toivanen P, Eerola E. Bacterial PCR in the diagnosis of joint infection. *Ann Rheum Dis* 2001;**60**:287–9.
13. Von Essen R. Culture of joint specimens in bacterial arthritis. Impact of blood culture bottle utilization. *Scand J Rheumatol* 1997;**26**:293–300.
14. Yagupsky P, Press J. Use of the isolator 1.5 microbial tube for culture of synovial fluid from patients with septic arthritis. *J Clin Microbiol* 1997;**35**:2410–12.
15. Kortekangas P, Peltola O, Toivanen A, Aro HT. Synovial fluid L-lactic acid in acute arthritis of the adult knee joint. *Scand J Rheumatol* 1995;**24**:98–101.
16. Shmerling RH, Delbanco TL, Tosteson AN, Trentham DE. Synovial fluid tests. What should be ordered? *JAMA* 1990;**264**:1009–14.
17. Piriou P, Garreau DL, Wattincourt L, Judet T. Simple punction versus notch needle-biopsy for bacteriological diagnosis of osteoarticular infection. A prospective study on 54 cases. [French] *Rev Chir Orthop Reparatrice Appar Mot* 1998;**84**:685–8.
18. Stutz G, Kuster MS, Kleinstuck F, Gachter A. Arthroscopic management of septic arthritis: stages of infection and results. *Knee Surg Sports Traumatol Arthrosc* 2000;**8**:270–4.
19. Nord KD, Dore DD, Deeney VF *et al.* Evaluation of treatment modalities for septic arthritis with histological grading and analysis of levels of uronic acid, neutral protease, and interleukin-1. *J Bone Joint Surg Am* 1995;**77**:258–65.
20. Lidgren L. Joint prosthetic infections: A success story. *Acta Orthop Scand* 2001;**72**:553–6.
21. Berbari EF, Hanssen AD, Duffy MC *et al.* Risk factors for prosthetic joint infection: Case–control study. *Clin Infect Dis* 1998;**27**:1247–54.
22. Peersman G, Laskin R, Davis J, Peterson M. The Insall award paper: Infection in total knee replacement: A retrospective review of 6489 total knee replacements. *Clin Orthop* 2001;**392**:15–23.
23. Haley RW. Nosocomial infections in surgical patients: developing valid measures of intrinsic patient risk. *Am J Med* 1991;**91**(3B):145S-151S.
24. Costerton JW, Stewart PS, Greenberg EP. Bacterial biofilms: a common cause of persistent infections. *Science* 1999;**284**:1318–22.
25. van de Belt H, Neut D, Schenk W *et al.* Infection of orthopedic implants and the use of antibiotic-loaded bone cements. A review. *Acta Orthop Scand* 2001;**72**:557–71.
26. Kaplan EL, Meier P. Nonparametric estimation from incomplete observations. *J Am Stat Ass* 1958;**53**:457–81.
27. Cox DR. Regression models and life tables. *J R Stat Soc* 1972;**34**:187–220.
28. Coventry MB. Treatment of infections occurring in total hip surgery. *Orthop Clin N Amer* 1975;**6**:991–1003.
29. Zimmerli W, Widmer AF, Blatter M, Frei R, Ochsner PE. Role of rifampin for treatment of orthopedic implant-related staphylococcal infections: a randomized controlled trial. Foreign-Body Infection (FBI) Study Group. *JAMA* 1998;**279**:1537–41.
30. Tsukayama DT, Estrada R, Gustilo RB. Infection after total hip arthroplasty. A study of the treatment of one hundred and six infections. *J Bone Joint Surg Am* 1996;**78**:512–23.
31. Callaghan JJ, Katz RP, Johnston RC. One-stage revision surgery of the infected hip. A minimum 10–year followup study. *Clin Orthop* 1999;**369**:139–43.
32. Raut VV, Siney PD, Wroblewski BM. One-stage revision of total hip arthroplasty for deep infection. Long-term followup. *Clin Orthop* 1995;**321**:202–7.
33. Brandt CM, Sistrunk WW, Duffy MC *et al. Staphylococcus aureus* prosthetic joint infection treated with debridement and prosthesis retention. *Clin Infect Dis* 1997;**24**:914–19.
34. Blaser J, Vergeres P, Widmer AF, Zimmerli W. In vivo verification of in vitro model of antibiotic treatment of device-related infection. *Antimicrob Agents Chemother* 1995;**39**:1134–9.
35. Fisman DN, Reilly DT, Karchmer AW, Goldie SJ. Clinical effectiveness and cost-effectiveness of 2 management strategies for infected total hip arthroplasty in the elderly. *Clin Infect Dis* 2001;**32**:419–30.
36. Josefsson G, Gudmundsson G, Kolmert L, Wijkstrom S. Prophylaxis with systemic antibiotics versus gentamicin bone cement in total hip arthroplasty. A 5-year survey of 1688 hips. *Clin Orthop* 1990;**253**:173–8.

37. Espehaug B, Engesaeter LB, Vollset SE, Havelin LI, Langeland N. Antibiotic prophylaxis in total hip arthroplasty. *J Bone Joint Surg Br* 1997;**79**:590–5.
38. Moller AM, Villebro N, Pedersen T, Tonnesen H. Effect of preoperative smoking intervention on postoperative complications: A randomized clinical trial. *Lancet* 2002;**359**:114–17.
39. Bridges Jr SL, Lopez-Mendez A, Han KH, Tracy IC, Alarcon GS. Should methotrexate be discontinued before elective orthopedic surgery in patients with rheumatoid arthritis? *J Rheumatol* 1991;**18**:984–8.
40. Carpenter MT, West SG, Vogelgesang SA, Casey Jones DE. Postoperative joint infections in rheumatoid arthritis patients on methotrexate therapy. *Orthopedics* 1996;**19**:207–10.
41. Boulton AJ. The diabetic foot: a global view. *Diab Metab Res Rev* 2000;**16**(Suppl. 1): S2–S5.
42. Muller IS, de Grauw WJ, van Gerwen WH *et al.* Foot ulceration and lower limb amputation in type 2 diabetic patients in Dutch primary health care. *Diab Care* 2002;**25**:570–4.
43. Eneroth M, Larsson J, Apelqvist J. Deep foot infections in patients with diabetes and foot ulcer: an entity with different characteristics, treatments, and prognosis. *J Diab Complic* 1999;**13**:254–63.
44. Tomas MB, Patel M, Marwin SE, Palestro CJ. The diabetic foot. *Br J Radiol* 2000;**73**:443–50.
45. Boyko EJ, Ahroni JH, Stensel V *et al.* A prospective study of risk factors for diabetic foot ulcer. The Seattle Diabetic Foot Study. *Diab Care* 1999;**22**:1036–42.
46. Peters EJ, Lavery LA. Effectiveness of the diabetic foot risk classification system of the International Working Group on the Diabetic Foot. *Diab Care* 2001;**24**:1442–7.
47. Grayson ML, Gibbons GW, Balogh K, Levin E, Karchmer AW. Probing to bone in infected pedal ulcers. A clinical sign of underlying osteomyelitis in diabetic patients. *JAMA* 1995;**273**:721–3.
48. Bonham P. A critical review of the literature: part I: diagnosing osteomyelitis in patients with diabetes and foot ulcers. *J Wound Ostomy Continence Nurs* 2001;**28**:73–88.
49. Howard CB, Einhorn M, Dagan R, Yagupski P, Porat S. Fine-needle bone biopsy to diagnose osteomyelitis. *J Bone Joint Surg Br* 1994;**76**:311–14.
50. Snyder RJ, Cohen MM, Sun C, Livingston J. Osteomyelitis in the diabetic patient: diagnosis and treatment. Part 1: Overview, diagnosis, and microbiology. *Ostomy Wound Manage* 2001;**47**:18–30.
51. Pittet D, Wyssa B, Herter-Clavel C *et al.* Outcome of diabetic foot infections treated conservatively: A retrospective cohort study with long-term follow up. *Arch Intern Med* 1999;**159**:851–6.
52. Lipsky BA. Evidence-based antibiotic therapy of diabetic foot infections. *FEMS Immunol Med Microbiol* 1999;**26**:267–76.
53. Stengel D, Bauwens K, Sehouli J, Ekkernkamp A, Porzsolt F. Systematic review and meta-analysis of antibiotic therapy for bone and joint infections. *Lancet Infect Dis* 2001;**1**:175–88.
54. Norden CW, Bryant R, Palmer D, Montgomerie JZ, Wheat J. Chronic osteomyelitis caused by *Staphylococcus aureus*: controlled clinical trial of nafcillin therapy and nafcillin-rifampin therapy. *South Med J* 1986;**79**:947–51.
55. Senneville E, Yazdanpanah Y, Cazaubiel M *et al.* Rifampicin-ofloxacin oral regimen for the treatment of mild to moderate diabetic foot osteomyelitis. *J Antimicrob Chemother* 2001;**48**:927–30.
56. de Lalla F, Pellizzer G, Strazzabosco M *et al.* Randomized prospective controlled trial of recombinant granulocyte colony-stimulating factor as adjunctive therapy for limb-threatening diabetic foot infection. *Antimicrob Agents Chemother* 2001;**45**:1094–8.
57. Pinzur MS, Smith D, Osterman H. Syme ankle disarticulation in peripheral vascular disease and diabetic foot infection: the one-stage versus two-stage procedure. *Foot Ankle Int* 1995;**16**:124–7.
58. Mason J, O'Keeffe C, McIntosh A *et al.* A systematic review of foot ulcer in patients with Type 2 diabetes mellitus. I: prevention. *Diabet Med* 1999;**16**:801–12.
59. Mason J, O'Keeffe C, Hutchinson A *et al.* A systematic review of foot ulcer in patients with Type 2 diabetes mellitus. II: treatment. *Diabet Med* 1999;**16**:889–909.
60. Chantelau E, Tanudjaja T, Altenhofer F *et al.* Antibiotic treatment for uncomplicated neuropathic forefoot ulcers in diabetes: A controlled trial. *Diabet Med* 1996;**13**:156–9.
61. Leslie CA, Sapico FL, Ginunas VJ, Adkins RH. Randomized controlled trial of topical hyperbaric oxygen for treatment of diabetic foot ulcers. *Diab Care* 1988;**11**:111–15.
62. Veves A, Falanga V, Armstrong DG, Sabolinski ML. Graftskin, a human skin equivalent, is effective in the management of noninfected neuropathic diabetic foot ulcers: A prospective randomized multicenter clinical trial. *Diab Care* 2001;**24**:290–5.

4

Infective endocarditis

Scott D Halpern, Elias Abrutyn, Brian L Strom

Case presentation

A 47-year-old man presents to the emergency room with a 1-week history of fever, malaise, and back pain. The patient's symptoms began insidiously, but have been severe enough to keep him home from work for the past 2 days. The patient was previously healthy, but reports having been told he had a heart murmur caused by mitral valve prolapse. He has no significant family history of medical illness. Further questioning reveals that the patient had a tooth extracted 5 weeks prior to presentation. He does not recall having taken antibiotics prior to the extraction (or at any time during the past 2 months). He denies having ever used intravenous drugs.

Physical examination reveals a temperature of 38·3°C (101·8°F), pulse of 90 per minute, and blood pressure of 120/80 mmHg. Diffuse petechiae are seen on the sublingual oral mucosa, and a grade III/VI holosystolic regurgitant murmur is most audible at the apex. Initial lab results are significant for a hemoglobin of 115 g/liter (11·5 mg/dL) and an erythrocyte sedimentation rate of 70 mm per hour. Urinalysis shows microscopic hematuria. An ELISA for antibodies to HIV is negative.

You admit the patient with a presumptive diagnosis of infective endocarditis, and arrange for three sets of blood cultures to be obtained, spaced so that 12 hours may pass between drawing the first and last set. You wonder whether this patient should be further examined by transthoracic or transesophageal echocardiography.

Diagnosis

There are generally five steps to determining whether a particular patient has infective endocarditis (IE).

Epidemiology

The clinician should consider, prior to obtaining any information from diagnostic studies, the probability that any patient with similar demographic and clinical characteristics would develop the disease (i.e., the prior probability of disease). Because IE is an incident disease, it is best to consider probabilities expressed as incidence, rather than prevalence, so as to gauge a patient's risk of developing IE over time.

Reported incidence rates of IE range from 1·6 to 11·6 cases per 100 000 person-years.[1–7] Much of the variation is attributable to the proportion of people who have prosthetic valves, the proportion who use intravenous drugs, and the population's age distribution (older patients having higher incidences of IE (Figure 4.1).[3,6]

For this patient, the most applicable estimate to consider – that specific to cases of community-acquired, native-valve IE – is 3·56–4·81 cases per 100 000 person-years.[5] Although this chapter focuses on suspected cases of community-acquired, native-valve endocarditis, it is important to note that the risk for IE is higher

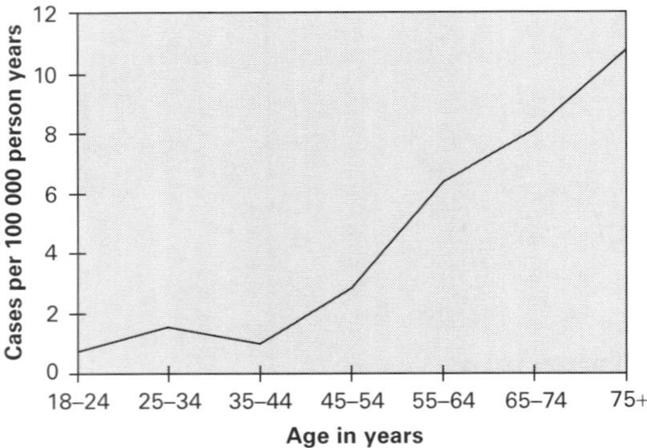

Figure 4.1 Age-specific person-years* of community native valve non-IVDU cases residing in six contiguous counties† during 27-month‡ recruitment period.[5]

*Person-years of follow up were calculated by multiplying the population in each age stratum by the 27 months/12 = 2·25 years of case accrual.
†Philadelphia, Delaware, Montgomery, Bucks, Chester Counties (PA), and Camden County (NJ).
‡August 1988–October 1990

among patients with prosthetic valves, those who use intravenous drugs,[8] and those at risk for nosocomial infections. These differences in the prior probability of IE may influence decisions regarding the appropriate use of diagnostic criteria and tests in these populations.

Physical examination and medical history

The second step in diagnosing IE involves both a careful physical exam, with special evaluation for the common cardiac, neurologic, vascular, and immunologic manifestations of the disease (many of which are listed in Box 4.1), and a medical history focused on whether the patient has any known risk factors for developing IE. With regard to this patient, it is known that patients with mitral-valve prolapse (MVP), are 8–19 times more likely to develop IE than patients without MVP.[9,10] By contrast, it is useful to know that this patient was HIV-negative, as patients infected with HIV are approximately five times more likely to develop IE (independent of

Box 4.1 The Duke Criteria* for diagnosis of infective endocarditis (IE)

Major Criteria

I Positive blood culture for infective endocarditis

A. Typical micro-organism for IE from two separate blood cultures

- *Streptococcus viridans* (including nutritionally variant strains), *Streptococcus bovis*, HACEK† group, *or*
- Community-acquired *Staphylococcus aureus* or enterococci, in the absence of a primary focus, *or*

B. Persistently positive blood culture, defined as recovery of a micro-organism consistent with IE from:

- Blood cultures drawn more than 12 hours apart, *or*
- All of three or a majority of four or more separate blood cultures, with first and last drawn at least 1 hour apart

II Evidence of endocardial involvement

A. Positive echocardiogram for IE

- Oscillating intracardiac mass, on valve or supporting structures, *or* in the path of regurgitant jets, *or* on implanted material, in the absence of an alternative anatomic explanation, *or*
- Abscess, *or*
- New partial dehiscence of prosthetic valve, *or*

B. New valvular regurgitation (increase or change in pre-existing murmur not sufficient)

Minor Criteria

I Predisposition: predisposing heart condition or intravenous drug use

- Fever: ≥ 38·0°C (100·4°F)
- Vascular phenomena: major arterial emboli, septic pulmonary infarcts, mycotic aneurysm, intracranial hemorrhage, conjunctival hemorrhages, Janeway lesions

- Immunologic phenomena: glomerulonephritis, Osler's nodes, Roth spots, rheumatoid factor
- Microbiologic evidence: positive blood culture but not meeting major criterion as noted previously,[‡] *or* serologic evidence of active infection with organism consistent with IE
- Echocardiogram: consistent with IE but not meeting major criterion as noted previously

*Adapted from Durack *et al.*[15] The diagnosis of "definite endocarditis" is made on pathological grounds when appropriate pathologic specimens from surgery or autopsy reveal positive histology and/or culture. The diagnosis of "definite endocarditis" is made on clinical grounds when two major criteria, one major and three minor criteria, or five minor criteria are met. The diagnosis of "possible endocarditis" is given when patients present with findings consistent with IE, but fall short of the requirements for definite endocarditis. The diagnosis of endocarditis is "rejected" if there is a firm alternative diagnosis to explain the clinical manifestations, if there is resolution of the manifestations suggesting IE with ≤ 4 days of antibiotic therapy, or if no pathologic evidence of IE is found at surgery or autopsy, in patients who received ≤ 4 days of antibiotic therapy.

[†]HACEK, *Hemophilus* spp., *Actinobacillus actinomycetemcomitans, Cardiobacterium hominis, Eikenella* spp., and *Kingella kingae.*

[‡]Excluding single positive cultures for coagulase-negative staphyloccoci and organisms that do not cause IE.

intravenous drug use),[8] with the precise risk being related to the level of immunodeficiency.[11] Other risk factors for IE that have been documented in case–control studies include congenital heart disease,[9] prior cardiac valvular surgery,[9] rheumatic fever,[9] heart murmur without other known cardiac abnormalities,[9] previous episodes of IE,[9] severe kidney disease,[12] diabetes mellitus,[12] and prior skin infections [12] or wounds.[13]

Blood culture

Third, clinicians should arrange for blood cultures to be obtained prior to the initiation of empiric antimicrobial treatment. Proper timing and technique of blood cultures remain the keys to accurate diagnosis; unfortunately, errors remain common.[14] Multiple blood cultures should be obtained over time so as to demonstrate persistent bacteremia if culturable organisms are present. Valid use of the Duke Criteria (see below) requires that three independent sets of blood cultures (independent venepunctures) be obtained, with at least 12 hours separating the first and last.[15] More than 99% of cases of true bacteremia or fungemia can be detected with three venepunctures.[16,17] Ideally, each venepuncture should yield at least 15 ml of blood,[17] although some culture systems may have different requirements. Organisms commonly associated with community-acquired, native-valve IE are listed in Table 4.1.

Echocardiography

The fourth diagnostic step to be considered is echocardiography. Many studies evaluating patients with confirmed or rejected IE, based on pathologic specimens or long-term follow up, have firmly established that transesophageal echocardiography (TEE) has better operating characteristics than transthoracic echocardiography (TTE). For example, in two case series, the sensitivity of TEE for diagnosing IE (in the absence of other clinical information) was 94–100%, and the specificity was 100%.[18,19] By contrast, the sensitivity of TTE in these two series was 44–50%, and the specificity was 93–98%,

Table 4.1 **Common etiologic agents of community-acquired, native-valve of endocarditis***

Organism	Proportion of cases (%)
Streptococcus species	50
S. viridans, alpha-hemolytic	35
S. bovis	12
Other streptococci	< 5
Staphylococcus species	30
S. aureus	25
Coagulase-negative	5
Enterococcus species	7
HACEK† group	< 5
gram-negative bacilli	< 5
Other bacteria/polymicrobial	< 5
Fungi	< 5
Culture-negative	5

*These proportions are approximations based on data from a large number of series. Observed proportions may vary considerably based on features of the local population, including the proportion of intravenous drug users, patients with prosthetic valves, and age distribution.

†HACEK, *Hemophilus* spp., *Actinobacillus actinomycetemcomitans, Cardiobacterium hominis, Eikenella* spp., and *Kingella kingae.*

when the same echocardiographic findings were required for diagnosis.[18,19]

TEE is also superior for detecting specific lesions, such as vegetations, perivalvular abscesses, valvular aneurysms, and valvular perforations, that are commonly associated with both the presence of IE and the patient's prognosis.[20–29] In addition, despite early concerns about safety, the procedure carries a very low risk of complications.[30]

Despite the superiority of TEE, there are two reasons why it should not be routinely used as a first-line diagnostic test for every patient suspected of having IE. First, among patients with very high or very low probabilities of IE based on history and physical exam, TTE and TEE yielc highly concordant diagnostic classifications.[31] Although incorporating the results of TEE improves the sensitivity of the Duke Criteria (see below) for diagnosing both culture-positive[32] and culture-negative[33] endocarditis compared to classifications based on TTE results, this improvement is largely confined to

- patients with intermediate probabilities of IE on clinical grounds
- patients with prosthetic valves.[31,32]

The second reason to limit the use of TEE is that it is only cost-effective as a first-line test in these same two groups of patients.[34] Indeed, a detailed decision analysis suggests that among patients with very low (e.g. < 2%) probabilities of IE, short-term treatment of bacteremia in the absence of echocardiography is warranted, whereas, among patients with high probabilities of disease (e.g., > 60%, as might be observed among patients with persistently positive bacteremia without another known cause), it is most cost-effective to treat empirically for endocarditis, regardless of echocardiographic results.[34] This analysis recommends the use of TEE as a first-line test for patients with intermediate probabilities of disease, though initial use of TTE, followed by TEE in the event of negative or inconclusive results, remains a recommended strategy.[35]

Regardless of the probability of IE, echocardiography retains an important role in the identification of patients who have complications of IE, such as perivalvular abscess, aneurysm, and valvular perforation. Because TEE is clearly superior to TTE in identifying such complications, it ought to be used whenever complications are suspected, or whenever there is a need to rule them out.[21,27] TEE is also indicated for defining underlying structural abnormalities that predispose patients to future IE.[35]

Diagnostic criteria

Another reason to use echocardiography is that it enables formal diagnosis of "definite", "possible," or "rejected" IE using the well-established Duke Criteria (Box 4.1).[15] Incorporating clinical, laboratory, and echocardiographic information, the Duke Criteria have been shown repeatedly[36–40] to have more favorable operating characteristics than the earlier Beth Israel criteria.[41] A retrospective evaluation of 410 patients also showed that the Duke Criteria had good agreement (72–90%) with expert clinical judgment.[42]

The operating characteristics of the Duke Criteria are best determined using studies, or subgroups within studies, for which the diagnosis of endocarditis was eventually proven or rejected by surgery, autopsy, and/or long-term follow up. Considering only such studies, and grouping "definite" *and* "possible" categorizations as positive tests, the sensitivity of the Duke Criteria is 98–100%,[15,36,38–40,43] and the specificity is 93%.[44] If only a "definite" categorization on the Duke Criteria is considered as a positive test, the sensitivity drops to 72–80%[15,38,39,43] (69% in elderly patients),[40] while the specificity rises to 99%.[44]

The Duke Criteria are also valid for diagnosing culture-negative endocarditis, with one study of 49 patients with pathologically proven or rejected IE showing a sensitivity of 72%, and specificity of 100% when serial blood cultures are negative.[33] In light of this reduced sensitivity with retained specificity, several authors have recently proposed modifications to the Duke Criteria.[43,45,46] However, we cannot recommend the routine use of any of these proposed modifications until further investigation of their comparative value is available. For example, these studies are uniform in suggesting that the sensitivity of the Duke Criteria might be improved, without sacrificing specificity, by adding the serologic diagnosis of Q fever (caused by *Coxiella burnetii*) as a major criterion.[45–47] However, the incremental value of such modifications may only be realized in geographic areas where Q fever accounts for an important proportion of IE cases.

These estimates of sensitivity and specificity are more robust than corresponding estimates of positive and negative predictive values because the latter are strongly influenced by the underlying prevalence of disease in a given population. None the less, predictive values answer the more clinically relevant question of whether a patient with a positive (or negative) categorization using the Duke Criteria does (or does not) have IE. One study of the negative predictive value of the Duke Criteria suggested it was at least 92% when both "definite" and "possible" categorizations are considered positive tests.[48] Presently, the positive predictive value of the Duke Criteria can only be estimated by jointly considering the results of several small, independent samples of patients with pathologically confirmed diagnoses. On the basis of these reports on heterogeneous patient samples, the positive predictive value appears to be ≥ 85% for diagnosing both culture-positive and culture-negative IE in patients with native or prosthetic valves.[32,33,36]

Proper diagnosis of the presented patient should therefore be based on the Duke Criteria, incorporating information obtained from a thorough history and physical examination, three sets of blood cultures, and TEE. If the blood cultures are negative, and the patient is classified as "possible IE" according to the Duke Criteria, further diagnostic tests, reviewed elsewhere,[33,49–53] may be warranted.

Case presentation (continued)

After overnight incubation, Gram stains of blood culture specimens obtained at two of the three separate venepunctures reveal gram-positive cocci in chains. The following day, these cultures grow *Streptococcus viridans*, and are found to be highly susceptible to penicillin (MIC ≤ 0·1 micrograms/mL) on day 3. Transesphageal echocardiography reveals a moderate sized, mobile mass attached to the atrial surface of the anterior leaflet of a prolapsed mitral valve, and color Doppler study shows mitral regurgitation with no evidence of extension of the intracardiac lesion. The patient appears hemodynamically stable, and has no evidence of renal dysfunction. Evaluation for signs of congestive heart failure reveals only 1+ edema in the lower extremities. No rales are appreciated, no S3 is audible, and the jugular veins are not distended. A chest *x* ray film is clear. While deciding upon the most appropriate course of antibiotics, you wonder whether evaluation for mitral valve replacement is warranted.

Antimicrobial management

This patient meets two major criteria in the Duke classification – isolation of a typical organism for IE and echocardiographic detection of an oscillating mass attached to a valvular leaflet – and is thus classified as having "definite endocarditis". Determination of the most appropriate antibiotic regimen requires consideration of the appropriate agent(s), their dose, route of administration, duration of treatment, and whether such treatment requires prolonged hospitalization.

A working group of the American Heart Association has provided thorough treatment recommendations for IE caused by both typical[54] and atypical[49] organisms. Few randomized trials of these regimens have been conducted because the disease itself is rare, and specific etiologies are rarer still. Recruiting sufficient numbers of patients with IE caused by specific bacteria is therefore difficult. Furthermore, the excellent efficacy of known regimens that would be used in control subjects makes type II errors likely in all but extremely large trials. We will limit our discussion to reviewing the best available evidence on regimens for treating the most common causes of native-valve IE in non-drug users, *Streptococcus viridans* and *S. bovis*.

With few trials to guide treatment recommendations, decisions must be guided by case series documenting the efficacy of various regimens against streptococcal species. The *Streptococcus viridans* group includes several species, such as *S. mutans*, *S. sanguis*, *S. oralis* (*mitis*), and *S. salivarius*. The treatment of penicillin-susceptible *S. bovis*, a non-enterococcal, group D streptococcus, is similar, and is often grouped with viridans species in these series.

Four weeks of antimicrobial treatment is traditionally recommended for IE caused by penicillin-sensitive streptococci.[54] Typical regimens include parenteral penicillin, either alone or in tandem with an aminoglycoside. More recently, a single daily dose of intravenous or intramuscular ceftriaxone (2 g per day) for 4 weeks has been shown to be effective in treating endocarditis caused by sensitive strains of streptococci.[55–57] One small randomized trial showed that both this 4-week regimen, as well as a modified regimen of 2 weeks of parenteral ceftriaxone followed by 2 weeks of oral amoxicillin, were curative in all 15 patients receiving each regimen (one possible relapse was noted among the group receiving 4 weeks of ceftriaxone).[55] However, this trial was not adequately powered to determine whether clinically important differences exist in the efficacy of these regimens.

The efficacy of shorter courses (2 weeks) of antimicrobial therapy (typically for patients without longstanding symptoms) has been suggested by uncontrolled studies for 50 years.[58,59] Penicillin alone was initially used in sensitive isolates,[58] although more recent series have shown lower relapse rates when an aminoglycoside was added.[59,60] This is attributable to synergistic bactericidal activity between the agents.

Single daily doses of ceftriaxone (2 g per day intravenously) plus netilmicin (4 mg/kg per day intravenously) for 2 weeks have recently been shown to be effective, achieving clinical cure in 89% of patients, and microbiologic cure in 100% of patients with documented streptococcal endocarditis.[61] In a randomized trial of 51 evaluable patients, Sexton *et al.* showed that a 2-week regimen of single daily doses of ceftriaxone (2 g per day intravenously) plus gentamicin (3 mg/kg per day intravenously) produced the same 96% cure rate as a 4-week regimen of ceftriaxone alone.[57]

Despite these promising results with 2-week therapy, and the tremendous benefits they afford in reducing length of stay in the hospital, several important considerations may limit their widespread use. First, more extensive evaluation of the efficacy of single daily doses of aminoglycosides is needed. Second, clinicians may be reluctant to add an aminoglycoside for patients at high risk for nephrotoxicity or ototoxicity. Lastly, although isolates of penicillin-tolerant *Streptococcus viridans* and *S. bovis* remain uncommon, they have been noted in several recent series.[62] Four weeks of treatment is a prudent option in such cases.[62]

Case series suggest that for selected patients with susceptible isolates of the *S. viridans* group, no evidence of hemodynamic instability, and no other complications of IE, several of these regimens can be safely administered on an outpatient basis.[55,56] However, there have been no published trials directly comparing inpatient versus outpatient antimicrobial therapy for IE. Such trials seem unlikely because they would need to be extremely large to detect small, but clinically important differences in the rates of treatment failure. In the absence of such comparative evidence, physicians must weigh, for each individual patient, the risks and costs of remaining in the hospital versus the risks for having IE complications unattended to in the outpatient setting.[63]

In summary, there are several viable options for treating patients with penicillin-susceptible, *Streptococcus viridans* or *S. bovis* IE on native valves. These are listed in Table 4.2. If the isolates show relative penicillin resistance (0·1 micrograms/ml^{-1} < MIC < 0·5 micrograms/ml), 4 weeks of penicillin (18 million units per 24 hours intravenously) should be combined with gentamicin (1 mg/kg intramuscularly or intravenously every 8 hours) for at least the first 2 weeks.[54,64] For patients allergic to β-lactam antibiotics, vancomycin hydrochloride (30 mg/kg per 24 hours intravenously in two equally divided doses) should be used for 4 weeks.[54]

Case presentation 1 (continued)

You start the patient on intravenous penicillin (18 million units per 24 hours), plus intravenous gentamicin 1 mg/kg every 8 hours. You planned treatment for 2 weeks, but after 2 days, the patient becomes progressively dyspneic at rest. Pulse oximetry reveals an oxygen saturation of 89% on room air. Jugular venous distension is evident at 8 cm above the sternal notch, and rales are auscultated bilaterally. A second chest *x* ray film reveals patchy infiltrates in the lower lung fields bilaterally.

Surgical intervention

Indications for cardiac surgery

Traditional indications for cardiac surgery in IE include: moderate to severe heart failure, severe

Table 4.2 Suggested therapeutic regimens for the treatment of native-valve endocarditis due to penicillin-susceptible (MIC < 0·1 micrograms/mL *Streptococcus viridans and S. bovis*.*

Antibiotic regimen	Dosage and route	Duration (weeks)
Aqueous crystalline penicillin G sodium	12–18 million units per 24 hours IV,	
	continuously or in six equally divided doses	4
Ceftriaxone sodium	2 g once daily IV or IM	4
Aqueous crystalline	12–18 million units per 24 hours IV,	2
penicillin G sodium	continuously or in six equally divided doses	
with gentamicin sulfate	1 mg / kg IM or IV every 8 hours	
Ceftriaxone sodium	2 g once daily IV or IM	2
with netilmicin	4 mg / kg daily IV	

*Modified from Wilson et al.[54]

valvular dysfunction, perivalvular abscesses, multiple embolic events, prosthetic valve endocarditis, fungal infection, persistent bacteremia despite theoretically adequate antibiotic treatment, and, possibly, the echocardiographic detection of large, mobile vegetations.[65] Although 35 years of clinical experience supports the adherence to these indications, the lack of controlled studies makes it difficult to determine the validity or relative strengths of each. In deciding whether to proceed to surgery for an individual patient, careful (and perhaps separate) evaluation of hemodynamic and infectious disease considerations is warranted.

Timing of surgical intervention

Whether proceeding to surgery early (i.e. during the active stage of IE)[66] confers an additional risk for recurrence or mortality remains controversial. There are no randomized trials of the timing of surgical intervention. Clinicians should therefore be mindful that the results of the available cohort studies may be biased if patients with more severe disease, and hence poorer prognosis, were preferentially selected for earlier surgical intervention.

Ankari and colleagues reported that among patients with mitral-valve IE, proceeding to surgery before sterilizing the diseased valve with antimicrobial therapy was not associated with a poorer postoperative prognosis.[67] By contrast, among patients with aortic valve IE, delaying operation until the initial IE had healed was associated with more favorable outcomes.[68] Other series show no association between surgery in active IE and poorer prognosis, regardless of the valve involved.[69,70]

Several retrospective cohort studies indicate that early surgical intervention may improve short- and/or long-term outcomes in patients with *Staphylococcus aureus* IE,[66,71–73] and in any patient with IE complicated by CHF.[73,74] There remains no evidence indicating a benefit to early surgical intervention in patients with uncomplicated streptococcal IE. However, a prospective, randomized trial of medical versus early surgical intervention among patients with uncomplicated IE would be needed to overcome the selection biases that likely influence the foregoing conclusions. Unfortunately, such a trial would still be limited by the inability to blind patients to their received treatment.

Decisions to proceed to surgery must therefore be tailored to the individual patient, and should be based on consideration of at least three groups of factors.

- Physicians should consider the patient's risks for operative mortality.
- Physicians should consider the patient's risks for post-surgical complications such as relapse (resumption of the clinical picture of endocarditis, including isolation of the same micro-organism, within 6 months of initial treatment), recurrence (development of a new clinical picture also consistent with endocarditis, but with a different micro-organism or occurring more than 6 months after the initial episode), embolic events, worsening heart failure, need for subsequent valve replacement, and death.
- Physicians should consider the short- and long-term prognoses of patients managed surgically versus those managed medically.

Several case series have evaluated these prognostic issues.

Prognosis

Relapse and recurrence

Long-term (≥ 10 years) follow up of inception cohorts of non-intravenous drug users diagnosed with IE suggest that 0–3% of patients will have relapsing IE, and 6–12% will have recurrent IE.[29,70,75] Series of surgically managed patients show a higher (20–25%) incidence of recurrence,[76] although, again, the severity of disease may be higher among such patients. Recurrence is more likely in patients with initial IE on a prosthetic valve, those with positive valve cultures at the time of surgery, and in those with persistent fever more than 7 days postoperatively.[76] To monitor for relapses, which typically manifest within 4 weeks of the cessation of treatment, it is recommended that at least one set of blood cultures be obtained in the 8 weeks following completion of antimicrobial treatment.[54] However, the costs and benefits of different strategies have not been evaluated.

The need for subsequent valvular surgery

Several large case series indicate that approximately 10–20% of patients initially operated on for IE will need another valve replacement.[75,77,78] Patients at higher risk for requiring late valve replacement include those with recurrent IE,[75] those with initial endocarditis on a prosthetic valve,[75] those with initial involvement of the aortic valve,[70] and those with positive cultures of valvular material obtained intraoperatively.[78]

Embolic events

Embolic events, typically caused by the fragmentation and dislodging of valvular vegetations, have been reported to occur in 9–44% of patients after being diagnosed with IE;[79–81] many others will have already experienced embolic complications by the time of presentation.[81–82] The variability among these retrospective cohort studies is attributable to differing frequencies of early surgical intervention, heterogeneity in the underlying severity of disease among cohorts, and to whether or not computed tomography was used to detect silent emboli. Once appropriate antimicrobial therapy is initiated, the risk of embolic events decreases precipitously, particularly after the first week of therapy.[79,83] The most common sites for embolization are the central nervous system, spleen, lungs, kidneys, peripheral arteries, retinal artery, and coronary vessels.[79–81]

Because of the frequency and substantial morbidity associated with embolic events in IE, and the (untested) premise that early surgical intervention could prevent many embolic events, several investigators have conducted retrospective cohort studies to determine whether patients' risks for embolism could be predicted by echocardiography.[79–81,84–87] The results of these studies have been mixed, depending on the size of study samples, whether TTE or TEE was used, and whether or not computed tomography was used to detect silent emboli. The larger studies using TEE to evaluate vegetations have consistently found that vegetation size (> 10 mm) and mobility are each associated with an elevated risk for embolism.[81,85,87] However, the fact that embolism also occurs in many patients without detectable vegetations raises doubts as to the clinical usefulness of routinely screening patients for embolism risk using TEE.[88]

Congestive heart failure

Symptoms of CHF are found at presentation in more than half of patients with IE. Other patients will experience incident CHF or worsening CHF after the initial infection has healed with appropriate treatment. Patients with NVE are more likely to present with CHF symptoms than are those with PVE.[28] Although severe CHF is an indication for early surgery, intractable pulmonary edema and impaired left ventricular systolic function are independent predictors of operative mortality.[77]

Early and late mortality

Advances in the diagnosis and management of IE have had substantial impact on overall mortality, although it remains discouragingly high. Recent case series of consecutive patients with IE report survival rates of approximately 75% at 1 year, dropping to approximately 70% at 10 years.[29] Survival is significantly better among patients with initial NVE than among those with PVE.[29,89]

Among all patients with IE, risk factors for early mortality (typically defined as within 6 weeks of diagnosis) include older age[29] a variety of cardiac complications,[29,77,90] and neurologic complications.[82,91] Among patients managed surgically, early postoperative mortality (typically defined as occurring within 30 days of surgery or prior to discharge from the hospital, whichever comes second) occurs in 8–16%, depending on the preoperative clinical severity of the cohort.[28,69,77,89] Risk factors for early operative mortality include older age, *S. aureus* infection, perivalvular abscess with fistulization, worse preoperative heart failure, and preoperative renal failure.[28,69,77,92]

Late mortality appears to be greater among men,[75] older patients,[28,75] patients with *S. aureus* infection,[28] perivalvular abscess,[27,74,93] and those with initial IE on a prosthetic valve.[67]

Case presentation (continued)

Based on this patient's worsening CHF and risk for embolism, mitral valve replacement is performed on day 7 following admission. Six days later, the patient is stable and discharged to home, where arrangements have been made for him to complete his antibiotic course. Before leaving, the patient inquires as to whether he could have prevented this episode of endocarditis. He also asks what he should do in the future to prevent recurrence.

Antibiotic prophylaxis

Antibiotic prophylaxis against infective endocarditis continues to be recommended for high-risk patients, including those who, like this patient, have MVP and regurgitation, before they undergo many dental, genitourinary, and gastrointestinal procedures.[94] However, the value of this recommendation has been repeatedly questioned,[9,95–97] and there is evidence that many physicians do not follow it.[14,98]

The low incidence of IE makes it unlikely that a randomized, controlled trial of prophylactic efficacy will be undertaken to resolve this question definitively. As a result, several groups have used alternative methods to provide insights into the potential usefulness of prophylaxis. Three case–control studies have directly evaluated the efficacy of antibiotic prophylaxis.[13,99,100] The first reported that prophylaxis provides clinically and statistically significant protection against IE.[99] However, this analysis was based on only eight patients who developed IE and 24 controls, and misclassification of just one of the cases would nullify the results entirely.[99] Furthermore, selective recall of having taken antibiotic prophylaxis among patients with cardiac lesions who did not develop IE may have inflated the observed efficacy. The second and third studies of efficacy, both of which were larger, found no significant benefit of prophylaxis.[13,100]

Another approach to quantifying the potential value of prophylaxis is to determine whether procedures known to induce transient bacteremia occur more commonly among patients who develop endocarditis than among those who do not. One hospital-based case–control study,[13] and one population-based case-control study[9] have evaluated these risk factors. Both studies found that dental treatments were not associated with an increased risk for IE,[9,13] even among patients with known cardiac lesions.[9] Because such patients represent those for whom prophylaxis is recommended,[94] the lack of an association between dental treatments and IE in this group suggests that even strict adherence to these recommendations would yield little benefit.

Finally, investigators have conducted formal decision analyzes considering both the incidence of IE in patients with MVP who undergo dental procedures, and the incidence of adverse drug reactions following prophylaxis.[101,102] These analyzes indicate that prophylaxis is extremely unlikely to produce a net health benefit, and that it could not plausibly provide such a benefit at a cost that society might consider reasonable.

These findings are, perhaps, to be expected considering that only 10·6% of patients who develop IE would have been targets of prophylaxis by virtue of having both a pre-existing cardiac lesion and a dental procedure.[9] Therefore, not only does there exist no good evidence supporting the efficacy of known prophylactic regimens, but there is substantial evidence to suggest that prophylaxis could not prevent a sizeable number of IE cases, even if a uniformly effective regimen were developed.

Case presentation (continued)

This patient should therefore be told that his episode of IE was an unfortunate occurrence that could not have (reasonably) been prevented with known interventions. Maintaining good oral hygiene with regular flossing may be beneficial.[12] The patient should also be told that his risk for IE is now markedly increased due to his having had both IE in the past and a prosthetic mitral valve.[9] Formal evaluation of the costs and benefits of prophylaxis in such a high-risk population is needed to guide the patient in preventing future episodes.

References

1. Smith RH, Radford DJ, Clark RA, Julian DJ. Infective endocarditis: a survey of cases in the South-East region of Scotland. *Thorax* 1976;**31**:373–9.
2. Hickey AJ, MacMahon SW, Wilcken DEL. Mitral valve prolapse and bacterial endocarditis: when is antibiotic prophylaxis necessary? *Am Heart J* 1985;**109**:431–5.
3. Griffin MR, Wilson WR, Edwards WD, O'Fallon WM, Kurland LT. Infective endocarditis, Olmsted County, Minnesota, 1950 through 1981. *JAMA* 1985;**254**:1199–202.
4. King JW, Nguyen VQ, Conrad SA. Results of a prospective statewide reporting system for infective endocarditis. *Am J Med Sci* 1988;**295**:517–27.
5. Berlin JA, Abrutyn E, Strom BL, *et al.* Incidence of infective endocarditis in the Delaware Valley, 1988–1990. *Am J Cardiol* 1995;**76**:933–6.

6. Hogevick H, Olaison L, Andersson R, Lindeberg J, Alestig K. Epidemiologic aspects of infective endocarditis in an urban population: A 5-year prospective study. *Medicine* (Baltimore) 1995;**74**:324–39.
7. Bouza E, Menasalvas A, Munoz P, Vasallo FJ, Del Mar Moreno M, Fernandez MAG. Infective endocarditis – A prospective study at the end of the twentieth century. *Medicine* (Baltimore) 2001;**80**:298–307.
8. Spijkerman IJB, van Ameijden EJC, Mientjes GHC, Coutinho RA, van den Hoek A. Human immunodeficiency virus infection and other risk factors for skin abscesses and endocarditis among injection drug users. *J Clin Epidemiol* 1996;**49**:1149–54.
9. Strom BL, Abrutyn E, Berlin JA, *et al.* Dental and cardiac risk factors for infective endocarditis: a population-based case-control study. *Ann Intern Med* 1998;**129**: 761–9.
10. Clemens J, Horwitz R, Jaffe C, Feinstein A, Stanton B. A controlled evaluation of the risk of bacterial endocarditis in persons with mitral-valve prolapse. *N Engl J Med* 1982;**307**:776–81.
11. Manoff SB, Vlahov D, Herskowitz A, *et al.* Human immunodeficiency virus infection and infective endocarditis among injecting drug users. *Epidemiology* 1996;**7**:566–70.
12. Strom BL, Abrutyn E, Berlin JA, *et al.* Risk factors for infective endocarditis: Oral hygiene and nondental exposures. *Circulation* 2000;**102**:2842–8.
13. Lacassin F, Hoen B, Leport C, *et al.* Procedures associated with infective endocarditis in adults. A case control study. *Eur Heart J* 1995;**16**:1968–74.
14. Delahaye F, Rial M-O, de Gevigney G, Ecochard R, Delaye J. A critical appraisal of the quality of the management of infective endocarditis. *J Am Coll Cardiol* 1999;**33**:788–93.
15. Durack DT, Lukes AS, Bright DK. New criteria for diagnosis of infective endocarditis: utilization of specific echocardiographics findings. *Am J Med* 1994;**96**:200–9.
16. Washington JA, II. Blood cultures: principles and techniques. *Mayo Clin Proc* 1975;**50**:91–8.
17. Weinstein M, Reller L, Murphy J, Lichtenstein K. Clinical significance of positive blood cultures: a comprehensive analysis of 500 episodes of bacteremia and fungemia in adults. I. Laboratory and epidemiologic observations. *Rev Infect Dis* 1983;**5**:35–53.
18. Pedersen WE, Walker M, Olsen JD, *et al.* Value of transesophageal echocardiography as an adjunct to transthoracic echocardiography, in evaluation of native and prosthetic valve endocarditis. *Chest* 1991;**100**: 351–6.
19. Shively BK, Gurule FT, Roldan CA, Leggett JH, Schiller NB. Diagnostic value of transesophageal echocardiography compared with transthoracic echocardiography in infective endocarditis. *J Am Coll Cardiol* 1991;**18**: 391–7.
20. Birmingham GD, Rahko PS, Ballantyne F. Improved detection of infective endocarditis with transesophageal echocardiography. *Am Heart J* 1992;**123**:774–81.
21. De Castro S, d'Amati G, Cartoni D, *et al.* Valvular perforation in left-sided infective endocarditis: a prospective echocardiographic evaluation and clinical outcome. *Am Heart J* 1997;**134**:656–64.
22. Daniel WG, Mugge A, Martin RP, *et al.* Improvement in the diagnosis of abscesses associated with endocarditis by transesophageal echocardiography. *N Engl J Med* 1991;**324**:795–800.
23. Daniel WG, Schroeder E, Nonnast-Daniel B, Lichtlen PR. Conventional and transesophageal echocardiography in the diagnosis of infective endocarditis. *Eur Heart J* 1987;**8**(Suppl. J):303–6.
24. Erbel R, Rohmann S, Drexler M, *et al.* Improved diagnostic value of echocardiography in patients with infective endocarditis by transesophageal approach: a prospective study. *Eur Heart J* 1988;**9**:43–53.
25. Taems MA, Gussenhoven EJ, Bos E, *et al.* Enhanced morphological diagnosis in infective endocarditis by transesophageal echocardiography. *Br Heart J* 1990;**63**: 109–13.
26. Shapiro SM, Young E, De Guzman S, *et al.* Transesophageal echocardiography in diagnosis of infective endocarditis. *Chest* 1994;**105**:377–82.
27. Blumberg EA, Karalis DA, Chandrasekaran K, *et al.* Endocarditis-associated paravalvular abscesses: do clinical parameters predict the presence of abscess? *Chest* 1995;**107**:898–903.
28. Choussat R, Thomas D, Isnard R, *et al.* Perivalvular abscesses associated with endocarditis: clinical features and prognostic factors of overall survival in a series of 233 cases: Perivalvular Abscess French Multicenter Study. *Eur Heart J* 1999;**20**:232–41.

29. Castillo JC, Anguita MP, Ramirez A, *et al.* Long term outcome of infective endocardit s in patients who were not drug addicts: a 10 year study. *Heart* 2000;**83**:525–30.
30. Daniel WG, Erbel R, Kaspar W, *et al.* Safety of transesophageal echocardiography, a multicenter survey of 10,419 examinations. *Circulation* 1993;**83**:817–21.
31. Lindner JR, Case RA, Dent JM, Abbott RD, Scheld WM, Kaul S. Diagnostic value of echocardiography in suspected endocarditis: an evaluation based on the pretest probability of disease. *Circulation* 1996;**93**:730–6.
32. Roe MT, Abramson MA, Li J, *et al.* Clinical information determines the impact of transesophageal echocardiography on the diagnosis of infective endocarditis by the Duke Criteria. *Am Heart J* 2000;**139**:945–51.
33. Kupferwasser LI, Darius H, Muller AM, *et al.* Diagnosis of culture-negative endocarditis: the role of the Duke criteria and the impact of transesophageal echocardiography. *Am Heart J* 2001;**142**:146–52.
34. Heidenreich PA, Masoudi FA, Maini B, *et al.* Echocardiography in patients with suspected endocarditis: a cost-effectiveness analysis. *Am J Med* 1999;**107**:198–208.
35. Cheitlin MD, Alpert JS, Armstrong WF, *et al.* ACC/AHA Guidelines for the Clinical Application of Echocardiography: A Report of the American College of Cardiology/ American Heart Association Task Force on Practice Guidelines (Committee on Clinical Application of Echocardiography) Developed in Collaboration With the American Society of Echocardiography. *Circulation* 1997;**95**:1686–744.
36. Bayer AS, Ward JI, Ginzton LE, Shapiro SM. Evaluation of new clinical criteria for the diagnosis of infective endocarditis. *Am J Med* 1994;**96**:211–19.
37. Hoen B, Selton-Suty C, Danchin N, *et al.* Evaluation of the Duke Criteria versus the Beth Israel Criteria for the diagnosis of infective endocarditis. *Clin Infect Dis* 1995;**21**:905–9.
38. Cecchi E, Parrini A, Chinaglia F, *et al.* New diagnostic criteria for infective endocarditis. *Eur Heart J* 1997;**18**:1149–56.
39. Heiro M, Nikoskelainen J, Hartiala JJ, Saraste MK, Kotilainen PK. Diagnosis of infective endocarditis. Sensitivity of the Duke vs. von Reyn criteria. *Arch Intern Med* 1998;**158**:18–24.
40. Gagliardi JP, Nettles RE, McCarthy DE, Sanders LL, Corey GR, Sexton DJ. Native valve infective endocarditis in elderly and younger adult patients: comparison of clinical features and outcomes with use of Duke Criteria and the Duke Endocarditis Database. *Clin Infect Dis* 1998;**26**: 1165–8.
41. von Reyn CF, Levy BS, Arbeit RD, Friedland G, Crumpacker CS. Infective endocarditis: an analysis based on strict case definitions. *Ann Intern Med* 1981;**94**: 505–17.
42. Sekeres MA, Abrutyn E, Berlin JA, *et al.* An assessment of the usefulness of the Duke criteria for diagnosing active infective endocarditis. *Clin Infect Dis* 1997;**24**:1185–90.
43. Lamas CC, Eykyn SE. Suggested modifications to the Duke criteria for the clinical diagnosis of native valve and prosthetic valve endocarditis: analysis of 118 pathologically proven cases. *Clin Infect Dis* 1997;**25**: 713–9.
44. Hoen B, Beguinot I, Rabaud C, *et al.* The Duke criteria for diagnosing infective endocarditis are specific: analysis of 100 patients with acute fever of unknown origin. *Clin Infect Dis* 1996;**23**:298–302.
45. Fournier P-E, Casalta J-P, Habib G, Messana T, Raoult D. Modification of the diagnostic criteria proposed by the Duke Endocarditis Service to permit improved diagnosis of Q Fever endocarditis. *Am J Med* 1996;**100**:629–33.
46. Li JS, Sexton DJ, Mick N, *et al.* Proposed modifications to the Duke criteria for the diagnosis of infective endocarditis. *Clin Infect Dis* 2000;**30**:633–8.
47. Habib G, Derumeaux G, Avierinos J-F, *et al.* Value and limitations of the Duke criteria for the diagnosis of infective endocarditis. *J Am Coll Cardiol* 1999;**33**:2023–2029.
48. Dodds GAI, Sexton DJ, Durack DT, *et al.* Negative predictive value of the Duke Criteria for infective endocarditis. *Am J Cardiol* 1996;**77**:403–7.
49. Bayer AS, Bolger AF, Taubert KA, *et al.* Diagnosis and management of infective endocarditis and its complications. *Circulation* 1998;**98**:2936–48.
50. Mylonakis E, Calderwood SB. Infective endocarditis in adults. *N Engl J Med* 2001;**345**:1318–30.
51. Hoen B, Selton-Suty C, Lacassin F, *et al.* Infective endocarditis in patients with negative blood cutltures: analysis of 88 cases from a one-year nationwide survey in France. *Clin Infect Dis* 1995;**20**:501–6.
52. Fournier PF, Raoult D. Non-culture laboratory methods for diagnosis of infective endocarditis. *Curr Infect Dis Rep* 1999;**1**:136–141.

53. Brouqi P, Raoult D. Endocarditis due to rare and fastidious bacteria. *Clin Microbiol Rev* 2001;**14**:177–207.
54. Wilson WR, Karchmer AW, Dajani AS, *et al.* Antibiotic treatment of adults with infective endocarditis due to Streptococci, Enterococci, Staphylococci, and HACEK microorganisms. *JAMA* 1995;**274**:1706–13.
55. Stamboulian D, Bonvehi P, Arevalo C, *et al.* Antibiotic management of outpatients with endocarditis due to penicillin-susceptible streptococci. *Rev Infect Dis* 1991;**13**:S160–3.
56. Francioli PF, Etienne J, Hoigne R, Thys J, Gerber A. Treatment of streptococcal endocarditis with a single daily dose of ceftriaxone sodium for 4 weeks. Efficacy and outpatient treatment feasibility. *JAMA* 1992;**267**:264–7.
57. Sexton DJ, Tenenbaum MJ, Wilson WR, *et al.* Ceftriaxone once daily for four weeks compared with ceftriaxone plus gentamicin once daily for two weeks for treatment of endocarditis due to penicillin-susceptible streptococci. *Clin Infect Dis* 1998;**27**:1470–4.
58. Hamburger M, Stein L. Streptococcus viridans subacute bacterial endocarditis. Two week treatment schedule with penicillin. *JAMA* 1952;**149**:542–5.
59. Tan JS, Kaplan S, Terhune CA, Jr., Hamburger M. Successful two-week treatment schedule for penicillin-susceptible streptococcus viridans endocarditis. *Lancet* 1971;**2**:1340–3.
60. Wilson WR, Thompson RL, Wilkowske CJ, *et al.* Short-term therapy for streptococcal infective endocarditis: combined intramuscular administration of penicillin and streptomycin. *JAMA* 1981;**245**:360–3.
61. Francioli PF, Ruch W, Stamboulian D, and the International Infective Endocarditis Study Group. Treatment of Streptococcal endocarditis with a single dose of ceftriaxone and netilmicin for 14 days: A prospective multicenter study. *Clin Infect Dis* 1995;**21**:1406–10.
62. Hoen B. Special issues in the management of infective endocarditis caused by Gram positive cocci. *Infect Dis Clin North Amer* 2002;**16**:437–52.
63. Andrews M-M, von Reyn CF. Patient selection criteria and management guidelines for outpatient parenteral antibiotic therapy for native valve infective endocarditis. *Clin Infect Dis* 2001;**33**:203–9.
64. Working Party of the British Society for Antimicrobial Therapy. Antibiotic treatment of Streptococcal, Enterococcal, and Staphylococcal endocarditis. *Heart* 1998;**79**:207–10.
65. Olaison L, Pettersson G. Current best practices and guidelines: indications for surgical intervention in infective endocarditis. *Infect Dis Clin North Am* 2002;**16**:453–75.
66. Bishara J, Leibovici L, Gartman-Israel D, *et al.* Long-term outcome of infective endocarditis: the impact of early surgical intervention. *Clin Infect Dis* 2001;**33**:1636–43.
67. Aranki SF, Adams DH, Rizzo RJ, *et al.* Determinants of early mortality and late survival in mitral valve endocarditis. *Circulation* 1995;**92**(9 Suppl.):II143–9.
68. Aranki SF, Santini F, Adams DH, *et al.* Aortic valve endocarditis. Determinants of early survival and late morbidity. *Circulation* 1994;**90(5pt2)**:II175–82.
69. Jault F, Gandjbakhch I, Rama A, *et al.* Active native valve endocarditis: determinants of operative death and late mortality. *Ann Thorac Surg* 1997;**63**:1737–41.
70. Tornos MP, Permanyer-Miralda G, Olona M, *et al.* Long-term complications of native valve infective endocarditis in non-addicts. *Ann Intern Med* 1992;**117**:567–72.
71. Malquarti V, Saradarian W, Etienne J, *et al.* Prognosis of native valve infective endocarditis: a review of 253 cases. *Eur Heart J* 1984;**5**(Suppl. C):11–20.
72. Delahaye F, Ecochard R, de Gevigney G, *et al.* The long term prognosis of infective endocarditis. *Eur Heart J* 1995;**16**(Suppl. B):48–53.
73. Richardson JV, Karp RB, Kirklin JW, Dismukes WE. Treatment of infective endocarditis: a 10-year comparative analysis. *Circulation* 1978;**58**:589–97.
74. Croft CH, Woodward W, Elliott A, Commerford PJ, Barnard CN, Beck W. Analysis of surgical versus medical therapy in active complicated native valve endocarditis. *Am J Cardiol* 1983;**51**:1650–5.
75. Mansur AJ, Dal Bo CMR, Fukushima JT, Issa VS, Grinberg M, Pomerantzeff PMA. Relapses, recurrences, valve replacements, and mortality during the long-term follow up after infective endocarditis. *Am Heart J* 2001;**141**:78–86.
76. Renzulli A, Carozza A, Romano G, *et al.* Recurrent infective endocarditis: a multivariate analysis of 21 years of experience. *Ann Thorac Surg* 2001;**72**:39–43.
77. Alexiou C, Langley SM, Stafford H, Lowes JA, Livesey SA, Monro JL. Surgery for active culture-positive endocarditis: determinants of early and late outcome. *Ann Thorac Surg* 2000;**69**:1448–54.
78. Renzulli A, Carozza A, Marra C, *et al.* Are blood and valve cultures predictive for long-term outcome following

surgery for infective endocarditis? *Eur J Cardiothorac Surg* 2000;**17**:228–33.

79. Steckelberg JM, Murphy JG, Ballard D, *et al.* Emboli in infective endocarditis: the prognostic value of echocardiography. *Ann Intern Med* 1991;**114**:635–40.
80. De Castro S, Magni G, Beni S, *et al.* Role of transthoracic and transesophageal echocardiography in predicting embolic events in patients with active infective endocarditis involving native cardiac valves. *Am J Cardiol* 1997;**80**:1030–4.
81. Di Salvo G, Habib G, Pergola V, *et al.* Echocardiography predicts embolic events in infective endocarditis. *J Am Coll Cardiol* 2001;**37**:1069–1076.
82. Heiro M, Nikoskelainen J, Engblom E, Marttila R, Kotilainen P. Neurologic manifestations of infective endocarditis: a 17-year experience in a teaching hospital in Finland. *Arch Intern Med* 2000;**160**:2781–7.
83. Alestig K, Hogevick H, Olaison L. Infective endocarditis: a diagnostic and therapeutic challenge for the new millenium. *Scand J Infect Dis* 2000;**32**:343–56.
84. Heinle S, Wilderman N, Harrison K, *et al.* Value of transthoracic echocardiography in predicting embolic events in active infective endocarditis. *Am J Cardiol* 1994;**74**:799–801.
85. Mugge A, Daniel WG, Frank G, Lichtlen PR. Echocardiography in infective endocarditis: reassessment of the prognostic implications of vegetation size determined by the transthoracic and the transesophageal approach. *J Am Coll Cardiol* 1989;**14**:631–8.
86. Sanfilippo AJ, Picard MH, Newell JB, *et al.* Echocardiographic assessment of patients with infectious endocarditis: prediction of risk for complications. *J Am Coll Cardiol* 1991;**18**:1191–9.
87. Rohmann S, Erbel R, Gorge G, *et al.* Clinical relevance of vegetation localization by transoesophageal echocardiography in infective endocarditis. *Eur Heart J* 1992;**13**:446–52.
88. Shapiro S, Kupferwasser LI. Echocardiography predicts embolic events in infective endocarditis. *J Am Coll Cardiol* 2001;**37**:1077–9.
89. Delay D, Pellerin M, Carrier M, *et al.* Immediate and long-term results of valve replacement for native and prosthetic valve endocarditis. *Ann Thorac Surg* 2000;**70**:1219–23.
90. Meine TJ, Nettles RE, Anderson DJ, *et al.* Cardiac conduction abnormalities in endocarditis defined by the Duke Criteria. *Am Heart J* 2001;**142**:280–5.
91. Roder BL, Wandall DA, Espersen F, Frimodt-Moller N, Skinhoj P, Rosdahl VT. Neurologic manifestations in *Staphylococcus aureus* endocarditis: A Review of 260 bacteremic cases in nondrug addicts. *Am J Med* 1997;**102**:379–86.
92. Bauernschmitt R, Jakob HG, Vahl C-F, Lange R, Hagl S. Operation for infective endocarditis: Results after implantation of mechanical valves. *Ann Thorac Surg* 1998;**65**:359–64.
93. Aguado JM, Gonzalez-Vilchez F, Martin-Duran R, Arjona R, Vazquez de Prada JA. Perivalvular abscesses associated with endocarditis. Clinical features and diagnostic accuracy of two-dimensional echocardiography. *Chest* 1993;**104**:88–93.
94. Dajani AS, Taubert KA, Wilson W, *et al.* Prevention of Bacterial Endocarditis: Recommendations by the American Heart Association. *Circulation* 1997;**96**:358–66.
95. Durack DT, Kaplan EL, Bisno AL. Apparent failures of endocarditis prophylaxis: analysis of 52 cases submitted to a national registry. *JAMA* 1983;**250**:2318–22.
96. Levison ME, Abrutyn E. Infective endocarditis: current guidelines on prophylaxis. *Curr Infect Dis Rep* 1999;**1**:119–25.
97. Roberts GJ. Dentists are innocent! 'Everyday' bacteremia is the real culprit: a review and assessment of the evidence that dental surgical procedures are a principle cause of bacterial endocarditis in children. *Pediatr Cardiol* 1999;**20**:317–35.
98. Seto TB, Kwiat D, Taira DA, Douglas PS, Manning WJ. Physicians' recommendations to patients for use of antibiotic prophylaxis to prevent endocarditis. *JAMA* 2000;**284**:68–71.
99. Imperiale TF, Horwitz RI. Does prophylaxis prevent postdental infective endocarditis? A controlled evaluation of protective efficacy. *Am J Med* 1990;**88**:131–6.
100. van der Meer JTM, van Wijk W, Thompson J, Vandenbroucke JP, Valkenburg HA, Michel MF. Efficacy of anitbiotic prophylaxis for prevention of native-valve endocarditis. *Lancet* 1992;**339**:135–9.
101. Bor DH, Himmelstein DU. Endocarditis prophylaxis for patients with mitral valve prolapse. *Am J Med* 1984;**76**:711–17.
102. Clemens J, Ransohoff DF. A quantitative assessment of pre-dental antibiotic prophylaxis for patients with mitral-valve prolapse. *J Chronic Dis* 1984;**37**:531–44.

5

Meningitis and encephalitis

Carolyn V Gould, Ebbing Lautenbach

Meningitis

> **Case presentation 1**
>
> A 30-year-old male presents to the emergency department with a 24-hour history of fever and headache. The patient's symptoms began abruptly and have worsened steadily over the last day. His wife reports that in the last 6 hours he has become somewhat confused. He has no significant past medical or surgical history. He takes no medications and denies alcohol, tobacco, and drug use. His family history is likewise non-contributory.
>
> Physical examination reveals a temperature of 38·5°C, a pulse of 110 beats per minute, and a blood pressure of 130/70 mmHg. He does not demonstrate photophobia or neck stiffness. His neurologic exam is non-focal but he is orientated only to person. Initial laboratory evaluation is remarkable for a white blood cell count of $21{\cdot}4 \times 10^9$/liter.
>
> You admit the patient with the presumptive diagnosis of meningitis, order two sets of blood cultures, and plan to perform a lumbar puncture (LP). You wonder whether to order a computed tomography (CT) scan prior to the LP to rule out an intracranial mass lesion, as well as whether antibiotics can be withheld until after the CT and LP have been performed.

Diagnosis

Epidemiology

The acute meningitis syndrome may be caused by a wide variety of infectious pathogens as well as by non-infectious diseases and syndromes (Box 5.1).[1–4] Given its frequency and clinical impact, this chapter will focus specifically on acute bacterial meningitis. The annual incidence of bacterial meningitis varies by geographic region, from approximately 3 per 100 000 in the United States (US), to 45·8 per 100 000 in Brazil, to 500/100 000 in Africa.[5–8] The incidence of bacterial meningitis has been profoundly affected by the introduction of the *Haemophilus influenzae* vaccine in 1987. Previously isolated in nearly 50% of cases of bacterial meningitis in the US,[8] *H. influenzae* now accounts for only about 7% of cases.[9] Comparable reductions in the incidence of *H. influenzae* meningitis have also been noted in countries in which the use of the vaccine is less comprehensive, suggesting herd immunity may be enhanced by the vaccine.[10]

Since the incidence of bacterial meningitis due to non-*Haemophilus influenzae* pathogens has remained constant during this time period, the net result of introduction of the *H. influenzae* vaccine has been a marked reduction in the overall incidence of bacterial meningitis.[9] Furthermore, the vaccine has also changed the age distribution of meningitis; the median age of persons with bacterial meningitis increased from 15 months in 1986 to 25 years in 1995,[9] such that bacterial meningitis in the US is now predominantly a disease of adults rather than children. This chapter thus focuses on bacterial meningitis in the adult population.

Box 5.1 Differential diagnosis of acute meningitis

Bacteria
- *Streptococcus pneumoniae*
- *Neisseria meningitidis*
- *Listeria monocytogenes*
- *Hemophilus influenzae*
- *Streptococcus agalactiae*
- *Escherichia coli*
- *Klebsiella pneumoniae*
- *Pseudomonas aeruginosa*
- *Salmonella* spp.
- *Nocardia* spp.
- *Mycobacterium tuberculosis*

Rickettsiae
- *Rickettsia rickettsii*
- *Rickettsia prowazekii*
- Rickettsiae typhi
- *Ehrlichia* spp.

Spirochetes
- *Treponema pallidum*
- *Borrelia burgdorferi*
- *Leptospira* spp.

Protozoa and helminths
- *Naegleria fowleri*
- *Angiostrongylus cantonensis*
- *Strongyloides stercoralis*
- *Toxoplasma gondii*
- *Plasmodium falciparum*

Viruses
- Nonpolio enteroviruses

Echoviruses

Coxsackieviruses

- Mumps virus
- Arboviruses
- Herpesviruses
- Lymphocytic choriomeningitis virus
- Human immunodeficiency virus
- Adenovirus
- Parainfluenza viruses 2 and 3
- Influenza virus
- Measles virus

Fungi
- *Cryptococcus neoformans*
- *Coccidioides immitis*
- *Histoplasma capsulatum*
- *Blastomyces dermatitidis*
- *Paracoccidioides brasiliensis*
- *Candida* spp.
- *Aspergillus* spp.
- *Sporothrix schenckii*

Neoplastic diseases
- Lymphomatous meningitis
- Carcinomatous meningitis
- Leukemia

Intracranial tumors and cysts
- Craniopharyngioma
- Dermoid/epidermoid cyst
- Teratoma

Medications
- Antimicrobial agents *
- Non-steroidal anti-inflammatory agents
- OKT3
- Azathioprine
- Cytosine arabinoside
- Immune globulin
- Ranitidine

Systemic illnesses
- Systemic lupus erythematosus
- Vogt–Koyanagi–Harada syndrome
- Sarcoidosis
- Behçet's disease
- Rheumatoid arthritis
- Polymyositis
- Wegener's granulomatosis
- Familial Mediterranean fever
- Kawasaki's syndrome

Miscellaneous
- Seizures
- Migraine
- Serum sickness
- Heavy metal poisoning

Adapted from references 1–4.

*Trimethoprim, sulfamethoxazole, ciprofloxacin, penicillin, cephalosporin, metronidazole, isoniazid, pyrazinamide.

Table 5.1 Empiric treatment of bacterial meningitis*

Patient population	Likely pathogens	Antimicrobial	Dosage and route	Duration§
Immunocompetent Age 18–50 years	*S. pneumoniae* *N. meningitidis*	Cefotaxime Ceftriaxone	2 g i.v. every 6 hours, or 2 g i.v. every 12 hours	10–14 days
Immunocompetent Age > 50 years	*S. pneumoniae* Gram-negative bacilli *L. monocytogenes*	Cefotaxime Ceftriaxone Ampicillin	2 g i.v. every 6 hours, or 2 g i.v. every 12 hours, plus 2 g i.v. every 4 hours	14–21 days
Impaired cellular immunity	*L. monocytogenes* Gram-negative bacilli	Ampicillin Ceftazidime	2 g i.v. every 4 hours, plus 5–100 mg/kg every 8 hours†	14–21 days
Head trauma, neurosurgery, cerebrospinal shunt	Staphylococci Gram-negative bacilli *S. pneumoniae*	Vancomycin Ceftazidime	15 mg/kg every 6 hours‡, plus 50–100 mg/kg every 8 hours†	21 days
Geographic region with high prevalence of penicillin-resistant *S. pneumoniae*	Multi-resistant *S. pneumoniae*	Cefotaxime Ceftriaxone Vancomycin	2 g i.v. every 6 hours, or 2 g i.v. every 12 hours, plus 15 mg/kg every 6 hours ‡	10–14 days

*Modified from references 30, 31.
†up to a total of 2 g every 8 hours.
‡up to a total of 2 g per day.
§Suggested duration of therapy for specific pathogens: *N. meningitidis* (7 days), *S. pneumoniae* (10–14 days), *L. monocytogenes* (14–21 days), gram-negative bacilli and staphylococci (21 days).

Etiology of bacterial meningitis

In an extensive surveillance project of 13 974 cases of bacterial meningitis, 80% of cases were accounted for by *Streptococcus pneumoniae, Neisseria meningitidis*, and *H. influenzae*.[8] More recent series of adult bacterial meningitis have also noted the prevalence of specific organisms: *S. pneumoniae* (20–53%) *N. meningitidis* (3–56%), *Listeria monocytogenes* (6–13%), and *H. influenzae* (4–8%).[11–13] The most likely causative organism depends on several factors including age, immunocompromise, preceding head trauma, recent neurosurgery, and site of acquisition (community-acquired *v* nosocomial) (Table 5.1).[2]

While this chapter will focus on community-acquired meningitis, nosocomial meningitis is also a significant problem. The National Nosocomial Infection Surveillance System (NNIS) noted an incidence of 5·6 non-surgical, nosocomial infections of the central nervous system (CNS) for every 100 000 patients discharged from the hospital between 1986–1993 with meningitis accounting for 91% of cases.[14] Unlike community-acquired meningitis, the most common pathogens in nosocomial meningitis are Gram-negative bacilli and staphylococci.[13]

Clinical presentation

Given the documented association between early institution of antimicrobial therapy and reduced mortality in meningitis,[15] rapid recognition and diagnosis of meningitis is imperative. The relative sensitivity of any given sign or symptom has varied across selected studies published within the past decade (Table 5.2). Fever is found in over 85% of cases, although it

Table 5.2 Symptoms and signs associated with bacterial meningitis in adults

Author/year [ref]	N*	Fever (%)	Neck stiffness (%)	Altered MS (%)	Headache (%)	Nausea/ vomiting (%)	Focal neurological signs (%)	Rash (%)
Durand 1993 [13]	259	95	88	78	NR	NR	29	11
Sigurdardottir 1997 [12]	127	97	82	66	NR	NR	10	52
Andersen 1997 [20]†	174	99	99	8	NR	52	NR	74
Hussein 2000 [11]	100	97	87	56	66	55	23	10
Rasmussen 1992 [53]	48 ‡	79	54	69	46	29	21	4

N*, number of patients (279 patient episodes in 275 patients[13]; 103 episodes in 100 patients[11]; 132 cases in 127 patients[12]).

MS, mental status

†Limited to cases of *N. meningitidis*.

‡6 cases of *Mycobacterium tuberculosis* included.

is rarely the only presenting symptom or sign.[13] Rash, particularly petechiae or purpura, are most common in meningococcal meningitis, but may also be observed in patients with meningitis caused by *S. pneumoniae*, *H. influenzae*, and *L. monocytogenes*.[13]

The classic clinical presentation of acute meningitis consists of the triad of fever, neck stiffness, and an altered mental status. Although recent reviews have found that only between 51% and 67% of patients with bacterial meningitis present with this classic triad,[11–13] 99–100% of patients have at least one of these findings.[12,13] It has thus been suggested that the diagnosis of bacterial meningitis may be effectively eliminated in a patient who presents without any of these findings.[16]

Cerebrospinal fluid culture

If the diagnosis of bacterial meningitis is a consideration, a lumbar puncture (LP) should be performed promptly. Routine morphologic and chemical analysis of the cerebrospinal fluid (CSF) in suspected bacterial meningitis should include a cell count, white blood cell differential count, glucose concentration, protein concentration, Gram stain, and bacterial culture.[2]

The appearance of the CSF in bacterial meningitis is typically turbid and/or discolored with an opening pressure ranging from 200–500 mm H_2O (Table 5.3).[2] The white blood cell count usually ranges from 1000 to 5000/mm $^{-3}$ with greater than 80% neutrophils.[2] Protein and glucose concentrations are usually 0·1–0·5 g/liter (100–500 mg/dL) and < 2·2 mol/liter (40mg/dL), respectively.[2] Recent large series of adult meningitis have noted that between 48–60% of CSF Gram stains from adults with bacterial meningitis were positive while CSF culture was positive in 65–80% of patients (Table 5.3).[11–13]

Patients partially treated with antibiotics may be less likely to have a positive CSF culture or Gram stain result, but such therapy has minimal effect on CSF indices such as leukocyte count.[17] Even after institution of appropriate antibiotics for meningitis, the CSF picture usually remains abnormal for at least 48–72 hours.[18] On the other hand, CSF pleocytosis, low CSF glucose, and elevated CSF protein may be found even in the absence of infection. Finally, the Gram stain of CSF from patients with Gram-negative bacillary or post-neurosurgery meningitis is less often as positive as for pneumococcal and meningococcal meningitis.[19]

Table 5.3 Cerebrospinal fluid analysis in bacterial meningitis in adults

Author/year [ref]	N*	Opening pressure > 300 mm H_2O (%)	Leukocyte count > 1000/mm³ (%)	Percent neutrophils ≥ 80%	Protein > 0·2 g/ liter (%)	Glucose ≤ 2·8 mol/ liter (%)	Gram stain positive (%)	CSF culture positive (%)
Durand 1993 [13]	259	39	28 (> 5000/mm³)	79	56	50 (> 2·2 mol/liter)	46	83
Sigurdardottir 1997 [12]	127	48	20	88	85 (> 0·5 g/liter)	89 (< 0·5 mol/liter)	57	80
Hussein 2000 [11]	100	NR	56	74	67	72	48	65

N*, number of patients (279 patient episodes in 275 patients[13]; 103 episodes in 100 patients[11]; 132 cases in 127 patients[12]).

Blood culture

Blood cultures should also be made in the evaluation of a patient with suspected bacterial meningitis, particularly if a CSF sample cannot be obtained prior to initiation of antibiotics (for example, when neuroimaging is planned prior to LP). Blood cultures in bacterial meningitis have been noted to be positive in 19–77% of patients.[12,15,20]

Other diagnostic modalities

Rapid bacterial antigen testing

The use of rapid bacterial antigen testing remains controversial. A recent review noted that of 478 CSF samples, 0·3% were positive by rapid antigen testing.[21] However, the false-positive rate exceeded the true positive rate, and therapy was not altered on the basis of any of the true-positive rapid antigen results. The false-positive results led to additional cost, prolonged hospitalisation, and some clinical complications. Furthermore, all true-positive CSF samples showed the causative micro-organisms by Gram stain.[21] In light of these and similar previous findings,[22] it has been suggested that the role of rapid antigen detection should be limited to those patients with suspected bacterial meningitis whose initial CSF Gram stain is negative and whose CSF culture is negative at 48 hours of incubation (for example, patients who received some period of antimicrobial therapy prior to examination of the CSF).[22,23] The role of antigen testing in this setting however requires further study.

Polymerase chain reaction

Polymerase chain reaction (PCR) of CSF has been used to detect microbial DNA in the CSF of patients with suspected bacterial meningitis. Primers have been developed that permit the simultaneous detection of the most common organisms, including *N. meningitidis*, *S. pneumoniae*, and *H. influenzae*. While a recent study demonstrated this technique to have good sensitivity (i.e. 89%) with no false positive results,[24] the time required to perform these tests was not noted. Future studies should help to clarify the role of this technology in the diagnostic approach to bacterial meningitis.

Another important role of PCR is in the detection of viral (specifically enteroviral) meningitis. In a recent multicenter study, 476 CSF specimens were collected from patients with suspected aseptic meningitis[25]: 68 samples were positive for enterovirus by PCR (14·4%), whereas 49 samples were positive by culture (10·4%). The sensitivity and specificity of the enterovirus PCR test (using viral culture as the "gold standard") were 85·7% and 93·9%, respectively. Rapid PCR-based detection of enteroviral meningitis would facilitate early decision-making regarding discontinuation of empiric antibacterial therapy as well as shortened hospitalization.

Neuroimaging

There exists controversy regarding the need to perform neuroimaging prior to the performance of the LP. Despite no supportive evidence, clinicians frequently perform computed tomography (CT) imaging prior to LP in order to rule out intracranial abnormalities which might increase the risk of brain herniation resulting from removal of cerebrospinal fluid during LP.[11,26] In a survey of 201 physicians who had ordered a CT prior to LP, stated reasons for this practice included suspicion that a focal brain abnormality was present (59%), belief that this practice was the standard of care (34%), and fear of litigation (5%).[27]

The risk of routine CT scanning prior to LP in patients with meningitis is that this practice is associated with a delay in performing LP and initiation of antimicrobial therapy.[27] This delay in initiation of antimicrobial therapy in turn increases the risk of a poor clinical outcome.[15]

In a study of 235 patients who underwent head CT prior to LP, clinical features associated with an abnormal finding on CT were age ≥ 60 years, immunocompromise, history of CNS disease, history of seizure within 1 week before presentation, as well as the following neurologic abnormalities: abnormal level of consciousness, inability to answer two consecutive questions correctly or to follow two consecutive comments, gaze palsy, abnormal visual fields, facial palsy, arm drift, leg drift, and abnormal language.[27] Of the 96 patients in whom none of these features was present, 93 had a normal CT scan. Although the negative predictive value of the approach was not 100%, the three patients who were misclassified underwent LP without subsequent brain herniation.[27] While these results should be validated in future studies, they suggest that a routine CT scan can safely be avoided in favor of careful evaluation of the clinical findings of patients with suspected meningitis.[28]

Possible indications for CT or magnetic resonance imaging (MRI) following initiation of therapy include persistent focal neurologic findings, persistently positive CSF cultures despite appropriate antimicrobial therapy, and persistent elevation of CSF polymorphonuclear leukocyte percentage after more than 10 days of therapy.[29] Neuroimaging is also indicated in patients with recurrent meningitis.

Therapy

Case presentation 1 (continued)

The patient undergoes LP without prior CT scanning. CSF reveals an opening pressure of 250 mm H_2O, and the patient is started on ceftriaxone 2 g i.v. every 12 hours. Subsequently, the CSF demonstrates a leukocyte count of 2400/mm^3 with 70% neutrophils, protein concentration of 0·32 g/liter (320 mg/dL), and a glucose concentration of 3·4 mol/liter (62 mg/dL). The Gram stain reveals Gram-positive cocci in pairs and chains.

Antimicrobials

Earlier initiation of antimicrobial therapy is essential in the approach to bacterial meningitis. Early diagnosis and therapy reduce morbidity and mortality, particularly if antimicrobial therapy is initiated before meningitis progresses to a high severity level.[13,15] If neuroimaging prior to LP is considered, antibiotics should not be delayed until neuroimaging is complete. In this situation, blood cultures should be obtained and antibiotics then administered. The choice of empiric antibiotic depends on which organisms are most likely causative, which in turn depends on several factors including age, immunocompromise, recent surgery or instrumentation, and local antimicrobial resistance patterns (Table 5.1).[30,31]

Corticosteroids

Adjunctive corticosteroid therapy for bacterial meningitis remains controversial. Animal studies of meningitis have shown that bacterial lysis resulting from antimicrobial therapy leads to inflammation in the subarachnoid space which in turn may contribute to poor outcomes.[32,33] These studies have also demonstrated that adjunctive corticosteroid therapy reduces cerebrospinal fluid inflammation and subsequent neurologic sequelae.[32,33] A number of randomized controlled trials have examined the possible role of corticosteroid therapy in pediatric meningitis but have come to differing conclusions. A meta-analysis of these trials showed a beneficial effect of adjunctive dexamethasone therapy in reducing severe hearing loss in children with *H. influenzae* type b meningitis and further suggested a similar benefit reducing hearing loss in those with pneumococcal meningitis.[34]

Recently, de *Gans et al.* reported the results of a multicenter trial of 301 adults with bacterial meningitis randomized to adjuvant dexamethasone vs placebo.[35] Administration of dexamethasone (10 mg) at 15 to 20 minutes before or with the first dose of antibiotic (and continued every 6 hours for 4 days) resulted in a statistically significant reduction in the risk of an unfavorable outcome (assessed with the Glasgow Outcome Scale[36]). Dexamethasone therapy was also associated with a statistically significant reduction in mortality, most pronounced for the subgroup of patients with meningitis due to *S. pneumoniae*. However, there was no significant beneficial effect of dexamethasone therapy on neurologic sequelae, including hearing loss.[35]

Given these recent results, routine adjunctive dexamethasone therapy has been recommended for those patients with suspected *S. pneumoniae* meningitis.[37] However, the ultimate role of dexamethasone in the treatment of meningitis needs to be clarified in future studies. In particular, future studies should focus on the possible impact of corticosteroids on penetration of certain antibiotics into the CNS. Dexamethasone reduces blood–brain barrier permeability and may impede the penetration of vancomycin into the subarachnoid space.[38] This issue has become increasingly important as the use of vancomycin for suspected bacterial meningitis increases because of concern regarding the continued emergence of penicillin-resistant *S. pneumoniae*.[31] Of note, while treatment with dexamethasone did not reduce vancomycin levels in the CSF in children with bacterial meningitis,[39] treatment failures have been reported in adults who received standard doses of vancomycin and adjunctive dexamethasone.[40]

Preventive therapy

H. INFLUENZAE

Currently available *H. influenzae* type b conjugate vaccines are highly immunogenic with more than 95% of infants developing protective antibody concentrations after a primary series of two or three doses. Use of this vaccine has been extremely effective at reducing the incidence of *H. influenzae* meningitis worldwide, often by more than 90%.[41] The American Academy of Pediatrics recommends that all infants should receive a primary series of *H. influenzae* vaccine beginning at 2 months of age.[42]

S. PNEUMONIAE

Use of the 23-valent pneumococcal vaccine to prevent bacteremic pneumococcal disease is recommended in certain high risk groups.[43] The efficacy of this vaccine against meningitis due to *S. pneumoniae* has never been proven, but has been suggested to be approximately 50%.[44,45] The more recently developed pneumococcal conjugate vaccine has been demonstrated to have excellent efficacy in the prevention of invasive pneumococcal disease in infants and children,[46] and its use is now recommended in all infants under 2 years of age.[47] Use of the conjugate vaccine is not, however, currently recommended in adults owing to limited experience in this population.

N. meningitidis

Routine vaccination with the currently available quadrivalent vaccine (covering meningococcal serotypes A, C, Y and W-135) is not recommended because of its poor immunogenicity in children under 2 years of age (i.e. the group at highest risk of sporadic meningococcal disease), and because of its relatively short duration of protection.[48,49] Use of the vaccine is recommended for certain groups:

- college freshmen, particularly those living in dormitories or residence halls
- military recruits
- persons who have terminal complement component deficiencies
- patients with anatomic or functional asplenia;
- research, industrial, and clinical laboratory personnel who are exposed routinely to *N. meningitidis*
- visitors to countries in which *N. meningitidis* is hyperendemic or epidemic (for example, the "meningitis belt" in sub-Saharan Africa).[49]

While sufficient experience exists to recommend vaccine for use in controlling outbreaks due to serogroup C meningococcal disease only, use of the vaccine may be applicable to control of outbreaks due to other vaccine preventable serogroups (A, Y, and W-135).[49] The applicability of the quadrivalent vaccine may be increased owing to recent changes in the epidemiology of meningococcus, particularly the increasing percentages of cases from serogroups covered by the vaccine.[50] Although the need for revaccination has not been determined, antibody levels decline rapidly over 2–3 years such that revaccination should be considered every 3–5 years if the patient remains at high risk.[49] The more recently developed meningococcal C conjugate vaccine has demonstrated superior immunogenicity when compared to the older polysaccharide vaccine.[51] While routine childhood immunization with the conjugate vaccine has been implemented in some countries,[52] data supporting its use in adults remains limited.

Prognosis

Case presentation 1 (continued)

The patient's CSF culture subsequently demonstrates growth of *S. pneumoniae*, which is resistant to penicillin but susceptible to ceftriaxone. The patient's fever, headache, and confusion resolve by day 3 of therapy, although the patient now complains of mild ataxia. He completes 14 days of therapy with ceftriaxone and his ataxia has resolved by the time of his hospital discharge.

While almost uniformly fatal in the pre-antibiotic era, the impact of bacterial meningitis remains great today. Mortality rates in meningitis in recent series have ranged from 17% to 37%.[11–13,15,53]

Several factors have been associated with increased mortality in patients with bacterial meningitis including advanced age,[12,13,15] obtunded mental state,[13,15] seizures,[13,15] hypotension,[15] and platelet count $< 100\,000/mm^3$.[20] Increased fatality was also associated with absence of typical symptoms and signs and was presumably due to a delay in diagnosis.[53] Indeed, despite the recognized association between delay in administration of antibiotics and mortality,[13,15] recent evidence notes that the median duration from initial presentation to administration of antibiotics was 4 hours, with 30% of patients waiting longer than 1 hour between performance of an LP and administration of antibiotics.[15]

Mortality rates also vary substantially across infecting organisms: *S. pneumoniae* (26–28%); *N. meningitidis* (10–16%), *L. monocytogenes* (32–38%), *H. influenzae* (11–17%), and culture negative (9–10%).[12,13]

CNS sequelae occur in up to 50% of previously healthy patients following meningitis, and include dizziness, tiredness, mild memory deficits, gait ataxia, cerebral edema, intracerebral hemorrhage, and hydrocephalus.[54,55] Systemic complications may include septic shock, adult respiratory distress syndrome, and disseminated intravascular coagulation.[55]

Encephalitis

Case presentation 2

A 64-year-old woman is brought to the emergency department by her daughter after a new onset seizure. The patient had been well until 48 hours prior when she had the abrupt onset of fever and headache. Over the next 2 days, she developed confusion and exhibited bizarre behaviour, and subsequently had a seizure. She has no significant past medical history. She takes no medications and does not use alcohol, tobacco, or drugs. The season is spring. The patient is retired and spends most of her time indoors and has not travelled recently. Her daughter recalls no animal exposures.

On physical examination, she has a temperature of 38·9°C, a pulse of 100 beats per minute, and a blood pressure of 140/64 mmHg. She is minimally responsive, without nuchal rigidity or focal neurologic findings. Her Glasgow Coma Scale score is 8. A serum white blood cell count is normal. A CT scan of the head reveals no intracranial mass lesions. Evaluation of CSF demonstrates a leukocyte count of 500 cells/mm^3 with lymphocyte predominance, an elevated protein concentration of 0·98 g/liter (980 mg/dL), and a normal glucose. You admit the patient with a diagnosis of acute encephalitis and institute intravenous acyclovir for the possibility of herpes simplex virus-1 encephalitis. You wonder what other diagnostic testing should be done.

Diagnosis

Epidemiology

Encephalitis indicates inflammation of the brain, and is distinguished from meningitis by the presence of abnormality of brain function, which may manifest as altered mental status, motor or sensory deficits, or movement disorders. The incidence of acute encephalitis varies according to geographical location but has been estimated at between 3·5 and 7·4 cases per 100 000 patient years,[56] with approximately 20 000 cases of encephalitis occurring annually in the US.[57]

While almost 100 agents have been associated with encephalitis, viruses are by far the most common cause, with the most life-threatening being herpes simplex virus (HSV) and arboviruses.[56] It is important to rule out other potentially treatable conditions that may mimic viral encephalitis (Box 5.2).

Box 5.2 Diseases that may mimic viral encephalitis*

- Abscess or subdural empyema
  - bacterial
  - listerial
  - fungal
  - mycoplasmal
- Tuberculosis
- Cryptococcus
- Rickettsia
- Toxoplasmosis
- Mucormycosis
- Meningococcal meningitis
- Tumor
- Subdural hematoma
- Systemic lupus erythematosus
- Adrenal leukodystrophy
- Toxic encephalopathy
- Reye's syndrome
- Vascular disease

* Adapted from [58]

Since clinical syndromes and routine laboratory tests are often non-specific, the diagnosis of viral encephalitis may be difficult. To aid in the diagnosis, certain epidemiological features should be elicited, including: time of year, location and prevalent diseases in the area, recent travel, occupational exposures, recreational activities (for example, caving or hiking), and animal contacts (for example, insect or animal bites).[58] This chapter will focus primarily on viral encephalitis in adults in the US.

Etiology of viral encephalitis

Encephalitis resulting from viral infection can manifest as two distinct disease entities:

- acute viral encephalitis – results from direct invasion of neurons by the virus, with subsequent inflammation and neuronal destruction
- postinfectious encephalomyelitis – may occur following a variety of viral infections, usually of the respiratory tract; perivascular inflammation and demyelination of the white matter are prominent.

The most common viruses causing acute encephalitis in the US are enteroviruses, followed by HSV and arboviruses (Box 5.3).[59] Less common viral etiologies include other herpesviruses, adenovirus, measles, mumps, and the human immunodeficiency virus (HIV). Rare causes of encephalitis such as rabies would be suspected based on exposure and occupational information.

Box 5.3 Causative agents for acute viral encephalitis in the United States

Arboviruses
- La Crosse virus
- Eastern equine encephalitis virus
- Western equine encephalitis virus
- St Louis encephalitis virus
- West Nile virus
- Venezuelan equine encephalitis virus
- Powassan virus
- Snowshoe Hare virus
- Jamestown Canyon virus

Enteroviruses
- Coxsackievirus A and B
- Echoviruses
- Poliovirus

Herpesviruses
- Herpes simplex type 1
- Herpes simplex type 2
- Cytomegalovirus
- Epstein–Barr virus
- Varicella–zoster virus
- Human herpesvirus 6
- Simian herpes B virus

Other viruses
- Measles virus
- Mumps virus
- Adenovirus
- Human immunodeficiency virus
- Influenza
- Rabies virus
- JC virus
- Lymphocytic choriomeningitis

Enteroviral infections (including coxsackieviruses, echoviruses, and polioviruses) peak in the summer and fall, and children and young adults are most commonly affected (Table 5.4).[57]

HSV type 1 is the most common cause of severe non-epidemic viral encephalitis in the US, accounting for about 10% of all cases of encephalitis.[57] It has a bimodal age distribution, with most cases occurring in patients under 20 or over 50 years of age.[58] The virus has no seasonal predilection, occurring at any time of the year.

Arthropod-borne viruses (arboviruses) are a heterogeneous group of viruses transmitted by the bite of arthropod vectors (mosquitoes and

Table 5.4 Seasonal preferences of selected viruses causing encephalitis

Time of year	Virus
Summer/fall	Enteroviruses
	West Nile virus
	La Crosse virus
	Eastern equine encephalitis virus
	Western equine encephalitis virus
	St Louis encephalitis
Winter/spring	Measles virus
	Mumps virus
	Varicella–zoster virus
Any season	Herpes simplex virus type 1
	Human immunodeficiency virus
	Rabies virus

ticks). They are a common cause of sporadic and epidemic encephalitis in the USA. Arboviral infections peak in late summer and early fall when exposure to vectors is highest. First documented in the USA in 1999, West Nile virus (WNV) is now the most common cause of epidemic viral encephalitis.[60] The next most common arboviruses causing encephalitis are the California encephalitis (CE) group (La Crosse virus) and the togaviruses: western equine encephalitis (WEE), eastern equine encephalitis (EEE), and St Louis encephalitis (SLE).[59,61] Venezuelan equine encephalitis (VEE) has also caused small epidemics in Florida, Louisiana, and Texas,[62,63] and Powassan virus, which is transmitted by ticks, has caused rare cases in New England.[64]

In August 1999, an outbreak of WNV encephalitis occurred in the New York City area, representing the first known presence of this virus in the Western Hemisphere.[65] Since then, the epizootic has reappeared every summer with a rapidly expanding geographic distribution, spreading to 45 states and the District of Columbia as of November 2002.[66] A wide variety of wild and domestic birds are the typical reservoirs, and Culex mosquitos are the vectors.[65]

Epidemiologic features may help narrow the diagnosis in arboviral infections, including:

- age of the patient
- location where the infection was acquired
- incidences of other cases of arboviral infections in the area (Table 5.5).

Two paramyxoviruses, measles and mumps viruses, are rarely seen now because of effective childhood vaccines, but were significant causes of encephalitis in the pre-vaccine era.[57] These infections usually occur in the winter and spring. A postinfectious encephalitis develops in approximately 1 in 1000 cases of measles[67] and typically 4–8 days after the rash, during convalescence.[56] Subacute sclerosing panencephalitis (SSPE) is a chronic degenerative disease that presents insidiously with myoclonus and seizure activity an average of 7 years after acute measles infection.[61] CNS disease from mumps, including encephalitis, complicates

Table 5.5 Epidemiologic features of encephalitis caused by arboviruses in the United States*

Virus	Geographical distribution	Age of typical patients	Mortality rate (%)
West Nile	East, mid-west, Gulf coast, southern USA	Adults, esp. elderly	4–12
La Crosse	Central, eastern USA	< 15 years	1
Eastern equine	East, Gulf coast, southern USA	Young children and > 50 years	> 30%
Western equine	West, mid west USA	Infants and > 50 years	2–3%
St Louis	Central, western, southern USA	> 50 years	10–20%
Powassan	New England	Any age	50

*Adapted references 58, 61.

about 1% of infections,[61] and usually occurs in older children or adults. It may occur before, during, or up to 2 weeks after parotid gland swelling or in the absence of parotitis.

Seroconversion to HIV infection and primary HIV disease has been associated with acute, self-limited encephalitis syndromes.[56] Patients with the acquired immunodeficiency syndrome (AIDS) can develop CNS disease from a number of unusual organisms, such as toxoplasma, pneumocystis, cryptococcus, cytomegalovirus, and JC polyoma virus (progressive multifocal leukoencephalopathy).[68]

Rabies is transmitted by the bite of an infected animal and is a rare cause of encephalitis in the USA. Most human disease in the USA is due to bat transmission, although a history of bat bite is uncommon.[69] Other animals that are most often infected include foxes, skunks, and raccoons.

Postinfectious encephalomyelitis is an acute inflammatory demyelinating disease that accounts for approximately 10–15% of cases of acute encephalitis in the USA.[56] It most commonly develops after an infection of the respiratory tract (particularly influenza), a viral exanthem such as measles or varicella, or in the past, immunisation with vaccinia virus.[57] Worldwide, measles is the most common etiological agent.[57] The pathogenesis is thought to be an autoimmune response triggered by the viral infection, with activation of lymphocytes against myelin.[70]

Clinical presentation

The triad of fever, headache, and altered level of consciousness is the clinical hallmark of acute viral encephalitis.[58] Additional clinical findings often include disorientation, disturbances in behaviour and speech, and focal or diffuse neurologic abnormalities such as hemiparesis and seizures.

Herpes simplex type 1

The onset of HSV-1 encephalitis (HSE) is usually abrupt, although a subacute prodrome of frontal headache and malaise may occur less commonly. Fever is present in 90% of cases, headache is prominent early in the course of disease, and the majority of patients have signs suggesting a localized lesion involving one or both temporal lobes.[56,71] These findings often include dramatic personality changes, which may be the first clinical manifestation. Following these behavioural changes, patients may develop aphasia, anosmia, temporal lobe seizures, and hemiparesis. Unlike with HSV-2 meningitis, mucocutaneous herpetic lesions are rarely seen with HSV-1 encephalitis.[61]

Arboviruses

The clinical spectrum of illness due to arboviruses is broad, ranging from a mild febrile illness to aseptic meningitis to fatal encephalitis.[72] The onset of encephalitis may be abrupt or subacute and begins with non-specific symptoms of fever, headache, nausea, and vomiting. CNS symptoms usually begin on day 2 or 3, and symptoms can range widely from only mild deficits to coma. Focal abnormalities such as hemiparesis, tremors, seizures, and cranial nerve palsies can occur.[61] EEE is the most virulent of the arboviral encephalitides and produces symptomatic disease with a high frequency in all age groups and a mortality of 30%.[72,73]

In most people, infection with WNV is subclinical or causes a self-limited febrile illness.[74] Only about 1 in 150 infections results in severe neurologic illness, and advanced age (50 years of age and older) is by far the greatest risk factor for this complication.[75] Encephalitis is more common than meningitis, and symptoms of severe muscle weakness or flaccid paralysis sometimes suggestive of Guillain–Barré syndrome may provide a clue to the diagnosis of WNV.

Enteroviruses

While most enteroviral encephalitides are mild, patients with agammaglobulinemia may develop a chronic, lethal form of enteroviral encephalitis.[76]

Other herpesviruses

Cytomegalovirus and Epstein–Barr virus can cause acute encephalitis syndromes.[77] Varicella–zoster virus (VZV) infection may also be complicated by encephalitis, which usually develops a week after the exanthem begins. Acute cerebellar ataxia is the most common complication of chickenpox.[57,61] An eruption of herpes zoster may be complicated by encephalomyelitis and granulomatous arteritis, the latter of which has been associated with zoster ophthalmicus.[57]

Rabies

The common presentation of rabies is one of agitation, delirium, and hydrophobia, which ultimately progresses to coma and death.[78] The incubation period usually ranges from days to months but may be as long as a year.

Postinfectious encephalomyelitis

The clinical presentation of postinfectious encephalomyelitis resembles that of an acute viral encephalitis, except that there is usually a history of an exanthem or non-specific respiratory or gastrointestinal illness about 5 days to 3 weeks prior to the onset of CNS disease.[61]

Laboratory findings

Peripheral white blood cell counts are rarely helpful because they may be normal, slightly elevated, or slightly low.[79] Evaluation of CSF in viral encephalitis reflects the inflammatory nature of the disease, typically demonstrating a mononuclear pleocytosis, ranging from 10 to 2000 cells/mm^3, an elevated protein level, and a normal or slightly low glucose. Polymorphonuclear cells may be present early in the disease, so it may be useful to repeat the lumbar puncture in 24 hours.[80] CSF PCR to detect viral nucleic acids is the superior diagnostic test in most cases of viral encephalitis; culture of CSF for isolation of viruses has only 14%–24% sensitivity compared with PCR.[81]

In HSE, CSF may be completely normal in 3–5% of patients.[71] The presence of red blood cells in the absence of a traumatic lumbar puncture is suggestive, but not diagnostic of, necrotizing HSV-1 infection.[61] The availability of CSF PCR techniques to detect HSV DNA has revolutionized the diagnosis of HSE, allowing for rapid, sensitive, and specific diagnosis.[59] In several series, PCR was found to have a sensitivity of greater than 95% with a specificity of 94% to 100%, and it can be positive as early as 1 day after disease onset.[81–83] Studies have found no effect on PCR yield during the first week of antiviral therapy, although the sensitivity of the test declines during the second week of treatment.[82]

Antibody titers in the CSF or serum are not helpful in establishing an early diagnosis of HSE, and viral cultures are insensitive.[60] HSV antigen is detected later than HSV DNA and has a sensitivity of only 33%.[83] The historical gold standard for diagnosis has been brain biopsy with demonstration of HSV in the brain tissue; however, the sensitivity has been reported to be only 60–70%, possibly because of sampling error or improper specimen handling.[83] For this reason, as well as the less invasive nature of lumbar puncture, PCR has largely replaced the need for brain biopsy.[60]

The diagnosis of arboviral infections is usually done by serologic assays for virus-specific IgM antibodies on serum and/or CSF. Both acute and convalescent (4 weeks) titers should be measured to confirm acute infection. Viral cultures and PCR testing of CSF, blood, or tissue samples are generally of low yield, except in the case of VEE where blood and throat cultures are frequently positive.[61]

A limitation of serologic tests is the possibility of cross-reactivity because of close antigenic relationships among the flaviviruses; for example, patients with WNV may test positive if they had recent infection with SLE or dengue, or vaccination for yellow fever or Japanese encephalitis.[75] A positive IgM test for WNV can be confirmed (eliminate positives caused by cross-reaction) by a WNV plaque-reduction neutralization antibody test (PRNT) titer of greater than 20.[60]

A case of WNV can be confirmed by any one of the following criteria:

- a 4-fold rise in the serum antibody titer
- isolation of virus, genomic sequences or antigen from tissue, blood, CSF, or other bodily fluids
- specific IgM antibody in CSF or serum by ELISA, confirmed by PRNT.[84]

When WNV infection is suspected, CSF should be obtained for PCR or IgM confirmed with PRNT, and PCR should be performed on peripheral blood if CSF is not available.[60]

The best diagnostic method for confirmation of rabies is detection of rabies virus RNA in saliva by reverse-transcriptase PCR.[58] Diagnosis may also be made by direct fluorescent antibody staining of viral antigens from a nuchal skin biopsy or brain tissue, isolation of rabies virus in a cell culture from CSF, saliva, or brain tissue, or a rabies neutralizing antibody titer of ≥ 5 in the CSF or serum in an unvaccinated person.[84]

The recommended laboratory tests for viral causes of encephalitis are listed in Table 5.6.

Other diagnostic modalities

Magnetic resonance imaging (MRI)

MRI with enhancement is superior to CT scan in detecting early lesions in the orbital–frontal and temporal lobes in HSE.[56] However, MRI has not been compared to PCR for confirmation of disease.[85] In varicella virus encephalitis, MRI may show ischemic or hemorrhagic infarctions or demyelinating lesions.[86] MRI is the most helpful test in distinguishing postinfectious encephalomyelitis from viral encephalitis since there is usually pronounced enhancement of multifocal white matter lesions.[86]

Electroencephalogram (EEG)

EEG is of value in diagnosing encephalitis, particularly in patients with HSE. Periodic high voltage spike wave activity and slow-wave complexes emanating from the temporal lobes at 2–3 second intervals are highly suggestive of HSE.[57,58,86]

Therapy

Case presentation 2 (continued)

You order PCR testing of the CSF for HSV. A MRI of the brain reveals enhancing lesions in both temporal lobes. An EEG shows diffuse slowing as well as bilateral periodic discharges in the temporal regions, suggestive of HSE.

Proven antiviral therapy is currently limited to HSV. In two separate trials comparing vidarabine to acyclovir in HSE, acyclovir was found to be superior.[87,88] The recommended dose is 10 mg/kg[1] intravenously every 8 hours for 10–14 days.[89] The dose should be adjusted in patients with renal

Table 5.6 Recommended laboratory tests in the diagnosis of viral encephalitis*

Aetiology	Diagnostic tests recommended
Herpes simplex virus type 1	PCR and cell culture of CSF and tissue
West Nile virus	PCR testing of CSF, IgM antibody of CSF and serum (with confirmation by neutralization antibody test)
Other arboviruses†	IgM and IgG antibody of serum and CSF, antigen detection and PCR (brain tissue) available for some viruses
Enterovirus	PCR and cell culture of CSF
Varicella–zoster virus	PCR and cell culture of CSF and tissue
Cytomegalovirus	PCR and cell culture of CSF and tissue
Epstein–Barr virus	PCR of CSF and tissue, serum antibody (often inconclusive)
Rabies	PCR of saliva or tissue, antigen testing of skin biopsy, brain tissue, or corneal impressions
JC polyoma virus (agent of progressive multifocal leukoencephalopathy)	PCR of CSF, PCR or in situ hybridisation of brain tissue
Colorado tick fever virus	Antibody (serum)
Human immunodeficiency virus	Laboratory tests not specific for central nervous system involvement
Herpes B virus	Cell culture or PCR of lesion (special biocontainment laboratory required)
Post-infectious encephalitis‡	Document recent infection at primary site outside CSF

*Adapted from references 59–61.

PCR, polymerase chain reaction; CSF, cerebrospinal fluid; IgM, immunoglobulin M; IgG, immunoglobulin G.

†Includes common arboviruses in North America including St Louis encephalitis, La Crosse encephalitis, eastern equine encephalitis, and western equine encephalitis.

‡Postinfectious encephalitis usually caused by measles virus, varicella–zoster virus, influenza virus, and vaccinia (pox) virus.

insufficiency. Both mortality and later sequelae can be substantially reduced if therapy is instituted before there is a major alteration in consciousness.[87] Therefore, early treatment is essential and should be initiated as soon as the diagnosis is suspected. Although several new antiviral drugs with activity against HSV are available in oral formulations with good bioavailability, none has been studied for HSV infections of the CNS.

Treatment of arboviral encephalitis is primarily supportive, as there are no proven therapies. Ribavirin and interferon-α2b have been shown to have activity against WNV *in vitro*, but no controlled trials have been done evaluating these agents.[90]

There is no specific antiviral agent for enteroviruses, but early studies of the agent pleconaril in animals have been promising.[91]

Treatment of postinfectious encephalomyelitis is largely supportive. The use of corticosteroids is often advocated, but no controlled trials have evaluated their efficacy and safety. There is no established treatment of rabies, short of supportive therapy, once symptoms have begun.

Preventive therapy

There are no human vaccines currently available for WNV. A live, attenuated Japanese encephalitis vaccine has been developed with a reported single-dose efficacy of > 99%, boding well for the possibility of a WNV vaccine in the future.[59,92] Prevention of arboviral infections rests on mosquito control and avoidance measures. The live attenuated measles and mumps vaccines, are extremely effective in preventing these infections. Recognition of a potential exposure to an animal infected with rabies should prompt prophylactic treatment with rabies vaccine and immune globulin.[78]

Prognosis

Case presentation 2 (continued)

The patient's CSF PCR for HSV is positive and she completes a 14-day course of intravenous acyclovir. She has a slow recovery over several weeks with no clinical evidence of relapse and is transferred to a rehabilitation facility. Six months after the encephalitis, she is living independently but functioning at a lower level than previously and has short-term memory impairment and anosmia.

In the absence of therapy, mortality from HSV-1 encephalitis exceeds 70%, with only 2·5% of patients overall regaining normal function.[57,58] Even with acyclovir therapy, morbidity and mortality remain high, with a mortality of 19% and 28% at 6 months and 18 months after therapy, respectively.[87] Poorer outcome was associated with older age, a Glasgow Coma Scale score of < than 6 at presentation, and the presence of encephalitis for > 4 days prior to initiation of therapy.[87]

Many patients who survive are left with severe, debilitating sequelae, including aphasia, anosmia, problems with cognitive function, and motor and sensory deficits.[93] Relapses may also occur after completion of therapy in a small percentage (i.e. 4–7%) of patients.[87,88,94] Retreatment with acyclovir alone or combined with vidaribine is recommended for relapse.[61] Although some authors advocate a longer course of acyclovir therapy (14–21 days) to prevent relapse,[94] no definitive evidence exists that a longer duration of therapy is associated with a decreased rate of relapse.

In cases of arbovirus encephalitis, mortality rates and the presence of neurologic sequelae depend on the specific organism and age of the patient, with the extremes of age having a worse outcome.[65,72] Case fatality rates among hospitalized patients with WNV infection have ranged from 4–12%,[75] with advanced age and diabetes identified as risk factors for mortality.[65,75] Finally, rabies is uniformly fatal in non-immunized patients.[61,78]

References

1. Tunkel AR, Scheld WM. Acute meningitis. In: Mandell GL, Bennett JE, Dolin R, eds. *Principles and Practice of Infectious Diseases. Vol. 5.* Philadelphia: Churchill Livingstone, 2000.
2. Tunkel AR. *Bacterial meningitis.* Philadelphia: Lippincott Williams & Wilkins, 2001.
3. Connolly KJ, Hammer SM. The acute aseptic meningitis syndrome. *Infect Dis Clin North Am* 1990;**4**:599–622.
4. Moris G, Garcia-Monco JC. The challenge of drug-induced aseptic meningitis. *Arch Intern Med* 1999;**159**:1185–94.
5. Bryan JP, de Silva HR, Tavares A, Rocha H, Scheld WM. Etiology and mortality of bacterial meningitis in northeastern Brazil. *Rev Infect Dis* 1990;**12**:128–35.
6. Scheld WM. Meningococcal diseases. In: Warren KS MA, ed. *Tropical and geographic medicine.* New York, NY: McGraw-Hill, 1990:798–814.
7. Tunkel AR, Scheld WM. Pathogenesis and pathophysiology of bacterial meningitis. *Clin Microbiol Rev* 1993;**6**: 118–36.
8. Schlech WF, Ward JI, Band JD, Hightower A, Fraser DW, Broome CV. Bacterial meningitis in the United States, 1978 through 1981. The National Bacterial Meningitis Surveillance Study. *JAMA* 1985;**253**:1749–54.
9. Schuchat A, Robinson K, Wenger JD, *et al.* Bacterial meningitis in the United States in 1995. Active Surveillance Team. *N Engl J Med* 1997;**337**:970–6.
10. Booy R, Kroll JS. Is Haemophilus influenzae finished? *J Antimicrob Chemother* 1997;**40**:149–53.
11. Hussein AS, Shafran SD. Acute bacterial meningitis in adults. A 12-year review. *Medicine* 2000;**79**:360–8.
12. Sigurdardottir B, Bjornsson OM, Jonsdottir KE, Erlendsdottir H, Gudmundsson S. Acute bacterial meningitis in adults. A 20-year overview. *Arch Intern Med* 1997;**157**:425.

13. Durand ML, Calderwood SB, Weber DJ, *et al.* Acute bacterial meningitis in adults. A review of 493 episodes. *N Engl J Med* 1993;**328**:21–8.
14. Farr BM, Scheld WM. Nosocomial meningitis. *Ochner Clin Rep* 1998;**10**:1–7.
15. Aronin SI, Peduzzi P, Quagliarello VJ. Community-acquired bacterial meningitis: risk stratification for adverse clinical outcome and effect of antibiotic timing. *Ann Intern Med* 1998;**129**:862–9.
16. Attia J, Hatala R, Cook DJ, Wong JG. The rational clinical examination. Does this adult patient have acute meningitis? *JAMA* 1999;**282**:175–81.
17. Conly JM, Ronald AR. Cerebrospinal fluid as a diagnostic body fluid. *Am J Med* 1983;**75**:102–8.
18. Blazer S, Berant M, Alon U. Bacterial meningitis: effect of antibiotic treatment on cerebrospinal fluid. *Am J Clin Pathol* 1983;**80**:386–7.
19. Mancebo J, Donmingo P, Blanch L, Coll P, Net A, Nolla J. Post-neurosurgical and spontaneous gram-negative bacillary meningitis in adults. *Scand J Infect Dis* 1986;**18**:533–8.
20. Andersen J, Backer V, Voldsgaard P, Skinhoj P, Wandall JH. Acute meningococcal meningitis: Analysis of features of the disease according to the age of 255 patients. *J Infect* 1997;**34**:227.
21. Perkins MD, Mirrett S, Reller LB. Rapid bacterial antigen detection is not clinically useful. *J Clin Microbiol* 1995;**33**:1486–91.
22. Maxson S, Lewno MJ, Schutze GE. Clinical usefulness of cerebrospinal fluid bacterial antigen studies. *J Pediatr* 1994;**125**:235–8.
23. Finlay FO, Witherow H, Rudd PT. Latex agglutination testing in bacterial meningitis. *Arch Dis Child* 1995;**73**:160–1.
24. Radstrom P, Backman A, Qian N, Kragsbjerg P, Pahlson C, Olcen P. Detection of bacterial DNA in cerebrospinal fluid by an assay for simultaneous detection of *Neisseria meningitidis*, *Haemophilus influenzae*, and streptococci using a seminested PCR strategy. *J Clin Microbiol* 1994;**32**:2738–44.
25. van Vliet KE, Glimaker M, Lebon P, *et al.* Multicenter evaluation of the Amplicor Enterovirus PCR test with cerebrospinal fluid from patients with aseptic meningitis. The European Union Concerted Action on Viral Meningitis and Encephalitis. *J Clin Microbiol* 1998;**36**:2652–7.
26. Archer BD. Computed tomography before lumbar puncture in acute meningitis: a review of the risks and benefits. *Can Med Ass J* 1993;**148**:961–5.
27. Hasbun R, Abrahams J, Jekel J, Quagliarello VJ. Computed tomography of the head before lumbar puncture in adults with suspected meningitis. *N Engl J Med* 2001;**345**:1727–33.
28. Steigbigel NH. Computed tomography of the head before a lumbar puncture in suspected meningitis – is it helpful? *N Engl J Med* 2001;**345**:1768–70.
29. Kline MW, Kaplan SL. Computed tomography in bacterial meningitis of childhood. *Pediatr Infect Dis J* 1988;**7**:855–7.
30. Saez-Llorens X, McCracken GH. Antimicrobial and anti-inflammatory treatment of bacterial meningitis. *Infect Dis Clin North Am* 1999;**13**:619–36.
31. Quagliarello VJ, Scheld WM. Treatment of bacterial meningitis. *N Engl J Med* 1997;**336**:708–16.
32. Touber MG, Khayam-Bashi H, Sande MA. Effects of ampicillin and corticosteroids on brain water content, cerebrospinal fluid pressure, and cerebrospinal fluid lactate levels in experimental pneumococcal meningitis. *J Infect* Dis 1985;**151**:528–34.
33. Scheld WM, Dacey RG, Winn HR, Welsh JE, Jane JA, Sande MA. Cerebrospinal fluid outflow resistance in rabbits with experimental meningitis: alterations with penicillin and methylprednisolone. *J Clin Invest* 1980;**66**:243–53.
34. McIntyre PB, Berkey CS, King SM, *et al.* Dexamethasone as adjunctive therapy in bacterial meningitis. A meta-analysis of randomized clinical trials since 1988. *JAMA* 1997;**278**:925–31.
35. de Gans J, van de Beek D. Dexamethasone in Adults with Bacterial Meningitis. *N Engl J Med* 2002;**347**:1549–56.
36. Jennett B, Teasdale G. *Management of head injuries. Contemporary Neurology. Vol. 20.* Philadelphia: FA Davis, 1981.
37. Tunkel AR, Scheld WM. Corticosteroids for everyone with meningitis? *N Engl J Med* 2002;**347**:1613–5.
38. Coyle PK. Glucocorticoids in central nervous system bacterial infection. *Arch Neurol* 1999;**56**:796–801.
39. Klugman KP, Friedland IR, Bradley JS. Bactericidal activity against cephalosporin-resistant Streptococcus pneumoniae in cerebrospinal fluid of children with acute bacterial meningitis. *Antimicrob Agents Chemother* 1995;**39**:1988–92.

40. Viladrich PF, Gudiol F, Linares J, *et al.* Evaluation of vancomycin for therapy of adult pneumococcal meningitis. *Antimicrob Agents Chemother* 1991;**35**:2467–72.
41. Peltola H. Worldwide Haemophilus influenzae type b disease at the beginning of the 21st century: global analysis of the disease burden 25 years after the use of the polysaccharide vaccine and a decade after the advent of conjugates. *Clin Microbiol Rev* 2000;**13**: 302–17.
42. American Academy of Pediatrics, Committee on Infectious Diseases. Recommended childhood immunization schedule – United States, January-December 2000. *Pediatrics* 2000;**105**:148–51.
43. Centers for Disease Control and Prevention. Prevention of pneumococcal disease: recommendations of the Advisory Committee on Immunization Practices (ACIP). *MMWR* 1997;**46**:1–23.
44. Bolan G, Broome CV, Facklam RR, Plikaytis BD, Fraser DW, Schlech WF. Pneumococcal vaccine efficacy in selected populations in the United States. *Ann Intern Med* 1986;**104**:1–6.
45. Butler JC, Breiman RF, Campbell JF, Lipman HB, Broome CV, Facklam RR. Pneumococcal polysaccharide vaccine efficacy. An evaluation of current recommendations. *JAMA* 1993;**270**:1826–31.
46. Black S, Shinefield H, Fireman B, *et al.* Efficacy, safety and immunogenicity of heptavalent pneumococcal conjugate vaccine in children. *Pediatr Infect Dis J* 2000;**19**:187–95.
47. American Academy of Pediatrics, Committee on Infectious Diseases. Policy statement: recommendations for the prevention of pneumococcal infections, including use of pneumococcal conjugate vaccine (Prevnar), pneumococcal polysaccharide vaccine, and antibiotic prophylaxis. *Pediatrics* 2000;**106**:362–6.
48. Zangwill KM, Stout RW, Carlone GM, *et al.* Duration of antibody response after meningococcal polysaccharide vaccination in US Air Force personnel. *J Infect Dis* 1994;**169**:847–52.
49. Advisory Committee on Immunization Practices. Prevention and control of meningococcal disease. *MMWR* 2000;**49**:1–32.
50. Rosenstein NE, Perkins BA, Stephens DS, *et al.* The changing epidemiology of meningococcal disease in the United States, 1992–1996. *J Infect* Dis 1999;**180**:1894–901.
51. Campagne G, Garba A, Fabre P, *et al.* Safety and immunogenicity of three doses of a Neisseria meningitidis A + C diphtheria conjugate vaccine in infants from Niger. *Pediatr Infect Dis J* 2000;**19**:144–50.
52. Public Health Laboratory Service. Vaccination program for group C meningococcal infection is launched. *Commun Dis Rep CDR Weekly* 1999;**9**:261–4.
53. Rasmussen HH, Sorensen HT, Moller-Petersen J, Mortensen FV, Nielsen B. Bacterial meningitis in elderly patients: clinical picture and course. *Age Ageing* 1992;**21**:216–20.
54. Bohr V, Paulson OB, Rasmussen N. Pneumococcal meningitis. Late neurologic sequelae and features of prognostic impact. *Arch Neurol* 1984;**41**:1045–9.
55. Pfister HW, Feiden W, Einhaupl KM. Spectrum of complications during bacterial meningitis in adults. Results of a prospective clinical study. *Arch Neurol* 1993;**50**:575–81.
56. Johnson RT. Acute encephalitis. *Clin Infect Dis* 1996; **23**:219–26.
57. Whitley RJ. Viral encephalitis. *N Engl J Med* 1990; **323**:242–50.
58. Whitley RJ, Gnann JW. Viral encephalitis: familiar infections and emerging pathogens. Lancet 2002;**359**:507–14.
59. Redington JJ, Tyler KL. Viral infections of the nervous system, 2002: update on diagnosis and treatment. *Arch Neurol* 2002;**59**:712–8.
60. Thomson RB, Bertram H. Laboratory diagnosis of central nervous system infections. *Infect Dis Clin North Am* 2001;**15**:1047–71.
61. Gluckman SJ, DiNubile MJ. Infections of the central nervous system: acute viral infections. In: Weiner WJ, Shulman LM, eds. *Emergent and Urgent Neurology.* Philadelphia: Lippincott Williams & Wilkins, 1999.
62. Ventura AK, Buff EE, Ehrenkranz NJ. Human Venezuelan equine encephalitis virus infection in Florida. *Am J Trop Med Hyg* 1974;**23**:507–12.
63. Zehmer RB, Dean PB, Sudia WD, Calisher CH, Sather GE, Parker RL. Venezuelan equine encephalitis epidemic in Texas, 1971. 1974. *Health Services Reports* 1974;**89**: 278–82.
64. Embil JA, Camfield P, Artsob H, Chase DP. Powassan virus encephalitis resembling herpes simplex encephalitis. *Arch Intern Med* 1983;**143**:341–3.

65. Nash D, Mostashari F, Fine A, *et al.* The outbreak of West Nile virus infection in the New York City area in 1999. *N Engl J Med* 2001;**344**:1807–14.
66. Centers for Disease Control and Prevention. West Nile virus activity – United States, November 7–13, 2002. *MMWR* 2002;**51**:1026–7.
67. Johnson RT, Griffin DE, Hirsch RL, *et al.* Measles encephalomyelitis–clinical and immunologic studies. *N Engl J Med* 1984;**310**:137–41.
68. Simpson DM, Tagliati M. Neurologic manifestations of HIV infection. *Ann Intern Med* 1994;**121**:769–85.
69. Centers for Disease Control and Prevention. Human rabies – Texas and New Jersey, 1997. *MMWR* 1998;**47**:1–5.
70. Johnson RT. The pathogenesis of acute viral encephalitis and postinfectious encephalomyelitis. *J Infect* Dis 1987;**155**:359–64.
71. Whitley RJ, Soong SJ, Linneman C, Liu C, Pazin G, Alford CA. Herpes simplex encephalitis. Clinical Assessment. *JAMA* 1982;**247**:317–20.
72. Tsai TF. Arboviral infections in the United States. *Infect Dis Clin North Am* 1991;**5**:73–102.
73. Przelomski MM, O'Rourke E, Grady GF, Berardi VP, Markley HG. Eastern equine encephalitis in Massachusettes: A report of 16 cases, 1970–1984. *Neurology* 1988;**38**: 736–9.
74. Marfin AA, Gubler DJ. West Nile Encephalitis: an emerging disease in the United States. *Clin Infect Dis* 2001;**33**:1713–9.
75. Peterson LR, Marfin AA. West Nile virus: a primer for the clinician. *Ann Intern Med* 2002;**137**:173–9.
76. McKinney RE Jr, Katz SL, Wilfert CM. Chronic enteroviral meningoencephalitis in agammaglobulinemic patients. *Rev Infect Dis* 1987;**9**:334–56.
77. Whitley RJ, Cobbs CG, Alford CA Jr, *et al.* Diseases that mimic herpes simplex encephalitis: diagnosis, presentation, and outcome. *JAMA* 1989;**262**:234–9.
78. Fishbein DB, Robinson LE. Rabies. *N Engl J Med* 1993;**329**:1632–8.
79. Griffin DE. Encephalitis, Myelitis, and Neuritis. In: Mandell GL, Bennett JE, Dolin R, eds. *Principles and practice of infectious diseases.* Philadelphia: Churchill Livingstone, 2000.
80. Feigin RD, Shackelford PG. Value of repeat lumbar puncture in the differential diagnosis of meningitis. *N Engl J Med* 1973;**289**:571–4.
81. Zunt JR, Marra CM. Cerebrospinal fluid testing for the diagnosis of central nervous system infection. *Neurol Clin* 1999;**17**:675–89.
82. Lakeman FD, Whitley RJ. Diagnosis of herpes simplex encephalitis: application of polymerase chain reaction to cerebrospinal fluid from brain-biopsied patients and correlation with disease. *J Infect* Dis 1995;**171**:857–63.
83. Guffond T, Dewilde A, Lobert PE, Caparros-Lefebvre D, Hober D, Wattre P. Significance and clinical relevance of the detection of herpes simplex virus DNA by the polymerase chain reaction fluid from patients with presumed encephalitis. *Clin Infect Dis* 1994;**18**:744–9.
84. Centers for Disease Control and Prevention. Case definitions for infectious conditions under public health surveillance. *MMWR* 1997;**46**:1–55.
85. Zimmerman RD, Haimes AB. The role of MR imaging in the diagnosis of infections of the central nervous system. *Curr Clin Top Infect Dis* 1989;**10**:82–102.
86. Roos KL. Encephalitis. *N Engl J Med* 1990;**323**:242–50.
87. Whitley RJ, Alford CA, Hirsch MS *et al.* Vidarabine versus acyclovir therapy in herpes simplex encephalitis. *N Engl J Med* 1986;**314**:144–9.
88. Skoldenberg B, Forsgren M, Alestig K, *et al.* Acyclovir versus vidarabine in herpes simplex encephalitis. Randomized multicenter study in consecutive Swedish patients. *Lancet* 1984;**2**:707–11.
89. Whitley RJ, Lakeman F. Herpes simplex infections of the central nervous system: therapeutic and diagnostic considerations. *Clin Infect Dis* 1995;**20**:414–20.
90. Anderson JF, Rajal JJ. Efficacy of interferon alpha-2b and ribavirin against West Nile virus in vitro. *Emerg Infect Dis* 2002;**8**:107–8.
91. Pevear DC, Tull TM, Seipel ME, Groarke JM. Activity of pleconaril against enteroviruses. *Antimicrob Agents Chemother* 1999;**43**:2109–15.
92. Bista MB, Banerjee MK, Shin SH, *et al.* Efficacy of single-dose SA 14–14–2 vaccine against Japanese encephalitis: a case control study. *Lancet* 2001;**358**:791–5.
93. McGrath N, Anderson NE, Corxson M, Powell KF. Herpes simplex encephalitis treated with acyclovir: diagnosis and long term oucome. *J Neurol Neurosurg Psychiatry* 1997;**63**:321–6.
94. VanLandingham KE, Marsteller HB, Ross G, Hayden FG. Relapse of herpes simplex encephalitis after conventional acyclovir therapy. *JAMA* 1988;**259**:1051–3.

6 Community-acquired pneumonia

David C Rhew

Case presentation

A 63-year-old man presents to your office with complaints of fever and cough productive of sputum. His symptoms began 3 days ago. He has hypertension and is being treated with an angiotensin-converting enzyme (ACE) inhibitor. He does not smoke and has had no recent travel or ill contacts. Does this patient have pneumonia, in which case you would want to treat with antibiotics, or does the patient have a viral upper respiratory infection, in which case you may wish to hold on antibiotic treatment?

Burden of illness/relevance to clinical practice

Community-acquired pneumonia (CAP) is a major cause of mortality worldwide. According to the World Health Organization (1998), acute respiratory infection including pneumonia and influenza results in 3·5 million deaths each year and is the leading cause of death owing to infection.[1] In the USA, pneumonia and influenza-related illness is the most common cause of death from infection in persons age 60 and older, and the fourth most common cause of death overall for persons aged 80 and older.[2] A meta-analysis (N = 33,148) of 122 studies published between 1966 and 1995 demonstrates that the mortality rate for CAP ranges from 5·1% (including ambulatory patients) to 36·5% (in ICU patients), with an overall rate of 13·7%.[3] The economic impact of CAP is also significant. In the UK, the annual direct healthcare cost of CAP is £441 million at 1992–1993 prices.[4] In the USA, $8·5 billion is spent annually treating patients with CAP, with the majority of this cost ($4·8 billion) spent in the treatment of patients 65 and older.[5]

Clinical management decisions in CAP often impact mortality and cost. For example, large retrospective analyzes of US Medicare patients hospitalized with CAP have demonstrated that early administration of antibiotics is associated with lower 30-day mortality rates.[6,7] Also, prediction rules have been developed to assist the practitioner in determining eligibility for admission to the hospital.[8] In the UK and USA, hospitalization accounts for 87%[4] and 89%[5] of the total cost of treating pneumonia, respectively, and application of pneumonia prediction rules may help to decrease admissions to the hospital safely.[9] Treating patients in accordance with practices that are supported by the medical evidence (i.e., evidence-based medicine) may ultimately improve patient care and reduce costs.[10,11] The objective of this chapter is to review the clinical evidence for the management of patients with CAP and to report the highest level of evidence published in the peer-reviewed literature as it pertains to CAP management issues.

A search of the MEDLINE, EMBASE, Best Evidence, and Cochrane Systematic Review databases from January 1966 through December 2003 was performed using search terms specific to the following topics:

- diagnosis (history and physical examination, chest *x* ray film, sputum Gram's stain and/or culture, blood cultures, serology. [*Mycoplasma pneumoniae*, *Chlamydia pneumoniae*, *Legionella* spp.], legionella urine antigen)
- admission decision
- empiric antibiotic choice
- duration of treatment
- prevention (pneumococcal vaccine, influenza vaccine).

Also, a hand search of the American College of Physicians (ACP) Journal Club issues and the 2001-2003 BMJ *Clinical Evidence* textbook was performed to identify additional references. Articles were excluded if they were non-English language; addressed primarily hospital- or nursing home-acquired pneumonia; applied primarily to pediatrics; or were animal or *in vitro* studies. If several articles were identified that addressed the same topic, then articles were selected in the following preferential order: meta-analysis of randomized controlled trials (RCTs) > systematic review of RCTs > RCT > meta-analysis of non-RCTs (± RCTs) > systematic review of non-RCTs (± RCTs) > non-randomized trial or retrospective trial (with greater emphasis placed on studies with larger numbers of patients enrolled). This selection process was adapted from previously described evidence-based methodologies.[12,13] Data from RCTs were presented in addition to meta-analyses and/or systematic reviews when the RCTs were not included in the meta-analysis or systematic review *and* had results that conflicted with or were not included in the results from the meta-analysis or systematic review.

Case presentation (continued)

Upon physical examination, the patient has a temperature of 38°C (100·4°F), a respiratory rate of 32 breaths per minute, a pulse of 100 beats per minute, and a systolic blood pressure of 145 mmHg with a diastolic pressure of 90 mmHg. His lung examination is normal. Based on the presenting history, you suspect that the patient has CAP. However, his lung examination demonstrates no abnormalities. Does a normal lung examination rule out CAP? How confident are you that he has CAP based on the history alone? Should you order a chest *x* ray film?

Clinical history and physical examination

The above case is a common scenario that clinicians face in the outpatient setting. How much information can the history and physical examination provide in making the diagnosis of CAP? A 1997 review[14] identified four prospective studies[15–18] that applied an independent, blind comparison with a "gold" standard to assess the *accuracy of clinical history* in diagnosing CAP (Table 6.1). The same four studies also assessed the *accuracy of physical examination* in diagnosing CAP[14] (Table 6.2). The overall conclusion was that no individual element of history or physical examination possesses a likelihood ratio high or low enough to rule CAP in or out. This finding was also supported by a 2003 review of testing strategies in CAP in which the authors reported the ranges of calculated likelihood ratios for studies reporting statistically significant results. [19]

The combination of various elements from the history and physical examination has also been evaluated in terms of its ability to accurately predict pneumonia. Diehr *et al.*[15] assigned points based on the presence of each of the following findings: rhinorrhoea (– 2 points); sore throat (– 1 point); night sweats (+ 1 point); myalgias (+ 1 point);

Table 6.1 Diagnosing community-acquired pheumonia from patient history

	Sensitivity	Specificity	Positive LR	Negative LR	Reference
Symptoms					
Fever (temperature ≥ 37·8° C [100 °F])	0·44	0·80	2·1	0·71	Diehr, 1984[15]
(Temperature > 37·8 °C [100 °F])	0·63	0·63	1·7	0·59	Heckerling, 1990[18]
Cough	0·83	0·54	1·8	0·31	Singal, 1989[17]
Night sweats	0·33	0·81	1·7	0·83	Diehr, 1984[15]
Chills	0·51	0·70	1·7	0·70	Heckerling, 1990[18]
	0·32	0·80	1·6	0·85	Diehr, 1984[15]
	0·63	0·52	1·3	0·72	Gennis, 1988[16]
Dyspnea	0·63	0·55	1·4	0·67	Gennis, 1988[16]
Sputum production	0·78	0·40	1·3	0·55	Diehr, 1984[15]
Myalgias	0·76	0·42	1·3	0·58	Diehr, 1984[15]
Rhinorrhea	0·67	0·14	0·78	2·4	Diehr, 1984[15]
Sore throat	0·57	0·27	0·78	1·6	Diehr, 1984[15]
Concurrent medical conditions					
Dementia	0·08	0·98	3·4	0·94	Heckerling, 1990[18]
Immunosuppression	0·24	0·89	2·2	0·85	Heckerling, 1990[18]
Asthma	0·08	0·24	0·10	3·8	Heckerling, 1990[18]

LR, likelihood ratio.

sputum production (+ 1 point); respiratory rate > 25 breaths per minute (+ 2 points); and temperature ≥ 37·8°C (100°F)(+ 2 points). Patients who had a score of – 1 or greater were considered to have pneumonia. A threshold score of – 1 was associated with a positive likelihood ratio (+ LR) of 1·5 and a negative likelihood ratio (– LR) of 0·22. A threshold score of + 1 was associated with a + LR of 5·0 and a – LR of 0·47, while a threshold score of + 3 had a + LR of 14·0 and a – LR of 0·82.

Singal *et al.*[17] estimated the probability of CAP based on the following formula:

$$1/(1 + \varepsilon^{-Y})$$

where Y = – 3·095 + (1·214, if cough present) + (1·007, if fever present) + (0·823, if crackles present). Heckerling *et al.*[18] estimated the probability of pneumonia by first determining how many of the following five findings were present:

- absence of asthma
- temperature > 37·8°C (100°F)
- decreased breath sounds
- crackles
- heart rate > 100 beats per minute.

The number of findings in combination with the prevalence (i.e. pretest probability) of pneumonia could then be applied to a nomogram provided by Heckerling *et al.*[18] to determine the post-test probability of pneumonia. The prediction rule by Heckerling *et al.*[18] demonstrated a receiver operating characteristic (ROC) area of 0·82 in the derivation cohort and ROC areas of 0·82 and 0·76 in the two validation cohorts. Gennis *et al.*[16]

Table 6.2 Diagnosing community-acquired pheumonia from physical examination

	Sensitivity	Specificity	Positive LR	Negative LR	Reference
Vital signs					
Temperature > 37·8 °C (100 °F)	0·27	0·94	4·4	0·78	Diehr, 1984[15]
	0·45	0·81	2·4	0·68	Singal, 1989[17]
	0·55	0·77	2·4	0·58	Heckerling, 1990[18]
	0·67	0·52	1·4	0·63	Gennis, 1988[16]
RR > 30	0·29	0·89	2·6	0·80	Gennis, 1988[16]
RR > 25	0·29	0·92	3·4	0·78	Diehr, 1984[15]
	0·40	0·74	1·5	0·82	Heckerling, 1990[18]
RR > 20	0·76	0·37	1·2	0·66	Gennis, 1988[16]
HR > 120	0·21	0·89	1·9	0·89	Gennis, 1988[16]
HR > 100	0·65	0·72	2·3	0·49	Heckerling, 1990[18]
	0·50	0·69	1·6	0·73	Gennis, 1988[16]
Any abnormal VS	0·97	0·20	1·2	0·18	Gennis, 1988[16]
Lung examination					
Asymmetric respirations	0·04	1·00	∞	0·96	Diehr, 1984[15]
Egophony	0·04	0·995	8·6	0·96	Diehr, 1984[15]
	0·28	0·95	5·3	0·76	Heckerling, 1990[18]
	0·08	0·97	2·0	0·96	Gennis, 1988[16]
Dullness to percussion	0·26	0·94	4·3	0·79	Heckerling, 1990[18]
	0·12	0·95	2·2	0·93	Gennis, 1988[16]
Bronchial BS	0·13	0·96	3·5	0·90	Heckerling, 1990[18]
Crackles	0·19	0·93	2·7	0·87	Diehr, 1984[15]
	0·50	0·81	2·6	0·62	Heckerling, 1990[18]
	0·41	0·76	1·7	0·78	Singal, 1989[17]
	0·35	0·78	1·6	0·83	Gennis, 1988[16]
Decreased BS	0·49	0·81	2·5	0·64	Heckerling, 1990[18]
	0·33	0·86	2·3	0·78	Gennis, 1988[16]
Rhonchi	0·35	0·77	1·5	0·85	Gennis, 1988[16]
	0·53	0·63	1·4	0·76	Heckerling, 1990[18]
Any chest finding	0·77	0·41	1·3	0·57	Gennis, 1988[16]

BS, breath sound; HR, heart rate; LR, likelihood ratio; RR, respiratory rate; T, temperature; VS, vital sign.

suggested that chest radiographs should be obtained if one or more of the following vital sign abnormalities was present: respiratory rate > 30 breaths per minute, heart rate > 100 beats per minute, and temperature ≥ 37·8°C (100°F). The presence of any these vital sign abnormalities was associated with a + LR of 1·2. The absence of all of these vital sign abnormalities was associated with a – LR of 0·18 for diagnosing pneumonia.

A national survey identified that 5% of patients with cough have pneumonia.[20] If we assumed that, prior to obtaining history, physical examination, or any other lab tests, the pretest probability of pneumonia for our patient was 5%, and we applied the above prediction rules to our patient, then the Diehr rule[15] would have suggested that our patient had a probability of CAP of 42%; the Singal rule[17] would have predicted a probability of 1/(1 + ε^{0874}) = 1/(1 + 2·71828^{0874}) = 1/(1 + 2·396477618) = 29%; the Heckerling rule[18] a probability of 3%, and the Gennis rule a probability of 6%. Thus, we are unable to make the diagnosis of pneumonia based solely on history and physical examination.

Chest radiograph

As to whether a chest *x* ray film (CXR) should be ordered, it is first necessary to determine if the CXR is sufficiently able to detect the presence of infiltrates, and if so, if the individual interpreting the CXR is sufficiently able to diagnose pneumonia and if the results from the CXR impact clinical management. A prospective study evaluated the ability of the CXR to detect infiltrates in 47 patients suspected of having CAP. Computed tomography (CT) of the chest was the gold standard for detecting infiltrates. The results demonstrated that the CXR had a sensitivity of 0·69 (18/26), a specificity of 1·00 (21/21), a positive LR of infinity, and a negative LR of 3·22 for detecting an infiltrate.[21] A retrospective study of 134 patients with diffuse infiltrative lung disease (DILD), of which interstitial pneumonia was one of several possible causes, demonstrated that high-resolution chest CT was superior to CXR in diagnosing interstitial lung disease.[22] These studies suggest that CT is better than CXR for detecting infiltrates. However, as the authors of the first study[22] point out, the presence of infiltrates in their study was not correlated with the presence of pneumonia, and the cost of CT was 6–7 times that of the CXR.

Three prospective blinded studies[23–25] assessed the interobserver variability of individuals in reading CXRs. In the study by Albaum *et al.*,[23] two staff radiologists agreed 79·4% of the time that an infiltrate was present, but only 6·0% of the time that an infiltrate was absent (κ = 0·37). In the study by Melbye *et al.*,[24] findings from an "expert panel" served as the gold standard for diagnosing pneumonia. The kappa-agreement between the expert panel and the Department of Radiology was 0·56, between the expert panel and chest consultant 0·59, and between the expert panel and residents 0·36. In the study by Young *et al.*,[25] findings from a panel of three radiologists served as the gold standard for diagnosing pneumonia. Agreement between the panel and the original radiologist was 87%, between the expert panel and first-year medical students 59%, between fourth-year medical students 54%, medical residents 66%, and attending staff 72%. Data from the above studies indicate that there is considerable interobserver variability in the diagnosis of CAP using CXR. Finally, a prospective randomized study of 1500 consecutive patients with acute cough (lasting < 1 month's duration) demonstrated that CXRs ordered by physicians resulted in potentially beneficial change in care for only 3% of patients.[26] Thus, the evidence suggests that the CXR can detect infiltrates (although less so than the CT), that there is considerable interobserver variability in the interpretation of CXR findings, and that, in clinical practice, the information provided by the CXR often does not impact management.

Case presentation (continued)

Admission decision

You decide to order a CXR, and the CXR demonstrates the presence of a left lower lung infiltrate without pleural effusion. Should you admit the patient to the hospital? Do you need to order any other tests to help you make this decision?

Admission decision

The decision whether to admit a patient to the hospital or to treat in the outpatient setting may be facilitated by applying a prediction rule. Prediction rules provide the clinician with the probability that a specific adverse outcome (for example, death) is likely to occur, based on the presence or absence of patient-specific data elements at the time of presentation. Patients deemed to be at low risk for adverse outcomes may be safely treated in the outpatient setting, while those considered to be at higher risk may require hospitalization.

The British Thoracic Society (BTS) has developed and validated two prediction rules.[27,28] The first rule, the BTS rule, specifies that patients with two or more of the following "core" risk factors upon admission have a 21-fold increased risk of death:

- respiratory rate ≥ 30 per minute
- diastolic blood pressure ≤ 60 mmHg
- blood urea > 7 mmol/liter.

The BTS rule has been derived from 453 inpatients and validated in a population of 246 inpatients.[27] The BTS rule[28] has been modified with the addition of a fourth "core" risk factor, presence of confusion on admission (as measured with a score of ≤ 8 on a 10 point scale). Studies comparing the BTS and the modified BTS rules have shown that the BTS modified rule is more sensitive and specific in terms of predicting in-hospital mortality than the BTS rule for persons aged 75 or older[29] and that, overall, the modified BTS rule has a higher sensitivity (66% *v* 52%) but a lower specificity (73% *v* 79%) compared with the BTS rule.[30]

The prediction rule that has been derived from and validated in the largest cohort of patients to date is the rule developed by Fine and colleagues.[8] This prediction rule (sometimes referred to as the Pneumonia Severity Index [PSI] or Fine Prediction rule) and the corresponding score (sometimes referred to as the Patient Outcomes Research Team [PORT] score) have been retrospectively derived from a cohort of 14 199 patients with CAP from the 1989 MedisGroups comparative hospital database, and prospectively validated in a cohort of 38 039 patients with CAP from the 1991 Pennsylvania MedisGroups database.

According to the PSI,[8] the presence or absence of risk factors for worsened outcomes are associated with a point score. Age is the most significant risk factor, with one point given for each year of age (minus 10 points if the patient is a women). Other risk factors receive individual scores ranging from 10 to 30 points. Risk factors include patient demographics, comorbid conditions, physical examination findings, and laboratory results. Patients who receive a score ≤ 70 (class I or II) have an attributable risk of death within 30 days of < 1% and are considered appropriate candidates for outpatient management. Patients who receive a score of 71–90 (class III) have an associated 30-day mortality rate of up to 2·8% and may be eligible for brief hospitalization, or, alternatively, outpatient management with close follow up.[9] Patients with scores 91–130 (class IV) have a 30-day risk of death of between 8·2% and 9·3%, and patients with score > 130 (class V) have a 30-day risk of death between 27·0% and 31·1%. It is recommended that class IV and V patients be treated in-hospital.[8] It should be noted that no RCTs have yet been performed that directly compare any of the admission decision rules (PSI, BTS, modified BTS).

Case presentation (continued)

Diagnostic tests

The complete blood count and serum chemistries are all within normal limits. You calculate that the patient has a PSI score of 83 (Class III) and contemplate admitting him to the hospital versus treating him in the outpatient setting. If you admit him to the hospital, what diagnostic tests should you order? Should you order a sputum Gram's stain and culture? What about blood cultures? Should you order tests to detect the presence of "atypical" pathogens (mycoplasma, chlamydia, legionella)?

Sputum Gram's stain and culture

To decide whether or not to order a diagnostic test, it is first necessary to understand the test's diagnostic characteristics (i.e. sensitivity, specificity, positive and negative likelihood ratios, ROC curves).[31] A 1996 meta-analysis evaluated the sensitivity and specificity of sputum Gram's stain in community-acquired pneumococcal pneumonia.[32] Inclusion criteria included: confirmed diagnosis of pneumococcal CAP, comparison to an independent reference standard, and all patients being properly accounted for (i.e. enough data provided to construct a 2×2 table of true positives, true negatives, false positives, and false negatives). Three blinded reviewers assessed the quality of the studies to determine eligibility for this review. A total of 12 studies published between 1966 and 1993 met inclusion criteria. These 12 studies enrolled a total of 1322 patients and evaluated 17 test characteristics. The results demonstrated that the sensitivity of sputum Gram's stain ranged between 15% and 100%, and the specificity ranged between 11% and 100%. In 10 of the 17 estimations, sputum culture was the reference standard. The authors noted a trend ($P = 0{\cdot}07$) for increased interpreter training and greater diagnostic accuracy. The conclusion of this study was that no single estimate of sensitivity and specificity could be determined for sputum Gram's stain in pneumococcal CAP, and that the results of sputum Gram's staining could be misleading, especially if the interpreter was not well trained.

Clinical studies have demonstrated conflicting results as to whether sputum Gram's stain and culture provide useful information in the management of patients hospitalized with CAP. In one prospective study[33] (N = 533), sputum samples of good quality were obtained from only 39% (210 of 533) of hospitalized patients. In another prospective study[34] (N = 74), sputum Gram's stain was unable to identify the pathogen affecting any of 74 hospitalized adult patients with non-severe CAP. This study also showed that sputum cultures identified pathogens in only 4 (5%) patients. A retrospective study[35] (N = 108) analyzed the diagnostic effectiveness of sputum cultures and sputum Gram's stains among inpatients with bacteremic pneumococcal pneumonia. The authors concluded that sputum Gram's stains had some diagnostic value when moderate or abundant Gram-positive diplococci were evident, but that the overall results of sputum cultures had limited impact on the diagnosis of pneumococcal pneumonia. Another retrospective study[36] (N = 184) examined the value of initial microbiologic studies (MBSs) in adults who were admitted for CAP and managed according to the 1993 ATS guidelines.[37] In this study, 14 patients with severe CAP had their antibiotic regimens changed owing to a non-response to their initial regimen. Three of these patients had their antibiotic regimens changed based on MBSs, while 11 had empiric antibiotic regimen changes. The mortality rate for patients whose antibiotics were changed based on MBSs was no different from that for patients who had antibiotics changed empirically (67% *v* 64%, respectively [*P* value not reported]). The authors concluded that initial MBSs were not warranted except in high-risk patients who were more likely to harbor resistant organisms.

Blood cultures

Clinical studies have demonstrated that the incidence of positive blood cultures in adult patients hospitalized with CAP ranges from 0% to 26·8%.[34,36,38–62] One prospective study has shown that the yield from blood cultures increases with worsening severity of illness (PSI Class I 5·3%; II 10·2%; III 10·3%; IV 16·1%; V 26·7%),[56] while another prospective study shows poor correlation between yield from blood cultures and severity of illness (PSI Class I and II 8·0%; III 6·2%; IV 4·6%; V 5·2%).[62] A retrospective study has found that the yield from patients who have received antibiotics prior to blood cultures is significantly lower than that from patients who have not (0%[0/23] *v* 16·6%[5/30] patients, respectively [$P < 0{\cdot}05$]).[63] The incidence of positive blood cultures in the outpatient setting is considerably lower than that seen in inpatients. According to a study of 1350 outpatients with a variety of infections, including CAP, the incidence of positive blood cultures is 1·8%.[64] In summary, these data suggest that blood cultures can provide information on the etiology of pneumonia for patients with CAP, especially for those who are hospitalized and sicker (for example requiring ICU care).

However, do blood culture results impact the clinical management of and improve patient outcomes for patients with CAP? A 1996 meta-analysis[3] has demonstrated that bacteremia is associated with an increased risk for death (OR 2·8; 95% CI 2·3, 3·6), and a large retrospective study (N = 14 069) has found an association between drawing of blood cultures prior to antibiotics (versus after antibiotics) and lower 30-day mortality rate (adjusted OR 0·92; 95% CI 0·82, 1·02; $P = 0{\cdot}10$).[6] Also, several studies have specifically addressed whether drawing versus not drawing blood cultures impacts clinical management. Two small studies have shown that blood culture results rarely result in a change in the initial antibiotic regimen.[63] Several other studies suggest that the results of positive blood cultures occasionally impact the management of patients with CAP, but are not associated with lower mortality rates as compared to empiric antibiotic changes.[36,51,56,65]

Serologies

Serologic tests for *Mycoplasma pneumoniae* include enzyme-linked immunosorbent assay (ELISA), complement fixation, and cold agglutinins; for *Chlamydia pneumoniae* they include microimmunofluorescence; and for *Legionella* spp. immunofluorescence assay.[66] However, results from serologic tests to diagnose "atypical" pathogens often return after the patient has been discharged and do not impact the treatment plan.[67] This is particularly challenging for SARS where real-time diagnosis is needed.

Urine *Legionella* antigen

The urine legionella antigen test identifies *Legionella pneumophila* serogroup I, which is the most common serogroup causing illness. The sensitivity of the test is 70%, specificity is 100%, and turn-around time is short.[68] A retrospective review of the increasing use of the test from 1995 to 1999 in Victoria, Australia, found that the urine legionella antigen test expedited the time to diagnosis of legionella by 5 days.[69]

Case presentation (continued)

Treatment

What empiric antibiotics should you order if you decide to treat your patient in the outpatient setting? How about the inpatient setting? If the patient is admitted and started on intravenous antibiotics, when is he stable enough to be switched from intraveneous to oral antibiotics and sent home?

Antibiotic treatment

Outpatients

A 1994 systematic review of the outpatient management of CAP has concluded that many studies of oral antibiotics in the outpatient treatment of CAP are limited by shortcomings in study design.[68] A 2002 meta-analysis of 13 RCTs (N = 5118) shows that oral fluoroquinoline treatment is modestly better than treatment with an oral macrolide or β-lactam antibiotic (intention to treat, OR 1·22; 95% CI 1·02, 1·47; $P = 0{\cdot}03$), and that the number needed to treat to prevent one therapeutic failure is 33 (95% CI 17, 362). Most patients enrolled in these studies were < 60 years of age and without comorbidities.[71] A 2001 meta-analysis of 18 RCTs (N = 1664) evaluating azithromycin in the treatment of lower respiratory tract infections identified that azithromycin reduced clinical failures by one-third (odds ratio 0·63, 95% CI 0·41, 0·95) as compared to other antibiotics.[72] To date, no RCTs have simultaneously compared multiple outpatient regimens to determine which is the most suitable.

One prospective, observational, multicenter, cohort study[73] (N = 864) characterized empiric antimicrobial outpatient CAP regimens with regards to compliance with the 1993 ATS guidelines,[37] and evaluated the association between the initial antibiotic choice and the following outcomes: mortality, subsequent hospitalization, medical complications, symptom resolution, return to work and usual activities, health-related quality of life, and antimicrobial costs. The results demonstrated no evidence of improved outcomes for patients receiving ATS-recommended antibiotics. In summary, evidence from clinical trials does not conclusively demonstrate which antibiotic or class of antibiotic is most appropriate for the outpatient treatment of CAP patients.

Inpatients

While many clinical trials have compared individual empiric antibiotic regimens, relatively few studies have simultaneously compared multiple different empiric regimens to identify an association between a certain regimen and a clinical outcome. One prospective, observational, multicenter, cohort study[74] (N = 2963) characterized empiric antimicrobial regimens, assessed their compliance with the 1993 ATS guidelines,[37] and evaluated associations between therapeutic choice and mortality and length of hospital stay (LOS), in patients admitted for presumed CAP. Compliance with ATS guidelines was 81% among patients with non-severe CAP, and 58% of those whose therapy was in compliance with the guidelines received a second- or third-generation cephalosporin or a β-lactam/β-lactamase inhibitor combination. Treatment with a second- or third-generation cephalosporin or a β-lactam/β-lactamase inhibitor combination with a macrolide was found to be independently associated with decreased mortality, according to multivariate logistic regression analysis (for non-severe CAP: OR 0·4; 95% CI 0·4, 0·8); $P = 0{\cdot}009$; the same treatment regimen produced a non-significant trend toward reduced mortality among ICU patients ($P = 0{\cdot}26$; OR 0·5; 95% CI 0·2, 1·6). A retrospective study (N = 213) of inpatient medical records at two hospitals assessed outcomes after non-pseudomonal third-generation cephalosporin treatment alone (group 1, N = 97) or in combination with a macrolide (group 2, N = 116) for the initial treatment of CAP.[75] There were no significant differences between groups in mortality rates (3·1% and 0·9% for groups 1 and 2, respectively), length of hospital stay (5·2 days for both), or duration of treatment with intravenous antibiotics (4·1 and 4·2 days for groups 1 and 2, respectively) between the two groups.

A secondary analysis of a prospective study (N = 385) investigated patients with "atypical"-pathogen pneumonia to identify associated clinical factors, rates of co-infection with other respiratory pathogens, and the relationship between mortality and macrolide-based treatment. Treatment for "atypical" agents (i.e. at least one dose of a macrolide or tetracycline) was provided for only seven (54%) of 13 patients with *Legionella pneumophila*, nine (57%) of 15 patients with *Chlamydia* spp., and two (66·7%) of three patients with *M. pneumoniae*. Furthermore, only four (9·3%) of 29 patients with "atypical" pathogens received at least 1 week of treatment for "atypical" agents. However, none of the 29 patients with "atypical" pneumonia died, including those who did not receive antibiotics with "atypical" activity.[67]

The largest evaluations of the relationship between the initial choice of antibiotics and clinical outcomes for patients with CAP have been performed using the USA Medicare (age 65 or older) database of patients. A retrospective study[76] (N = 10 069) of Medicare patients hospitalized in 10 Western USA states during 1993, 1995, and 1997 demonstrated an association between lower 30-day mortality and an initial empiric antibiotic regimen containing either a macrolide or fluoroquinolone. Another retrospective study[77] (N = 12 945) set as the reference standard a non-pseudomonal third-generation cephalosporin and demonstrated that the following antibiotic regimens were associated with significantly lower 30-day mortality rates compared with the reference standard: second-generation cephalosporin plus macrolide, third-generation cephalosporin (non-pseudomonal) plus macrolide, and quinolone alone; these results were obtained through multivariate and severity-adjusted analyzes. Results from these large retrospective analyzes[76,77] suggest that coverage for "atypical" pathogens with either a macrolide or an antipneumococcal quinolone is important in the treatment of inpatients with CAP.

In summary, data from RCTs do not conclusively demonstrate which antibiotic or class of antibiotic is most appropriate for the inpatient treatment of CAP patients. However, findings from large observational studies of USA Medicare patients suggest that coverage for "atypical" pathogens is associated with lower 30-day mortality rates for elderly patients hospitalized with CAP. It should also be noted that some RCTs have shown that patients hospitalized with CAP can be safely and effectively treated with oral antibiotic therapy.[78–80]

Duration of treatment

In several RCTs, duration of therapy ranges between 5 and 14 days.[81–86] The optimal duration of antibiotic therapy for CAP remains unestablished.

Prevention

Vaccines

Prevention of CAP may be possible by administering the pneumococcal and influenza vaccines for eligible patients. Four meta-analyses (published in 1994,[87] 1999,[88] 2000,[89] and 2001[90]) have evaluated the pneumococcal vaccine in adults. A 1994 meta-analysis by Fine and colleagues[87] evaluated nine randomized controlled trials and demonstrated that the pneumococcal vaccine reduces definitive (i.e. pathogen identified from normally sterile body fluid or tissue) pneumococcal pneumonia (OR 0·34; 95% CI 0·24–0·48); definitive pneumococcal pneumonia caused by *Streptococcus pneumoniae* strains included in the vaccine (OR 0·17; 95% CI 0·09–0·33); presumptive (for example, pathogen identified from sputum or nasal swab) pneumococcal pneumonia (OR 0·47; 95% CI 0·35–0·63); and presumptive pneumococcal pneumonia caused by *S. pneumoniae* strains only included in the vaccine (OR 0·39; 95% CI 0·26–0·59). Subgroup analysis demonstrated that the vaccine is not efficacious in high-risk patients. High risk is defined as older persons (mean age > 55 years), those with one or more chronic medical conditions (for example, chronic renal failure, diabetes mellitus, liver disease, COPD, cancer, or alcoholism), or those with immunosuppression. However, the authors noted that, results based on seroprevalence data showed the vaccine to be probably effective in elderly patients without chronic medical conditions, and they concluded that the pneumococcal vaccine appears to be effective for reducing bacteremic pneumococcal pneumonia in adults who are at low risk.

The 1999 meta-analysis by Hutchison and colleagues[88] evaluated 13 randomized controlled and "quasi-randomized" trials and demonstrated that the pneumococcal vaccine (vaccine valences 2–17) reduces all-cause pneumococcal pneumonia (OR 0·24–0·69) – with results significant in three studies – and reduces pneumococcal pneumonia covered by the valences (OR 0·08–0·85) – with eight of nine studies showing reduced risk and six studies significant results. Subgroup analyzes showed benefit in the elderly.

The 2000 meta-analysis by Moore and colleagues[89] evaluated 13 randomized controlled trials and demonstrated that the pneumococcal vaccine results in a significant reduction in pneumonia (RR 0·56, 95% CI 0·47, 0·66), pneumococcal pneumonia (RR 0·16, 95% CI

0·11, 0·23), pneumococal bacteremia (RR 0·18, 95% CI 0·09, 0·34), and pneumonia-related death (RR 0·70, 95% CI 0·50, 0·96) in the healthy. On the other hand, the pneumococcal vaccine does not significantly reduce pneumonia (RR 1·08, 95% CI 0·92, 1·27), pneumococcal pneumonia (RR 0·88, 95% CI 0·72, 1·07), pneumococal bacteremia (RR 0·53, 95% CI 0·14, 1·94), and pneumonia-related death (RR 0·93, 95% CI 0·72, 1·20) in the elderly.

The 2001 meta-analysis by Cornu and colleagues[90] analyzed data from 14 RCTs (N = 48 837) and concluded that the pneumococcal vaccine prevented both definitive (OR 0·29, 95% CI 0·20, 0·42) and presumptive (OR 0·6, 95% CI 0·37, 0·96) pneumococcal pneumonia, as well as mortality from pneumonia (OR 0·69, 95% CI 0·51, 0·93) in adults. However, the pneumococcal vaccine did not reduce all-cause mortality (OR 1·01, 95% CI 0·91, 1·12) or all-cause pneumonia (OR 0·80, 95% CI 0·59, 1·08).

In terms of the influenza vaccine, one randomized, double-blinded, placebo-controlled trial (N = 1838) demonstrated that influenza vaccine decreased the incidence of clinical influenza in adults aged 60 or older from 3% to 2% (RR, 0·53; 95% CI 0·39, 0·73).[91] Another randomized, double-blinded, placebo-controlled trial (N = 523) showed that adding intranasal live attenuated cold-adapted influenza A vaccine to inactivated influenza vaccine provided additional protection in preventing influenza A in elderly residents of long-term care institutions.[92]

Furthermore a 2002 meta-analysis of 15 non-RCTs shows that the influenza vaccine reduces mortality due to pneumonia and influenza by 47% (95% CI 25, 62) and hospitalizations due to pneumonia and influenza by 33% (95% CI 27, 38)[93] in persons aged 65 or older living in the community. A 1995 meta-analysis of non-RCTs demonstrated[94] that, in subjects aged 65 or older, pooled estimates from 20 cohort studies found the following influenza vaccine efficacies (1 minus odds ratio):

- 53% for the prevention of pneumonia (95% CI 35, 66)
- 56% for the prevention of respiratory illness (95% CI 39, 68)
- 50% for the prevention of hospitalization (95% CI 28, 65)
- 68% for the prevention of death (95% CI 56, 76).

Vaccine efficacy in the case–control studies exhibited the following ranges:

- 32–45% for the prevention of hospitalization owing to pneumonia
- 31–65% for the prevention of hospital deaths owing to pneumonia and all respiratory conditions
- 27–30% for the prevention of deaths owing to all causes.

In summary, data from meta-analyses of RCTs show that the pneumococcal vaccine reduces the incidence of definitive and presumptive pneumococcal pneumonia, but differ as to whether this benefit is seen in the elderly (i.e. 65 and older) or other high-risk patients. Also, data from RCTs demonstrate that the influenza vaccine reduces the incidence of clinical influenza in the elderly, while a meta-analysis of non-RCTs shows that the influenza vaccine reduces mortality and hospitalizations in the elderly.

References

1. World Health Organization. (http://www.who.int/infectious-disease-report/pages/graph5.html).
2. Centers for Disease Control and Prevention. *National vital statistics reports*. Hyattsville, Md: USA Dept of Health and Human Services, Centers for Disease Control and Prevention, National Center for Health Statistics, 1998.
3. Fine MJ, Smith MA, Carson CA *et al*. Prognosis and outcomes of patients with community-acquired pneumonia. A meta-analysis. *JAMA* 1996;**275**:134–41.

4. Guest JF, Morris A. Community-acquired pneumonia: the annual cost to the National Health Service in the UK. *Eur Resp J* 1997;**10**:1530–4.
5. Niederman MS, McCombs JS, Unger AN, Kumar A, Popovian R. The cost of treating community-acquired pneumonia. *Clin Therap* 1998;**20**:820–37.
6. Meehan TP, Fine MJ, Krumholz HM *et al.* Quality of care, process, and outcomes in elderly patients with pneumonia. *JAMA* 1997;**278**:2080–4.
7. Kahn KL, Rogers WH, Rubenstein LV *et al.* Measuring quality of care with explicit process criteria before and after implementation of the DRG-based prospective payment system. *JAMA* 1990;**264**:1969–73.
8. Fine MJ, Auble TE, Yealy DM *et al.* A prediction rule to identify low-risk patients with community-acquired pneumonia. *N Engl J Med* 1997; 1997;**336**:243–50.
9. Atlas SJ, Benzer TI, Borowsky LH *et al.* Safely increasing the proportion of patients with community-acquired pneumonia treated as outpatients: an interventional trial. *Arch Intern Med* 1998;**158**:1350–6.
10. Weingarten S. Translating practice guidelines into patient care: guidelines at the bedside. *Chest* 2000;**118**:4S–7S.
11. Grimshaw JM, Russell IT. Effect of clinical guidelines on medical practice: a systematic review of rigorous evaluations. *Lancet* 1993;**342**:1317–22.
12. BMJ Publishing Group. *Clinical Evidence.* London: BMJ Publishing Group, 2001.
13. Rhew DC, Goetz MB, Shekelle PG. Evaluating quality indicators for patients with community-acquired pneumonia. *Jr Comm J Qual Improv* 2001;**27**:575–590.
14. Metlay JP, Kapoor WN, Fine MJ. Does this patient have community-acquired pneumonia? Diagnosing pneumonia by history and physical examination. *JAMA* 1997;**278**:1440–5.
15. Diehr P, Wood RW, Bushyhead J, Krueger L, Wolcott B, Tompkins RK. Prediction of pneumonia in outpatients with acute cough – a statistical approach. *J Chronic Dis* 1984;**37**:215–25.
16. Gennis P, Gallagher J, Falvo C, Baker S, Than W. Clinical criteria for the detection of pneumonia in adults: guidelines for ordering chest roentgenograms in the emergency department. *J Emerg Med* 1989;**7**:263–8.
17. Singal BM, Hedges JR, Radack KL. Decision rules and clinical prediction of pneumonia: evaluation of low-yield criteria. *Ann Emerg Med* 1989;**18**:13–20.
18. Heckerling PS, Tape TG, Wigton RS *et al.* Clinical prediction rule for pulmonary infiltrates. *Ann Intern Med* 1990;**113**:664–70.
19. Metlay JP, Fine MJ. Testing strategies in the initial management of patients with community-acquired pneumonia. *Ann Intern Med* 2003;**138**(2):109–18.
20. Metlay JP, Stafford RS, Singer DE. National trends in the management of acute cough by primary care physicians. *J Gen Intern Med* 1997;**12**(Suppl.):77.
21. Syrjala H, Broas M, Suramo I, Ojala A, Lahde S. High-resolution computed tomography for the diagnosis of community-acquired pneumonia. *Clin Infect Dis* 1998;**27**:358–63.
22. Nishimura K, Izumi T, Kitaichi M, Nagai S, Itoh H. The diagnostic accuracy of high-resolution computed tomography in diffuse infiltrative lung diseases. *Chest* 1993;**104**:1149–55.
23. Albaum MN, Hill LC, Murphy M *et al.* Interobserver reliability of the chest radiograph in community-acquired pneumonia. PORT Investigators. *Chest* 1996;**110**:343–50.
24. Melbye H, Dale K. Interobserver variability in the radiographic diagnosis of adult outpatient pneumonia. *Acta Radiologica* 1992;**33**:79–81.
25. Young M, Marrie TJ. Interobserver variability in the interpretation of chest roentgenograms of patients with possible pneumonia. *Arch Intern Med* 1994;**154**:2729–32.
26. Bushyhead JB, Wood RW, Tompkins RK, Wolcott BW, Diehr P. The effect of chest radiographs on the management and clinical course of patients with acute cough. *Med Care* 1983;**21**:661–73.
27. Farr BM, Sloman AJ, Fisch MJ. Predicting death in patients hospitalized for community-acquired pneumonia. *Ann Intern Med* 1991;**115**:428–36.
28. Karalus NC, Cursons RT, Leng RA *et al.* Community acquired pneumonia: aetiology and prognostic index evaluation. *Thorax* 1991;**46**:413–18.
29. Lim WS, MacFarlane JT. Defining prognostic factors in the elderly with community acquired pneumonia: a case controlled study of patients aged > or = 75 yrs. *Eur Resp J* 2001;**17**:200–5.
30. Lim WS, Lewis S, MacFarlane JT. Severity prediction rules in community acquired pneumonia: a validation study. *Thorax* 2000;**55**:219–23.
31. Jaeschke R, Guyatt GH, Sackett DL. Users' guides to the medical literature. III. How to use an article about a

diagnostic test. B. What are the results and will they help me in caring for my patients? The Evidence-Based Medicine Working Group. *JAMA* 1994;**271**:703–7.

32. Reed WW, Byrd GS, Gates RHJ, Howard RS, Weaver MJ. Sputum gram's stain in community-acquired pneumococcal pneumonia. A meta-analysis. *West J Med* 1996;**165**:197–204.
33. Roson B, Carratala J, Verdaguer R, Dorca J, Manresa F, Gudiol F. Prospective study of the usefulness of sputum Gram-stain in the initial approach to community-acquired pneumonia requiring hospitalization. *Clin Infect Dis* 2000;**31**:869–74.
34. Theerthakarai R, El Halees W, Ismail M, Solis RA, Khan MA. Nonvalue of the initial microbiological studies in the management of nonsevere community-acquired pneumonia. *Chest* 2001;**119**:181–4.
35. Watanakunakorn C, Bailey TA. Adult bacteremic pneumococcal pneumonia in a community teaching hospital, 1992–1996. A detailed analysis of 108 cases. *Arch Intern Med* 1997;**157**:1965–71.
36. Sanyal S, Smith PR, Saha AC, Gupta S, Berkowitz L, Homel P. Initial microbiologic studies did not affect outcome in adults hospitalized with community-acquired pneumonia. *Am J Resp Crit Care Med* 1999;**160**:346–8.
37. Niederman MS, Bass JBJ, Campbell GD *et al.* Guidelines for the initial management of adults with community-acquired pneumonia: diagnosis, assessment of severity, and initial antimicrobial therapy. American Thoracic Society. Medical Section of the American Lung Association. *Am Rev Resp Dis* 1993;**148**:1418–26.
38. Lehtomaki K, Leinonen M, Takala A, Hovi T, Herva E, Koskela M. Etiological diagnosis of pneumonia in military conscripts by combined use of bacterial culture and serological methods. *Eur J Clin Microbiol Infect Dis* 1988;**7**:348–54.
39. McNabb WR, Shanson DC, Williams TD, Lant AF. Adult community-acquired pneumonia in central London. *J Royal Soc Med* 1984;**77**:550–5.
40. Ishida T, Hashimoto T, Arita M, Ito I, Osawa M. Etiology of community-acquired pneumonia in hospitalized patients: a 3-year prospective study in Japan. *Chest* 1998;**114**:1588–93.
41. Ostergaard L, Andersen PL. Etiology of community-acquired pneumonia. Evaluation by transtracheal aspiration, blood culture, or serology. *Chest* 1993;**104**:1400–7.
42. Marrie TJ. Bacteremic community-acquired pneumonia due to viridans group streptococci. *Clin Investigative Med* 1993;**16**:38–44.
43. Fang GD, Fine M, Orloff J *et al.* New and emerging etiologies for community-acquired pneumonia with implications for therapy. A prospective multicenter study of 359 cases. *Medicine* 1990;**69**:307–16.
44. Community-acquired pneumonia in adults in British hospitals in 1982–1983: a survey of aetiology, mortality, prognostic factors and outcome. The British Thoracic Society and the Public Health Laboratory Service. *Q J Med* 1987;**62**:195–220.
45. Venkatesan P, Gladman J, MacFarlane JT *et al.* A hospital study of community acquired pneumonia in the elderly. *Thorax* 1990;**45**:254–8.
46. Marrie TJ, Durant H, Yates L. Community-acquired pneumonia requiring hospitalization: 5-year prospective study. *Rev Infect Dis* 1989;**11**:586–99.
47. Porath A, Schlaeffer F, Lieberman D. The epidemiology of community-acquired pneumonia among hospitalized adults. *J Infect* 1997;**34**:41–8.
48. Marston BJ, Plouffe JF, File TMJ *et al.* Incidence of community-acquired pneumonia requiring hospitalization. Results of a population-based active surveillance Study in Ohio. The Community-Based Pneumonia Incidence Study Group. *Arch Intern Med.* 1997;**157**:1709–18.
49. Rello J, Quintana E, Ausina V, Net A, Prats G. A three-year study of severe community-acquired pneumonia with emphasis on outcome. *Chest* 1993;**103**:232–5.
50. Socan M, Marinic-Fiser N, Kraigher A, Kotnik A, Logar M. Microbial aetiology of community-acquired pneumonia in hospitalized patients. *Eur J Clin Microbiol Infect Dis* 1999;**18**:777–82.
51. Woodhead MA, Arrowsmith J, Chamberlain-Webber R, Wooding S, Williams I. The value of routine microbial investigation in community-acquired pneumonia. *Resp Med* 1991;**85**:313–17.
52. Bartlett JG, Mundy LM. Community-acquired pneumonia. *N Engl J Med* 1995;**333**:1618–24.
53. Levy M, Dromer F, Brion N, Leturdu F, Carbon C. Community-acquired pneumonia. Importance of initial noninvasive bacteriologic and radiographic investigations. *Chest* 1988;**93**:43–8.

54. Lim I, Shaw DR, Stanley DP, Lumb R, McLennan G. A prospective hospital study of the aetiology of community-acquired pneumonia. *Med J Aust* 1989;**151**:87–91.
55. Ruiz M, Ewig S, Marcos MA *et al.* Etiology of community-acquired pneumonia: impact of age, comorbidity, and severity. *Am J Resp Crit Care Med* 1999;**160**:397–405.
56. Waterer GW, Wunderink RG. The influence of the severity of community-acquired pneumonia on the usefulness of blood cultures. *Resp Med* 2001;**95**:78–82.
57. MacFarlane JT, Finch RG, Ward MJ, Macrae AD. Hospital study of adult community-acquired pneumonia. *Lancet* 1982;**2**:255–8.
58. Ewig S, Bauer T, Hasper E, Marklein G, Kubini R, Luderitz B. Value of routine microbial investigation in community-acquired pneumonia treated in a tertiary care center. *Respiration* 1996;**63**:164–9.
59. Mundy LM, Auwaerter PG, Oldach D *et al.* Community-acquired pneumonia: impact of immune status. *Am J Resp Crit Care Med* 1995;**152**:1309–15.
60. Leroy O, Santre C, Beuscart C *et al.* A five-year study of severe community-acquired pneumonia with emphasis on prognosis in patients admitted to an ICU. *Intens Care Med* 1995;**21**:24–31.
61. Moine P, Vercken JB, Chevret S, Gajdos P. Severe community-acquired pneumococcal pneumonia. The French Study Group of Community-Acquired Pneumonia in ICU. *Scand J Infect Dis* 1995;**27**:201–6.
62. Campbell SG, Marric TJ, Anstey R, *et al* for the Capital Study Investigators. The contribution of blood cultures to the clinical management of adult patients admitted to the hospital with community-acquired pneumonia: a prospective observational study. *Chest* 2003;**123**:1142–52.
63. Glerant JC, Hellmuth D, Schmit JL, Ducroix JP, Jounieaux V. Utility of blood cultures in community-acquired pneumonia requiring hospitalization: influence of antibiotic treatment before admission. *Resp Med* 1999;**93**:208–12.
64. Sturmann KM, Bopp J, Molinari D, Akhtar S, Murphy J. Blood cultures in adult patients released from an urban emergency department: a 15-month experience. *Acad Emerg Med* 1996;**3**:768–75.
65. Chalasani NP, Valdecanas MA, Gopal AK, McGowan JEJ, Jurado RL. Clinical utility of blood cultures in adult patients with community-acquired pneumonia without defined underlying risks. *Chest* 1995;**108**:932–6.
66. Bartlett J, Dowell S, Mandell L, File T, Musher D, Fine MJ. Practice guidelines for the management of community-acquired pneumonia in adults: guidelines from the Infectious Disease Society of America. *Clin Infect Dis* 2000;**31**:347–82.
67. Mundy LM, Oldach D, Auwaerter PG *et al.* Implications for macrolide treatment in community-acquired pneumonia. Hopkins CAP Team. *Chest* 1998;**113**:1201–6.
68. Stout JE, Yu VL. Legionellosis. *N Engl J Med* 1997;**337**: 682–7.
69. Formica N, Yates M, Beers M *et al.* The impact of diagnosis by legionella antigen test on the epidemiology and outcomes of legionnaires' disease. *Epidemiol Infect* 2001;**127**:275–80.
70. Pomilla PV, Brown RB. Outpatient treatment of community-acquired pneumonia in adults. *Arch Intern Med* 1994;**154**:1793–802.
71. Salkind AR, Cuddy PG, Foxworth JW. Fluoroquinolone treatment of community-acquired pneumonia in meta-analysis. *Ann Pharmacother* 2002;**36**(12):1938–43.
72. Countopoulos-Ioannidis DG, Ioannidis JP, Chew P, Lau J. Meta-analysis of randomized controlled trials on the comparative efficacy and safety of azithromycin against other antibiotics for lower respiratory tract infections. *J Antimicrob Chemother* 2001;**48**(5):691–703.
73. Gleason PP, Kapoor WN, Stone RA *et al.* Medical outcomes and antimicrobial costs with the use of the American Thoracic Society guidelines for outpatients with community-acquired pneumonia. *JAMA* 1997; **278**:32–9.
74. Dudas V, Hopefl A, Jacobs R, Guglielmo BJ. Antimicrobial selection for hospitalized patients with presumed community-acquired pneumonia: a survey of nonteaching US community hospitals. *Ann Pharmacother* 2000;**34**: 446–52.
75. Burgess DS, Lewis JS. Effect of macrolides as part of initial empiric therapy on medical outcomes for hospitalized patients with community-acquired pneumonia. *Clin Ther* 2000;**22**:872–8.
76. Houck PM, MacLehose RF, Niederman MS, Lowery JK. Empiric antibiotic therapy and mortality among medicare pneumonia inpatients in 10 western states: 1993, 1995, and 1997. *Chest* 2001;**119**:1420–6.
77. Gleason PP, Meehan TP, Fine JM, Galusha DH, Fine MJ. Associations between initial antimicrobial therapy and

medical outcomes for hospitalized elderly patients with pneumonia. *Arch Intern Med* 1999;**159**:2562–72.

78. Chan R, Hemeryck L, O'Regan M, Clancy L, Feely J. Oral versus intravenous antibiotics for community acquired lower respiratory tract infection in a general hospital: open, randomized controlled trial. *BMJ* 1995;**310**:1360–2.
79. Fredlund H, Bodin L, Back E, Holmberg H, Krook A, Rydman H. Antibiotic therapy in pneumonia: a comparative study of parenteral and oral administration of penicillin. *Scand J Infect Dis* 1987;**19**:459–66.
80. Castro-Guardiola A, Viejo-Rodriguez AL, Soler-Simon S *et al.* Efficacy and safety of oral and early-switch therapy for community-acquired pneumonia: a randomized controlled trial. *Am J Med* 2001;**111**:367–74.
81. Schonwald S, Gunjaca M, Kolacny-Babic L, Car V, Gosev M. Comparison of azithromycin and erythromycin in the treatment of atypical pneumonias. *J Antimicrob Chemother* 1990;**25**(Suppl A):123–6.
82. Kinasewitz G,.Wood RG. Azithromycin versus cefaclor in the treatment of acute bacterial pneumonia. *Eur J Clin Microbiol Infect Dis* 1991;**10**:872–7.
83. Vergis EN, Indorf A, File TMJ *et al.* Azithromycin vs cefuroxime plus erythromycin for empirical treatment of community-acquired pneumonia in hospitalized patients: a prospective, randomized, multicenter trial. *Arch Intern Med* 2000;**160**:1294–300.
84. File TMJ, Segreti J, Dunbar L *et al.* A multicenter, randomized study comparing the efficacy and safety of intravenous and/or oral levofloxacin versus ceftriaxone and/or cefuroxime axetil in treatment of adults with community-acquired pneumonia. *Antimicrob Agents Chemother* 1997;**41**:1965–72.
85. Sullivan JG, McElroy AD, Honsinger RW *et al.* Treating community-acquired pneumonia with once-daily gatifloxacin vs. once-daily levofloxacin. *J Resp Dis* 1999;**20**:S49–S59.
86. Siegel RE, Halpern NA, Almenoff PL, Lee A, Cashin R, Greene JG. A prospective randomized study of inpatient iv. antibiotics for community-acquired pneumonia. The optimal duration of therapy. *Chest* 1996;**110**:965–71.
87. Fine MJ, Smith MA, Carson CA *et al.* Efficacy of pneumococcal vaccination in adults. A meta-analysis of randomized controlled trials. *Arch Intern Med* 1994;**154**:2666–77.
88. Hutchison BG, Oxman AD, Shannon HS, Lloyd S, Altmayer CA, Thomas K. Clinical effectiveness of pneumococcal vaccine. Meta-analysis. *Canad Fam Phys* 1999;**45**:2381–93.
89. Moore RA, Wiffen PJ, and Lipsky BA. Are the pneumococcal polysaccharide vaccines effective? Meta-analysis of the prospective trials. *BMC Fam Pract* 2000;**1**.
90. Cornu C, Yzebe D, Leophonte P, Gaillat J, Boissel JP, Cucherat M. Efficacy of pneumococcal polysachharaide vaccine in immunocompetent adults: a meta-analysis of randomized trials. *Vaccine* 2001;**19**:4780–90.
91. Govaert TM, Thijs CT, Masurel N, Sprenger MJ, Dinant GJ, Knottnerus JA. The efficacy of influenza vaccination in elderly individuals. A randomized double-blind placebo-controlled trial. *JAMA* 1994;**272**:1661–5.
92. Treanor JJ, Mattison HR, Dumyati G *et al.* Protective efficacy of combined live intranasal and inactivated influenza A virus vaccines in the elderly. *Ann Intern Med* 1992;**117**:625–33.
93. Vu T, Farish S, Jenkins M, Kelly H. A meta-analysis of effectiveness of influenza vaccine in persons aged 65 years and over living in the community. *Vaccine* 2002;**20**:1831–6.
94. Gross PA, Hermogenes AW, Sacks HS, Lau J, Levandowski RA. The efficacy of influenza vaccine in elderly persons. A meta-analysis and review of the literature. *Ann Intern Med* 1995;**123**:518–27.

7
Tuberculosis

Manjula Datta, Marek Smieja

Case presentation 1

A 40-year-old man, who emigrated from India to Canada 2 years previously, presents with irregular fever and cough for several weeks. He is coughing up thick clear coin-like bits of sputum, sometimes streaked with blood. He had hemoptysis on one occasion. His fever is more marked in the evenings and he has cold sweats at night. He also has marked loss of appetite, and has lost some 10 kg of weight in the past 2 months. He smokes cigarettes but denies drinking alcohol. He works in the construction industry, but has been unable to work for a month.

On examination, the patient is thin, almost to the point of emaciation; the ribs stand out prominently, and the trachea is deviated to the right side. There is a hollow beneath the right clavicle. The skin feels hot and dry to the touch although there is no actual fever. There is dullness to percussion over the apex of the lung. Auscultation reveals moist crepitations and bronchial breathing over the same regions.

A chest radiograph reveals a dense opacity in the right apical region with a small cavity in the middle of the opacity. You admit him to hospital into a negative pressure, aerosol-isolation room, and order sputum examination for acid-fast bacilli (AFB) and mycobacterial culture. To your surprise, his first sputum examination is negative for AFB. You wonder whether polymerase chain reaction (PCR) for *Mycobacterium tuberculosis* would help to rapidly diagnose this man's suspected pulmonary tuberculosis.

Epidemiology

Tuberculosis (TB) is an infectious disease caused by the bacterium *Mycobacterium tuberculosis*, and remains a major cause of morbidity and mortality throughout the world. An estimated 1·7 billion people, or nearly one-third of the world's population, have been infected, and every year there are an estimated 8·4 million new cases and 1·7 million deaths.[1] TB was the seventh leading cause of death worldwide in 1990, and is projected to remain in seventh place in 2020.[2] Among adults, it is second only to HIV as a cause of infectious disease-related mortality. About 95% of the total burden of TB is in resource-poor countries, especially in south-east Asia and sub-Saharan Africa.[3]

In resource-poor nations, and particularly in sub-Saharan Africa, the HIV epidemic, poverty, large-scale displacement of populations caused by war or famine, and lack of comprehensive treatment and control programs have contributed to a resurgence of TB, prompting the World Health Organization to declare a Global Health Emergency in 1993. In India, which alone accounts for 2 million active TB cases and 0·5 millions deaths per year, a large-scale effort to improve laboratory services, drug supplies and standardized regimens, directly-observed therapy, and improved reporting methods resulted in a major improvement in the proportion of patients completing therapy. The authors of one report estimate that 200 000 deaths were prevented during the 10-year program.[4]

In contrast with resource-poor nations, with annual TB incidence rates of between 50 and 700 cases per 100 000,[1] the USA, Canada, and most industrialized countries have witnessed a steady decline in TB incidence through much of the 20th century. However, between 1985 and 1992, an unexpected increased incidence was observed. This has been attributed in part to the HIV epidemic, to an increased number of refugees from endemic countries, and to delayed recognition and control of inner-city outbreaks by under-funded public health departments.[5] With renewed government commitment, incidence has been declining since 1992, to 5·8 per 100 000 in the year 2000, with a 45% decline observed between 1992 and 2000.[6] In the year 2000, 22 of 50 American states reported an incidence of 3·5 cases per 100 000 or fewer, the interim goal for the new millennium set out in 1989 by the Advisory Council for the Elimination of Tuberculosis strategic plan of the Centers for Disease Control and Prevention (CDC).[7] These states, representing over one-quarter of the American population, are classified as "low-incidence states" and targeted for TB elimination. Over 50% of 3200 US counties reported no TB cases in the year 2000.[6] The Advisory Council for Elimination of Tuberculosis defined "eradication" as a level of less than 0·1 cases per 100 000 per year.[7]

Risk factors for infection and disease

The principal mode of transmission for *M. tuberculosis* is by air, and consequently the primary focus is in the lungs. Infection often does not manifest as disease, and depends on a number of contributing factors. The risk factors for developing TB can be divided into factors that increase the probability of exposure to infection (which is often asymptomatic), and factors that increase the probability of disease among those who become infected.

Given the low incidence of TB in industrialized countries, the major risk factor for exposure is previous habitation in endemic areas. Refugees and immigrants from TB-endemic areas of the world are at high risk of developing TB because of previous exposure, particularly in their first 5–10 years after arrival.[8,9] Initially, their TB incidence is similar to their country of origin, and after 5 years or more approaches that of their adopted country. Other groups at risk of TB exposure are household or institutional contacts of active TB cases, aboriginals, the homeless, injection drug users, and people in long-term institutions.[5,10–13] Many of the elderly were exposed to TB in their childhood, particularly if born outside of the USA and Canada, as TB was epidemic throughout Europe and most of the world at that time. The elderly with previous infection are at risk for reactivation, particularly if they have an abnormal chest *x* ray film and have never received "preventive treatment",[13] now termed treatment of latent TB infection (LTBI).[14]

Among those previously or concurrently exposed to *M. tuberculosis* infection, a number of risk factors have been shown to predispose to developing active disease. The strongest risk factors are concurrent HIV infection, associated with 50–200-fold increases in TB incidence.[15,16] The Centers for Disease Control and Prevention (CDC) recommend HIV testing in all patients diagnosed with TB.[15] Other risk factors include increasing age, malignancy, silicosis, liver or kidney disease, transplantation and other immunosuppression, chronic use of corticosteroids, alcoholism, malnutrition, gastrectomy, jejunoileal bypass, and diabetes mellitus.[14,17] New drugs such as tumor necrosis factor-alpha blockers, used for patients with severe rheumatoid arthritis, have been found to increase reactivation of TB.[18] In Mexico, indoor air pollution from traditional wood stoves was found to be strongly associated with developing TB (adjusted OR of 2·4).[19] Smoking is a newly recognized but extremely prevalent risk factor for TB infection.[20–24] In a retrospective study from India of 43 000 cases and 35 000 controls, smoking cigarettes (urban) or bidis (rural) was associated with increased TB mortality. The authors estimated that fully one-half of all TB cases in India, and half of all TB deaths, could be attributed to smoking.[21] A smaller nested case–control study, also from India, found a strong dose-response relationship between amount and duration of smoking, and development of pulmonary TB,[22] and a meta-analysis of 16 studies published between 1956 and 2002, found increased pulmonary and extrapulmonary TB among smokers and their children.[23]

Among new tuberculin skin test converters, 5% develop active TB within 2 years, and a further 5% are estimated to develop TB life-long.[25] These estimates are derived from studies in the 1950s and 1960s, when TB prevalence in the community was markedly higher than at present. Whether exposure to infection still carries the same risk today is unclear. Among patients with HIV, the risk following exposure to *M. tuberculosis* may be as high as 8% per year, or a cumulative 50% or higher risk of developing active TB.[16]

Diagnosis

Clinical presentation

The classic clinical features of active pulmonary TB include chronic cough, hemoptysis, expectoration of thick sputum, and constitutional symptoms such as fatigue or night sweats, anorexia, and weight loss. Although many case-series exist, there are few population-based studies that describe symptoms of TB. In a population-based study set in Los Angeles County, in which 12% of patients had HIV, the incidence of cough was 48%, fever 29%, weight loss 45%, and hemoptysis 21%.[26] Cough for 2 weeks or more was only present in 52% of patients with pulmonary TB, while fever of over 2 weeks' duration was present in only 29%. The other population-based study was from the Ivory Coast, where 44% of patients had HIV.[27] In this study, cough was present in 80%, fever in 69%, and weight loss in 74%. Other studies have shown variable results. In one case series from Chicago of 110 patients, where 44 patients had pulmonary TB, only one patient with TB did not have either an abnormal chest radiograph, 2 or more weeks of cough, sputum production, or weight loss.[28] Predictive models have been developed to help better predict who requires hospital isolation in patients with suspected TB.[29] However, although these models were more sensitive than the existing respiratory isolation policy (91% and 82% for two retrospective groups *v* 71% for isolation policy), the results are limited to smear-positive patients.

Chest radiograph

The diagnosis of pulmonary TB requires compatible changes on chest radiograph, accompanied by culture or other evidence of infection with *M. tuberculosis*. Radiographic changes depend on how recent the infection is, concomitant medical conditions (such as HIV or diabetes), and host reaction (fibrosis, calcification). Pulmonary TB can be primary or post-primary. Primary TB commonly occurs in the lower lung but may involve any lobe. In about 5% of cases, the primary lesion results in clinical pneumonia, which is seen as a lobar or segmental infiltrate with ipsilateral lymphadenopathy. Multiple lobes may also be involved with gross mediastinal lymph node enlargement with or without pleural effusion. Primary TB is increasingly found in adults with acute TB in outbreaks in Canada and other industrialized countries, as many people have had no prior exposure to TB.[30] The areas of consolidation in primary TB may undergo cavitation, referred to as "progressive primary disease". Occasionally, a completely normal *x* ray film may be seen in patients with small parenchymal or endobronchial lesions.

The predictive value and reproducibility of a radiograph system for screening of active TB was assessed in one study.[31] Inter-reader agreement using five broad categories was moderate (kappa values of 0·44–0·56). The adjusted odds of active TB, relative to normal or minor findings or granulomas, was 10·2 (95% CI 3·2–33) for fibronodular changes, 46·1 (95% CI 18–117) for parenchymal infiltrates, and 11·6 (95% CI 3·6–37) for pleural effusion.

Diabetics, compared with non-diabetics, more commonly had lower lobe disease and were more likely to have cavitation.[32] HIV-positive patients are more likely to have a primary pneumonia, pleural effusions, and multilobe disease. The *x* ray film was altered by immune status: among 135 HIV/TB co-infected patients, CD4-T-lymphocyte count of < 200 were more likely than those with counts > 200 to have hilar adenopathy, and less likely to have cavitation.[33]

Chest radiograph may be unable to distinguish active from inactive disease, or to exclude concomitant disease such as lung cancer. In such cases, high resolution CT or gallium scanning may be helpful. In a small case series, CT had 93% sensitivity and 100% specificity for detecting active pulmonary TB; gallium scanning had 100% sensitivity and 82% specificity.[34]

Immunologic testing

The tuberculin skin test, and gamma-interferon release by lymphocytes stimulated with mycobacterial antigen, can detect exposure to *M. tuberculosis*. Both tests are discussed extensively later in this chapter, under the heading of prevention of TB. For the diagnosis of active TB, the tuberculin skin test is often positive (> 5 mm in HIV or close contact to known active case, otherwise > 10 mm). However, due to false positives (from previous BCG or other mycobacteria) and false negatives (anergy from malnutrition, HIV, or other immune compromise), the skin test is only helpful if unequivocally pcsitive (> 20 mm). Even in such cases, lung disease may be due to other causes. At least 25% of patients with acute TB will have false-negative skin tests, although these may convert to positive as the patient is recovering.

The lymphocyte production of gamma-interferon assay has been shown to correlate well with the tuberculin skin test,[35] but its role in diagnosing active TB has not been adequately assessed. In one study, it was positive in 67% of patients with active TB, and did not change during treatment.[36] The diagnosis of active TB should generally require the isolation of organism, as detailed below, with immunologic tests playing only a supportive role.

Microbiologic testing

Confirmatory diagnosis of active TB requires demonstration of the pathogen in appropriately-stained smears together with PCR, or culture of the organism. Although TB can affect any part of the body, the lungs are by far the most commonly affected. Hence sputum, and in the case of children, gastric lavage, is the most commonly examined specimen. Early morning specimens are best, and at least three specimens should be collected. Bronchoscopy may be indicated if the patient cannot cough up sputum, although most such patients can be identified by inducing sputum production with hypertonic saline.[37] Bronchial washings, brushings, and biopsy specimens may be obtained, and sputum that is collected immediately after bronchoscopy is frequently positive. A variety of other specimens like urine, cerebrospinal fluid, pleural fluid, pus, or tissue biopsy specimens can be collected in suspected cases of extrapulmonary TB. Fresh or frozen tissue can be cultured for mycobacteria. Formalin-fixed tissue, while inappropriate for culture, may still be subjected to AFB stains followed by PCR to identify mycobacterial disease.

During specimen collection, patients produce an aerosol that may be hazardous to the healthcare worker or others in close proximity to the patient. For this reason, the workers should use protective masks while collecting the specimens. The specimens must be collected in an isolated, well-ventilated area. Sputum induction is particularly prone to generating aerosols that infect staff and other patients.

Smear examination

Mycobacteria are acid fast bacteria, which can be demonstrated in appropriately-prepared specimens by Ziehl–Neelsen (ZN) or related stains. At least 100 fields, which examine only 1% of the entire smear, must be examined under the oil immersion objective before a specimen is declared negative. To find one acid fast bacillus per field, there must be a minimum of 10^6 bacilli/ml of sputum; hence if there are 5000 bacilli/ml, there is only a 50% chance of finding the bacilli.[38] Thus the sensitivity of the smear examination is low. In surveys, the smear detects only about 50% of all culture positive cases. Sensitivity is increased using prestained ZN or auramine as compared to Kinyoun's cold carbol fuchsin method.[39] For laboratories doing high volume work, fluorescent microscopy has the further advantage of allowing more rapid specimen screening, although specialized instruments and skilled laboratory staff are required.[38]

Whereas a positive AFB smear may be diagnostic in an endemic country, fewer than 50% of AFB positive sputa in industrialized countries may be due to *M. tuberculosis*. The remainder are due to non-tuberculous mycobacteria, including *M. kansasii*, *M. avium intercellulare* complex, and *M. xenopii*. Thus, a positive AFB smear requires confirmation by culture, and, where available, by PCR. PCR has the advantage of providing a rapid result, whereas culture for non-tuberculous mycobacteria may take up to 8 weeks. PCR will be discussed separately.

Mycobacterial culture

As sputum AFB stain is insensitive, culture for mycobacteria will markedly improve detection of pulmonary TB. Results of culture by the conventional solid egg media take 2–8 weeks, whereas culture using the BACTEC radiometric system or other liquid media gives results in 4–14 days. After the colonies grow, they are identified by biochemical tests or, more rapidly, by nucleic acid hybridization. Drug susceptibility testing can only be performed once an organism has been cultured, and takes 1 more week. With current liquid broth methods, detection and drug susceptibility testing results are often available within 3–4 weeks. However, only sputum examination and PCR (see below) are available rapidly enough to influence the management of the acutely sick patient. Culture is estimated to be 80–85% sensitive, and 98–99% specific. Culture has an analytic sensitivity many times greater than sputum examination, and can detect as few as 10–100 bacilli/ml. However, suboptimal specimen collection or overly aggressive laboratory decontamination may result in false-negative cultures.

Nucleic acid amplification tests

Nucleic acid amplification tests such as PCR, whether in-house or commercially-produced, are increasingly used to rapidly diagnose TB. For AFB sputum-positive patients, PCR is 95% sensitive and 98–99% specific, and is used essentially as a rapid confirmatory test. In the setting of sputum positive *M. tuberculosis*, commercial assays have shown high sensitivity (94–96%) and very high specificity (99·7–100%).[40,41] Use of commercial assays obviates some of the quality control issues that affect in-house PCR assays.

In low-prevalence countries, AFB positive smears often represent non-tuberculous mycobacteria. PCR is able in such cases to rapidly exclude *M. tuberculosis*, with implications for treatment and infection control. PCR would not be cost-effective in high-prevalence areas, since AFB positive smears in such settings are virtually diagnostic. In either setting, PCR does not currently replace culture since the latter remains slightly more sensitive, and a cultured organism is required to determine drug susceptibilities and for molecular fingerprinting.

In contradistinction to its high sensitivity in AFB positive sputum samples, PCR is less sensitive in AFB-negative, culture-positive specimens. Estimates of sensitivity in this setting range from 9 to 100%, and specificity of 25 to 100%.[42] In this recent meta-analysis of 50 studies examining PCR in patients with sputum-negative, culture-positive pulmonary TB, Sarmiento and colleagues found major methodological deficiencies.[42] They concluded that PCR is not consistently accurate enough to be routinely recommended for the diagnosis of sputum-negative pulmonary TB, but that PCR of bronchial specimens may be useful in highly suspicious cases. They found that studies not reporting blinding probably overestimated accuracy of PCR. They recommend that studies evaluating PCR for pulmonary TB should be conducted by patient and type of respiratory specimen, appropriately blinded, and use an expanded reference standard of culture together with clinical criteria. A major problem remains the discordance between PCR positives and culture, probably attributable to false-positives for PCR.[43] Methods to minimize amplicon carry-over improve test specificity.[44] Using commercial assays, the sensitivity for detecting AFB-negative, culture-positive specimens was 50–60%, depending on the assay.[41]

Since PCR detects virtually all AFB-positive specimens, and a proportion of AFB-negatives, it is being investigated for routine initial specimen examination. However, as *M. tuberculosis* may present in only some 1% of specimens submitted to a laboratory in a low-prevalence country the routine use of PCR is not cost-effective. However, if there is high clinical suspicion of TB, PCR is recommended despite AFB-negative smears.[42]

PCR detection of *M. tuberculosis* has been demonstrated in various forms of pulmonary and extrapulmonary disease, in a variety of specimen types including pleural fluid, lymph nodes, cerebrospinal fluid, blood, and urine.[45–49] However, both false-positive and false-negative results occur, and further standardization and validation is required before the clinician can rely on PCR for routine diagnosis of extrapulmonary disease.

Molecular fingerprinting

In industrialized countries with a low prevalence of TB, reactivation of latent TB disease accounts for the majority of clinical cases of TB. The uniqueness of cultured isolates can be demonstrated by molecular fingerprinting methods such as IS6110 or spoligotyping.[50–53] The finding of clustered isolates strongly suggests recent transmission, and has been shown in several settings to be much more sensitive than conventional public health contact tracing for identifying community outbreaks. Thus, in an outbreak in Baltimore, only 30% of clustered isolates had been detected by contact tracing. National and international databases are being set up to look for temporal and spatial clustering of *M. tuberculosis* isolates, and will be particularly important in low prevalence countries for identifying otherwise-undetected outbreaks. The world-wide occurrence of a multidrug resistant “Beijing/W” strain was shown using molecular epidemiological methods to be present not only in Asia, but as far as New York, Cuba, and Estonia.[54]

Case presentation 1 (continued)

Your patient's second and third sputum samples are acid-fast positive for small numbers of characteristic bacilli. A nucleic acid amplification test confirms *M. tuberculosis* and you start him on isoniazid (INH), rifampicin (rifampin), pyrazinamide, and ethambutol. He consents to HIV antibody testing and tests negative. Two weeks later his culture confirms *M. tuberculosis*. One week later, his isolate is found to be fully susceptible to all first-line antituberculous drugs, and you discontinue his ethambutol.

You plan to treat him with three drugs for a total of 2 months, followed by a further 4 months of isoniazid and rifampicin. You warn him about potential drug side effects, and prescribe vitamin B6 to minimize his chance of neuropathy. You notify the local public health department to arrange contact tracing. You ask the department about the availability of directly observed therapy (DOT), and wonder about the need for DOT in this man.

Treatment

The aim of treatment is to cure patients, prevent relapses, and avert deaths. The treatment of pulmonary TB has been subjected to numerous randomized clinical trials, primarily in developing and high-prevalence countries, although no systematic review of such trials was identified. A number of studies conducted by the British Medical Research Council in Singapore, Hong Kong, India, and East Africa compared various durations and regimens,[55] and found that a combination of INH, rifampicin, and pyrazinamide for 2 months, followed by INH and rifampicin for a further 4 months, resulted in high (> 96%) cure rates. The CDC recommends these three drugs, together with ethambutol, for initial treatment of TB.[56]

For sputum-negative, culture-positive disease, randomized trials have demonstrated that 4 months or longer of therapy yielded very low relapse rates of 1–4% (depending on initial drug susceptibility).[57] Inclusion of sputum-negative, culture-negative patients with compatible chest radiographs in these trials, however, suggests that these may have fallen more in the category of treatment of "latent TB infection" rather than necessarily representing active TB.

In addition to examining the duration of therapy, randomized clinical trials have examined the efficacy of twice-weekly INH and rifampicin in the continuation phase versus daily therapy. A Cochrane Library systematic review found that intermittent therapy was as effective as daily therapy.[58] Of 399 patients, intermittent therapy cured 99·5% versus 100% in the daily treatment arm. Relapses were 2·5% and 0%, respectively. However, as only a single trial was identified, the authors conclude that larger studies are required to more precisely estimate long-term cure. Intermittent regimens may be particularly attractive as part of supervized programs in which all doses are administered and witnessed by medical personnel (DOT).

The effect of DOT remains unclear. There are cohort and before-after data to demonstrate the effectiveness of WHO's DOTS program, which utilizes DOT and short-course (6-month) therapy.[4,59] However, the program also emphasizes a number of other effective aspects of TB treatment including:

- appropriate laboratory facilities and training for microscopic diagnosis
- providing drugs and establishing conveniently located clinics
- appropriate record-keeping and follow up.

While this program, properly implemented, has clearly worked in areas such as India,[4] it remains unclear to what extent the direct supervision of pill-taking was responsible for the improvements.

In a meta-analysis of six randomized controlled trials of DOT or usual care, Volmink and Garner found no effect of DOT.[60] They note, however, that many of the DOT programs examined had poorly motivated staff and were inconvenient for patients to access. Furthermore, in many of the trials DOT was given at a site which was inconveniently located for patients. In one RCT of DOT in which patients were given a choice of treatment site, adherence was improved. The authors note that DOT is often more expensive than standard therapy, and requires a paternalistic model of medical care at variance with most other therapies. The authors note that an emphasis on incentives and enablers is probably as important as DOT. In many industrialized countries, DOT is used quite selectively for patients with multidrug resistant (MDR)-TB, or among homeless, injection drug users, or other groups at high risk of poor adherence.

Even with DOT, high adherence rates are not assured. Clinical trials of health education, monetary incentives, and reminders have found that monetary incentives were very effective at improving adherence to clinic visits among injection drug users on TB treatment.[61] In one randomized trial, a $5 incentive improved compliance two-fold compared with no intervention or education alone.[62]

Adjunctive therapies for TB that have been studied include corticosteroids and immunotherapy, with a large RCT demonstrating more rapid symptom control.[63] A meta-analysis of corticosteroid use concluded that, compared with placebo, steroids were associated with more rapid resolution of pulmonary infiltrates, and did not affect sputum conversion.[64] Steroids are indicated for tuberculous meningitis,[65] and showed some benefit for pericarditis.[66]

Immunotherapy with *Mycobacterium vaccae* has been studied in seven trials, and summarized in a systematic review.[67] Immunotherapy was ineffective in altering mortality (OR = 1·09; 95% CI 0·79–1·49), or in altering proportion with negative sputum smears or cultures. Immunotherapy was associated with increased local side effects including ulceration and scarring. The authors conclude that immunotherapy does not benefit TB patients.

The treatment of TB in the setting of HIV consists initially of standard therapies. However, three further interventions have demonstrated effectiveness. First, as TB is an AIDS-defining illness, all co-infected patients should be offered appropriate highly-active antiretroviral therapy (HAART). This has not been studied specifically in an RCT, but can be extrapolated from cohort studies indicating high death rates in TB/HIV co-infected patients in the pre-HAART era, and low mortality among AIDS patients taking appropriate antiretroviral medications (see Chapter 11). Second, secondary prevention with INH given to HIV/TB co-infected patients was more effective than placebo in preventing recurrent TB.[68] This study was undertaken in Haiti, and its results are probably generalizable to other developing nations with high prevalence of TB. However, secondary prevention is unlikely to be useful in low-prevalence settings, since re-infection rather than relapse was probably responsible for recurrent TB.[69] Third, HIV/TB co-infected patients have been shown to benefit from cotrimoxazole (trimethoprim/sulfamethoxazole). In an RCT, cotrimoxazole was more effective than placebo in preventing death and repeat hospitalization among co-infected patients.[70] However, CD4 lymphocyte counts were not available in that study, and are most likely a better method for stratifying risk among HIV/TB co-infected patients and for assessing the need for prophylaxis of opportunistic infections.

Multi-drug resistant TB

The World Health Organization reported in 2000 that globally 11% of *M. tuberculosis* strains are resistant to INH or rifampicin, and 1% are resistant to both. However, MDR-TB is at critical levels in specific regions of the world, including Estonia, Latvia, the Oblasts of Ivanovo and Tomsk in Russia, and the provinces of Henan and Zhejiang in China. MDR-TB is defined as strain-resistant to both INH and rifampicin, and has been associated with poorer response to therapy, higher mortality, and higher treatment costs.[71–74] While no randomized clinical trials of therapy are available to guide optimal management strategies, case series have demonstrated that choosing a minimum of three drugs to which the organism is sensitive, and treating for prolonged periods of time, are usually effective.[71,72,75,76] Second-line agents such as ofloxacin have been successfully used in these settings.[77,78] For pulmonary MDR-TB not responding to multiple chemotherapy, surgical resection has been demonstrated to be effective in a number of case series.[79,80]

Case presentation 1 (continued)

You treat your patient for a total of 6 months. At 1 and 2 months, his sputum smears and culture are negative, and he is unable to produce sputum thereafter. You see him monthly to assess symptoms and adherence. At 4 weeks, his transaminase levels rise to 3 times baseline. As he is asymptomatic, you continue his therapy and these normalize by week 8. He completes therapy and is asked to present 1 year later for *x* ray film follow up. Contact tracing reveals no immediate family or fellow workers with symptoms or a positive TB skin test. You reassure him and his wife that the chances of a future recurrence are very low, and quite treatable if recurrence does occur.

Prevention of TB

Case presentation 2

You are asked to see a 25-year-old asymptomatic woman who recently immigrated to Canada from the Philippines. Her screening intracutaneous 5-unit PPD test is positive at 13 mm of induration. She does not recall any previous skin testing. She received BCG vaccine as a young child and has had no known exposure to active TB among family, friends, or occupational contacts. She denies respiratory symptoms, has an unremarkable clinical examination, and has a normal chest radiograph. You diagnose latent TB infection (LTBI) and recommend INH treatment for 9 months. You measure baseline liver enzymes, and counsel her regarding potential side effects. You wonder whether the BCG vaccine is responsible for her TB skin test reactivity. You have read about a new blood test for TB and wonder if this would provide firmer evidence for *M. tuberculosis* exposure. Finally, you wonder whether a 6- or 9-month regimen of INH is preferred.

BCG vaccination

Prevention of active TB has focused on two strategies: vaccination of children with bacilli Calmette–Guerin (BCG), and tuberculin skin testing followed by treatment of LTBI. Childhood immunization with BCG has been studied in three separate meta-analyses, which pooled both randomized controlled trials and case–control studies.[81–83] BCG was shown to reduce miliary and meningeal TB by 75–86%, and pulmonary TB in children by 50%. However, great variation in efficacy was seen in different trials, and explained in part by distance from the equator.[84] The disadvantages of routine BCG vaccination include false-positive tuberculin skin tests (see below), which compromises contact tracing and initiation of INH treatment of LTBI; cutaneous abscesses; and occasional disseminated BCG.

The tuberculin skin test

The tuberculin skin test consists of injecting 5 units of purified protein derivative "S" (PPD-S) intracutaneously into the volar aspect of the forearm, and measuring the millimeters of induration in the transverse diameter 48–72 hours later. The tuberculin skin test is a well-validated measure of infection with *M. tuberculosis*. It is not, however, an optimal test for the diagnosis of active disease.

The test measures delayed type hypersensitivity to mycobacterial antigen. Conversion of the skin test may take 3 months after exposure to infection, and a change of 10 mm or more identifies patients who are at high risk for developing active TB (estimated at 5% in the next 2 years, and a further 5% lifelong).[25]

In the immunocompetent individual without acute symptoms of TB, the test approaches 100% sensitivity.[10] Among patients with acute TB, false negatives of 25% have been reported. Such anergy may be specific for *M. tuberculosis*, or there may be a general anergy to multiple antigens. Anergy is more common among HIV-positive and other immunocompromized patients, or among the malnourished. Although individuals anergic to multiple antigens can be identified by testing intracutaneous responses to Candida, tetanus, mumps, or other common antigens, these tests have poor reproducibility and are no longer recommended.[85]

False-positive tuberculin skin tests may result from previous BCG vaccination or from exposure to other mycobacteria. A meta-analysis has shown that, while BCG vaccination is associated with skin test positivity, the skin test is rarely > 15 mm, and the effects rarely persist beyond 15 years.[86] Other mycobacteria may also cause false-positive tuberculin skin tests, and the cut-off for "positivity" in such areas may need to be > 12 mm or > 15 mm of induration.

Various cut-off values for interpreting tuberculin skin test positivity have been recommended.[87,88] In India and many areas with high TB prevalence, > 12 mm is used as a cut-off for positivity. In the USA, the use of three different cut-off points has been recommended. For patients with HIV, recent contact with a patient with active TB, or signs of previous TB on chest radiograph, a skin test of > 5 mm identifies infection. For patients with other risk factors for infection, > 10 mm is used as a cut-off. These include immigrants from endemic countries and patients with silicosis, liver or kidney disease, gastrectomy or ileal bypass, the homeless, or aboriginals. In patients at low risk of infection or disease, > 15 mm is used. However, testing low-risk individuals with tuberculin skin tests are no longer generally recommended.[14] A fourth criterion for positivity is a change in induration by 10 mm between serial tests. For individuals undergoing screening prior to employment, a baseline tuberculin test may stimulate remote immunity due to previous BCG or *M. tuberculosis* infection. Such "boosting" of immunity is identified by the two-step tuberculin test, in which the skin test is repeated 1 week or more after the initial test. Detection of the boosted response prevents ascribing the boosted response to recent exposure, should the person be re-tested in the future.[89]

Tuberculin testing is recommended to aid diagnosis (see previous discussion) and to identify asymptomatic infected individuals who may be candidates for treatment of LTBI. When contacts of an active case are investigated, a skin test of > 5 mm indicates recent exposure and > 5% risk of active TB. Such patients have been shown to benefit from monotherapy with INH, as discussed later in this chapter.

Lymphocyte gamma-interferon release assays

Given the difficulties in interpreting the tuberculin skin test, and the need for the patient to return for a second visit, other tests for detecting immune responses to *M. tuberculosis* have been developed.[36,90–92] One such development is a blood-based assay in which whole blood is taken, and lymphocytes are stimulated with mycobacterial antigen. Gamma interferon production is then measured in blood. This test has been shown to correlate well with skin testing,[35] and was recently approved by the Food and Drug Administration (FDA) in the USA. Ideally, such a test would distinguish infection with *M. tuberculosis* from exposure to BCG. A variant of the above test, using *M. tuberculosis*-specific antigens such as ESAT-6 instead of PPD, may be more specific, but requires further validation.[90,93,94]

Treatment of LTBI

While the terms "chemoprophylaxis" or "preventive therapy" have been used in the past, the CDC recommends use of the term "treatment of latent TB infection" to describe the strategy of treating asymptomatic infected patients to prevent future active TB.[10] INH monotherapy for 6–12 months, rifampicin for 4 months, or rifampicin/pyrazinamide for 2 months, have all been studied in randomized clinical trials of LTBI. The comparator in these trials was either placebo, or INH.

Three meta-analyses for treatment of LTBI were identified. For non-HIV patients, Cochrane Reviewers identified 11 randomized trials of INH versus placebo, which enrolled 73 375 people between 1952 and 1994.[95] They calculated an overall efficacy for INH versus placebo to be a relative risk of 0·40 (95% CI 0·31–0·52, a relative risk reduction of 60%). INH also reduced extrapulmonary TB and TB deaths, whereas all-cause mortality was unchanged (RR = 1·10; 95% CI 0·94, 1·28). Durations of less than 6 months were no more effective than placebo. Both 6- and 12-month regimens were more effective than placebo, with relative risks of 0·44 (95% CI 0·27, 0·73) and 0·38 (95% CI 0·28, 0·50), respectively. Direct comparison of the efficacies of these two regimens is misleading, however, as heterogeneous study populations were randomized in the various studies. In the only direct randomized comparison of 6 versus 12 months,[96] relative efficacy was a 65% and 75% reduction, respectively (RR 1·4;95% CI 0·8, 2·4). The difference was not statistically significant. In subgroup analyzes, those who took 80% or more of their drug had efficacy of 93% with 12-months' treatment, versus 69% with the 6-month regimen. On the basis of this study, and a re-interpretation of the Alaskan US Public Health Service study,[97] the CDC has recommended 9 months of treatment for latent TB infection.[10]

In HIV-positive people, two meta-analyses have been published.[98,99] INH alone, rifampicin alone, or rifampicin with pyrazinamide were all more effective than placebo among tuberculin-positive patients, with a relative risk of 0·24 (95% CI 0·14–0·40). No effect was seen among skin-test negative or anergic individuals (RR = 0·87; 95% CI 0·56, 1·36), although the broad confidence intervals indicate that there is insufficient data to exclude a clinically important reduction. In spite of the reduction in subsequent active TB with preventive therapy, total mortality was not reduced (RR = 0·96; 95% CI 0·82–1·13), although a beneficial estimate.

Other effective regimens studied in randomized trials include rifampicin alone for 4 months, or rifampicin with pyrazinamide for 2 months. The combination of rifampicin with pyrazinamide has been studied in three RCTs, and shown to be at least as effective as INH with similar tolerability.[100–102] Subsequently, a case series reported a number of individuals with hepatotoxicity, including a number of deaths, secondary to the combination of rifampicin with pyrazinamide.[103] The CDC now recommends caution with this regimen,[104] and does not recommend this regimen for pregnant women.

Current ATS/CDC recommendations for treatment of LTBI are: 9 (preferred) or 6 months of INH, or 4 months of rifampicin. The 2-month regimen of rifampicin and pyrazinamide should only be considered if the risks justify the benefits. For latent MDR-TB infection, two drugs are recommended to which susceptibility has been demonstrated in the index case. These would usually include pyrazinamide and a quinolone, although one case series demonstrated that this combination is poorly tolerated.[105]

Case presentation 2 (continued)

Your patient is treated with daily INH and vitamin B6. She increasingly complains of tiredness and headaches, and difficulty concentrating on her university studies. After 5 months, she has decided that she will not continue with treatment. You convince her to complete 6 months of therapy, which you know to be an acceptable alternative to the full 9 months recommended by the CDC, and she agrees to this. You emphasize to her that treatment for latent TB infection is imperfect and that a small chance of future TB remains. You recommend that, should she ever develop symptoms compatible with TB, she will need to be investigated for this. You estimate that her baseline lifetime risk of TB reactivation was up to 5%, and following treatment, you have reduced this risk to 2% or less.

References

1. *Global tuberculosis control: WHO report 2001*. Geneva: World Health Organization, 2001.
2. Murray CJ, Lopez AD. Alternative projections of mortality and disability by cause 1990–2020: Global Burden of Disease Study. *Lancet* 1997;**349**:1498–504.
3. Kochi A. The global tuberculosis situation and the new control strategy of the WHO. *Tubercle* 1991;**72**:1–6.
4. Khatri GR, Frieden TR. Controlling tuberculosis in India. *N Engl J Med* 2002;**347**:1420–5.
5. Control of tuberculosis in the United States. Joint Statement of the American Thoracic Society, the Centers for Disease Control, and the Infectious Disease Society of America. *Respir Care* 1993;**38**:929–39.
6. Jereb JA. Progressing toward tuberculosis elimination in low-incidence areas of the United States. Recommendations of the Adviso Elimination of Tuberculosis. *MMWR* :
7. CDC. A strategic plan for the eliminat the United States. *MMWR* 1989;**38**(S-3).
8. Cowie RL, Sharpe JW. Tuberculosis among immigrants: interval from arrival in Canada to diagnosis. A 5-year study in southern Alberta. *CMAJ* 1998;**158**:599–602.
9. Marks GB, Bai J, Simpson SE, Sullivan EA, Stewart GJ. Incidence of tuberculosis among a cohort of tuberculin-positive refugees in Australia: reappraising the estimates of risk. *Am J Respir Crit Care Med* 2000;**162**:1851–4.
10. Revised treatment and testing guidelines for latent tuberculosis infection. *Rep Med Guidel Outcomes Res* 2000;**11**:9–10.
11. Prevention and control of tuberculosis among homeless persons. Recommendations of the Advisory Council for the Elimination of Tuberculosis. *MMWR Recomm Rep* 1992;**41**(RR-5):13–23.
12. Prevention and control of tuberculosis in U.S. communities with at-risk minority populations. Recommendations of the Advisory Council for the Elimination of Tuberculosis. *MMWR Recomm Rep* 1992;**41**(RR-5):1–11.
13. Prevention and control of tuberculosis in facilities providing long-term care to the elderly. Recommendations of the Advisory Committee for Elimination of Tuberculosis. *MMWR Recomm Rep* 1990;**39**(RR-10): 7–13.
14. Centers for Disease Control and Prevention. Targeted tuberculin testing and treatment of latent tuberculosis infection. *MMWR* 2000;**49**(No. RR-6):1–51.
15. Rose VL. CDC calls for tuberculosis screening and treatment for all patients with HIV infection. *Am Fam Physician* 1999;**59**:1682, 1687.
16. Selwyn PA, Hartel D, Lewis VA *et al.* A prospective study of the risk of tuberculosis among intravenous drug users with human immunodeficiency virus infection. *N Engl J Med* 1989;**320**:545–50.
17. Thulstrup AM, Molle I, Svendsen N, Sorensen HT. Incidence and prognosis of tuberculosis in patients with cirrhosis of the liver. A Danish nationwide population based study. *Epidemiol Infect* 2000;**124**:221–5.
18. Long R, Gardam M. Tumor necrosis factor-alpha inhibitors and the reactivation of latent tuberculosis infection. *CMAJ* 2003;**168**:1153–6.

19. Perez-Padilla R, Perez-Guzman C, Baez-Saldana R, Torres-Cruz A. Cooking with biomass stoves and tuberculosis: a case control study. *Int J Tuberc Lung Dis* 2001;**5**:441–7.
20. Yach D. Partnering for better lung health: improving tobacco and tuberculosis control. *Int J Tuberc Lung Dis* 2000;**4**:693–7.
21. Gajalakshmi V, Peto R, Kanaka TS, Jha P. Smoking and mortality from tuberculosis and other diseases in India: retrospective study of 43 000 adult male deaths and 35 000 controls. *Lancet* 2003;**362**:507–15.
22. Kolappan C, Gopi PG. Tobacco smoking and pulmonary tuberculosis. *Thorax* 2002;**57**:964–6.
23. Maurya V, Vijayan VK, Shah A. Smoking and tuberculosis: an association overlooked. *Int J Tuberc Lung Dis* 2002;**6**:942–51.
24. Tekkel M, Rahu M, Loit HM, Baburin A. Risk factors for pulmonary tuberculosis in Estonia. *Int J Tuberc Lung Dis* 2002;**6**:887–94.
25. Ferebee SH. Controlled chemoprophylaxis trials in tuberculosis: a general review. *Bibl Tuberc* 1970;**26**: 28–106.
26. Miller AG, Asch SM, Yu EI, *et al.* A population-based survey of tuberculosis symptoms: how atypical are atypical presentations? *Clin Infect Dis* 2000;293–9.
27. Gnaore E, Sassan-Morokro M, Kassim S *et al.* A comparison of clinical features in tuberculosis associated with infection with human immunodefiency viruses 1 and 2. *Trans Royal Soc Trop Med Hyg* 1993;**87**:57–9.
28. Cohen R, Muzaffar S, Capellan J, Azar H, Chinikamwala M. The validity of classic symptoms and chest radiograph configuration in predicting pulmonary tuberculosis. *Chest* 1996;**109**:420–3.
29. Tattevin P, Casalino E, Fleury L, *et al.* The validity of medical history, classic symptoms, and chest radiographs in predicting pulmonary tuberculosis. *Chest* 1996;**115**:1248–53.
30. Long R, Cowie R. Tuberculosis: 4. Pulmonary disease. *CMAJ* 1999;**160**:1344–8.
31. Graham S, Das GK, Hidvegi RJ, *et al.* Chest radiograph abnormalities associated with tuberculosis: reproducibility and yield of active cases. *Int J Tuberc Lung Dis* 2002;137–42.
32. Perez-Guzman C, Torres-Cruz A, Villarreal-Velarde H, Salazar-Lezama MA, Vargas MH. Atypical radiological images of pulmonary tuberculosis in 192 diabetic patients: a comparative study. *Int J Tuberc Lung Dis* 2001;**5**:455–61.
33. Perlman DC, el Sadr WM, Nelson ET, *et al.* Variation of chest radiographic patterns in pulmonary tuberculosis by degree of human immunodeficiency virus-related immuno-suppression. The Terry Beirn Community Programs for Clinical Research on AIDS (CPCRA). The AIDS Clinical Trials Group (ACTG). *Clin Infect Dis* 1997;**25**:242–6.
34. Lai FM, Liam CK, Paramsothy M, George J. The role of ^{67}gallium scintigraphy and high resolution computed tomography as predictors of disease activity in sputum smear-negative pulmonary tuberculosis. *Int J Tuberc Lung Dis* 1997;**1**:563–9.
35. Mazurek GH, LoBue PA, Daley CL, *et al.* Comparison of a whole-blood interferon-gamma assay with tuberculin skin testing for detecting latent Mycobacterium tuberculosis infections. *JAMA* 2001;**286**:1740–7.
36. Stuart RL, Olden D, Johnson PD, *et al.* Effect of anti-tuberculosis treatment on the tuberculin interferon-gamma response in tuberculin skin test (TST) positive health care workers and patients with tuberculosis. *Int J Tuberc Lung Dis* 2000;**4**:555–61.
37. Anderson C, Inhaber N, Menzies D. Comparison of sputum induction with fiber-optic bronchoscopy in the diagnosis of tuberculosis. *Am J Respir Crit Care Med* 1995;**152**(Pt 1):1570–4.
38. Laszlo A. Tuberculosis: 7. Laboratory aspects of diagnosis. *CMAJ* 1999;**160**:1725–9.
39. Somoskovi A, Hotaling JE, Fitzgerald M, *et al.* Lessons from a proficiency testing event for acid-fast microscopy. *Chest* 2001;**120**:250–7.
40. Eing BR, Becker A, Sohns A, Ringelmann R. Comparison of Roche Cobas Amplicor Mycobacterium tuberculosis assay with in-house PCR and culture for detection of M. tuberculosis. *J Clin Microbiol* 1998;**36**:2023–9.
41. Iinuma Y, Senda K, Fujihara N, *et al.* Comparison of the BDProbeTec ET system with the Cobas Amplicor PCR for direct detection of Mycobacterium tuberculosis in respiratory samples. *Eur J Clin Microbiol* Infect Dis 2003;**22**:368–71.
42. Sarmiento OL, Weigle KA, Alexander J, Weber DJ, Miller WC. Assessment by meta-analysis of PCR for diagnosis of smear-negative pulmonary tuberculosis. *J Clin Microbiol* 2003;**41**:3233–40.

43. Cartuyvels R, De Ridder C, Jonckheere S, Verbist L, Van Eldere J. Prospective clinical evaluation of Amplicor Mycobacterium tuberculosis PCR test as a screening method in a low-prevalence population. *J Clin Microbiol* 1996;**34**:2001–3.
44. Kunakorn M. Raksakai K, Pracharktam R, Sattaudom C. Overcoming the errors of in-house PCR used in the clinical laboratory for the diagnosis of extrapulmonary tuberculosis. *Southeast Asian J Trop Med Public Health* 1999;**30**:84–90.
45. Condos R, McClune A, Rom WN, Schluger NW. Peripheral-blood-based PCR assay to identify patients with active pulmonary tuberculosis. *Lancet* 1996; **347**:1082–5.
46. Kim SS, Chung SM, Kim JN, Lee MA, Ha EH. Application of PCR from the fine needle aspirates for the diagnosis of cervical tuberculous lymphadenitis. *J Korean Med Sci* 1996;**11**:127–32.
47. d'Arminio MA, Cinque P, Vago L, *et al.* A comparison of brain biopsy and CSF-PCR in the diagnosis of CNS lesions in AIDS patients. *J Neurol* 1997;**244**:35–9.
48. Ahmed N, Mohanty AK, Mukhopadhyay U, Batish VK, Grover S. PCR-based rapid detection of Mycobacterium tuberculosis in blood from immunocompetent patients with pulmonary tuberculosis. *J Clin Microbiol* 1998; **36**:3094–5.
49. Honore-Bouakline S, Vincensini JP, Giacuzzo V, Lagrange PH, Herrmann JL. Rapid diagnosis of extrapulmonary tuberculosis by PCR: impact of sample preparation and DNA extraction. *J Clin Microbiol* 2003; **41**:2323–9.
50. Hernandez-Garduno E, Kunimoto D, *et al.* Predictors of clustering of tuberculosis in Greater Vancouver: a molecular epidemiologic study. *CMAJ* 2002;**167**:349–52.
51. Kulaga S, Behr M, Musana K, *et al.* Molecular epidemiology of tuberculosis in Montreal. *CMAJ* 2002; **167**:353–4.
52. Kulaga S, Behr MA, Schwartzman K. Genetic fingerprinting in the study of tuberculosis transmission. *CMAJ* 1999;**161**:1165–9.
53. Murray MB. Molecular epidemiology and the dynamics of tuberculosis transmission among foreign-born people. *CMAJ* 2002;**167**:355–6.
54. Glynn JR, Whiteley J, Bifani PJ, Kremer K, van Soolingen D. Worldwide occurrence of Beijing/W strains of Mycobacterium tuberculosis: a systematic review. *Emerg Infect Dis* 2002;**8**:843–9.
55. Fox W, Ellard GA, Mitchison DA. Studies on the treatment of tuberculosis undertaken by the British Medical Research Council tuberculosis units, 1946–1986, with relevant subsequent publications. *Int J Tuberc Lung Dis* 1999;**3**(Suppl.2):S231–S279.
56. From the Centers for Disease Control and Prevention. Initial therapy for tuberculosis in the era of multidrug resistance: recommendations of the Advisory Council for the Elimination of Tuberculosis. *JAMA* 1993;**270**:694–8.
57. A controlled trial of 3-month, 4-month, and 6-month regimens of chemotherapy for sputum-smear-negative pulmonary tuberculosis. Results at 5 years. Hong Kong Chest Service/Tuberculosis Research Center, Madras/ British Medical Research Council. *Am Rev Respir Dis* 1989;**139**:871–6.
58. Mwandumba HC, Squire SB. Fully intermittent dosing with drugs for treating tuberculosis in adults (Cochrane Review). Chichester, UK: John Wiley & Sons, Ltd. *The Cochrane Library*, Issue 4, 2003.
59. Olle-Goig JE, Alvarez J. Treatment of tuberculosis in a rural area of Haiti: directly observed and non-observed regimens. The experience of Hospital Albert Schweitzer. *Int J Tuberc Lung Dis* 2001;**5**:137–41.
60. Volmink J, Garner P. Directly observed therapy for treating tuberculosis (Cochrane Review). Chichester, UK: John Wiley & Sons, Ltd. *The Cochrane Library*, Issue 4, 2003.
61. Volmink J, Garner P. Systematic review of randomized controlled trials of strategies to promote adherence to tuberculosis treatment. *BMJ* 1997;**315**:1403–6.
62. Tulsky JP, Pilot L, Hahn JA, *et al.* Adherence to isoniazid prophylaxis in the homeless: a randomized controlled trial. *Arch Intern Med* 2000;**160**:697–702.
63. Lee CH, Wang WJ, Lan RS, Tsai YH, Chiang YC. Corticosteroids in the treatment of tuberculous pleurisy. A double-blind, placebo-controlled, randomized study. *Chest* 1988;**94**:1256–9.
64. Smego RA, Ahmed N. A systematic review of the adjunctive use of systemic corticosteroids for pulmonary tuberculosis. *Int J Tuberc Lung Dis* 2003;**7**:208–13.
65. Prasad K, Volmink J, Menon GR. Steroids for treating tuberculous meningitis (Cochrane Review). Chichester, UK: John Wiley & Sons, Ltd. *The Cochrane Library*, Issue 4, 2003.

66. Ntsekhe M, Wiysonge C, Volmink JA, Commerford PJ, Mayosi BM. Adjuvant corticosteroids for tuberculous pericarditis: promising, but not proven. *QJM* 2003;**96**: 593–9.
67. de Bruyn G, Garner P. Mycobacterium vaccae immunotherapy for treating tuberculosis (Cochrane Review). Chichester, UK: John Wiley & Sons, Ltd. *The Cochrane Library*, Issue 4, 2003.
68. Fitzgerald DW, Desvarieux M, Severe P, *et al.* Effect of post-treatment isoniazid on prevention of recurrent tuberculosis in HIV-1 infected individuals: a randomized trial. *Lancet* 2000;**356**:1470–4.
69. van Rie A, Warren R, Richardson M, *et al.* Exogenous reinfection as a cause of recurrent tuberculosis after curative treatment. *N Engl J Med* 1999;**341**:1174–9.
70. Wiktor SZ, Sassan-Morokro M, Grant AD, *et al.* Efficacy of trimethoprim-sulphamethoxazole prophylaxis to decrease morbidity and mortality in HIV-1 infected patients with tuberculosis in Abidjan, Cote d'Ivoire: a randomized controlled trial. *Lancet* 1999;**353**:1469–75.
71. Geerligs WA, Van Altena R, De Lange WCM, van Soolingen D, Van Der Werf TS. Multidrug-resistant tuberculosis: long-term treatment outcome in the Netherlands. *Int J Tuberc Lung Dis* 2000;**4**:758–64.
72. Flament-Saillour M, Robert J, Jarlier V, Grosset J. Outcome of multi-drug-resistant tuberculosis in France: a nationwide case-control study. *Am J Respir Crit Care Med* 1999;**160**:587–93.
73. Singla R, Al Sharif N, Al Sayegh MO, Osman MM, Shaikh MA. Influence of anti-tuberculosis drug resistance on the treatment outcome of pulmonary tuberculosis patients receiving DOTS in Riyadh, Saudi Arabia. *Int J Tuberc Lung Dis* 2002;**6**:585–91.
74. Subhash HS, Ashwin I, Jesudason MV, *et al.* Clinical characteristics and treatment response among patients with multidrug-resistant tuberculosis: a retrospective study. *Indian J Chest Dis Allied Sci* 2003;**45**:97–103.
75. Fischl MA, Daikos GL, Uttamchandani RB, *et al.* Clinical presentation and outcome of patients with HIV infection and tuberculosis caused by multiple-drug-resistant bacilli. *Ann Intern Med* 1992;**117**:184–90.
76. Park SK, Kim CT, Song SD. Outcome of chemotherapy in 107 patients with pulmonary tuberculosis resistant to isoniazid and rifampin. *Int J Tuberc Lung Dis* 1998;**2**:877–84.
77. Yew WW, Chan CK, Chau CH *et al.* Outcomes of patients with multidrug-resistant pulmonary tuberculosis treated with ofloxacin/levofloxacin-containing regimens. *Chest* 2000;**117**:744–51.
78. Mangunnegoro H, Hudoyo A. Efficacy of low-dose ofloxacin in the treatment of multidrug-resistant tuberculosis in Indonesia. *Chemotherapy* 1999;**45**(Suppl.2):19–25.
79. Chiang CY, Yu MC, Bai KJ, *et al.* Pulmonary resection in the treatment of patients with pulmonary multidrug-resistant tuberculosis in Taiwan. *Int J Tuberc Lung Dis* 2001;**5**:272–7.
80. Sung SW, Kang CH, Kim YT, *et al.* Surgery increased the chance of cure in multi-drug resistant pulmonary tuberculosis. *Eur J Cardiothorac Surg* 1999;**16**:187–93.
81. Colditz GA, Brewer TF, Berkey CS, *et al.* Efficacy of BCG vaccine in the prevention of tuberculosis. Meta-analysis of the published literature. *JAMA* 1994;**271**:698–702.
82. Colditz GA, Berkey CS, Mosteller F, *et al.* The efficacy of bacillus Calmette-Guerin vaccination of newborns and infants in the prevention of tuberculosis: meta-analyses of the published literature. *Pediatrics* 1995;**96**(Pt 1):29–35.
83. Brewer TF. Preventing tuberculosis with bacillus Calmette-Guerin vaccine: a meta-analysis of the literature. *Clin Infect Dis* 2000;**31**(Suppl.3):S64–S67.
84. Wilson ME, Fineberg HV, Colditz GA. Geographic latitude and the efficacy of bacillus Calmette-Guerin vaccine. *Clin Infect Dis* 1995;**20**:982–91.
85. Anergy skin testing and tuberculosis [corrected] preventive therapy for HIV-infected persons: revised recommendations. Centers for Disease Control and Prevention. *MMWR Recomm Rep* 1997;**46**(RR-15):1–10.
86. Wang L, Turner MO, Elwood RK, Schulzer M, FitzGerald JM. A meta-analysis of the effect of Bacille Calmette Guerin vaccination on tuberculin skin test measurements. *Thorax* 2002;**57**:804–9.
87. Targeted tuberculin testing and treatment of latent tuberculosis infection. American Thoracic Society. *MMWR Recomm Rep* 2000;**49**(RR-6):1–51.
88. Duchin JS, Jereb JA, Nolan CM, Smith P, Onorato IM. Comparison of sensitivities to two commercially available tuberculin skin test reagents in persons with recent tuberculosis. *Clin Infect Dis* 1997;**25**:661–3.
89. Sepkowitz KA, Feldman J, Louther J, *et al.* Benefit of two-step PPD testing of new employees at a New York City hospital. *Am J Infect Control* 1997;**25**:283–6.

90. Arend SM, Engelhard AC, Groot G, *et al.* Tuberculin skin testing compared with T-cell responses to Mycobacterium tuberculosis-specific and nonspecific antigens for detection of latent infection in persons with recent tuberculosis contact. *Clin Diagn Lab Immunol* 2001;**8**:1089–96.
91. Boras Z, Juretic A, Rudolf M, Uzarevic B, Trescec A. Cellular and humoral immunity to purified protein derivative (PPD) in PPD skin reactive and nonreactive patients with pulmonary tuberculosis: comparative analysis of antigen-specific lymphocyte proliferation and IgG antibodies. *Croat Med J* 2002;**43**:301–5.
92. Mazurek GH, Villarino ME. Guidelines for using the QuantiFERON-TB test for diagnosing latent Mycobacterium tuberculosis infection. Centers for Disease Control and Prevention. *MMWR Recomm Rep* 2003;**52**(RR-2):15–18.
93. Arend SM, Andersen P, van Meijgaarden KE, *et al.* Detection of active tuberculosis infection by T cell responses to early-secreted antigenic target 6-kDa protein and culture filtrate protein 10. *J Infect Dis* 2000;**181**:1850–4.
94. Lalvani A, Pathan AA, Durkan H, *et al.* Enhanced contact tracing and spatial tracking of Mycobacterium tuberculosis infection by enumeration of antigen-specific T cells. *Lancet* 2001;**357**:2017–21.
95. Smieja MJ, Marchetti CA, Cook DJ, Smaill FM. Isoniazid for preventing tuberculosis in non-HIV infected persons (Cochrane Review). Chichester, UK: John Wiley & Sons, Ltd. *The Cochrane Library*, Issue 4, 2003.
96. Efficacy of various durations of isoniazid preventive therapy for tuberculosis: five years of follow up in the IUAT trial. International Union Against Tuberculosis Committee on Prophylaxis. *Bull World Health Organ* 1982;**60**:555–64.
97. Comstock GW. How much isoniazid is needed for prevention of tuberculosis among immunocompetent adults? *Int J Tuberc Lung Dis* 1999;**3**:847–50.
98. Wilkinson D. Drugs for preventing tuberculosis in HIV infected persons (Cochrane Review). Chichester, UK: John Wiley & Sons, Ltd. *The Cochrane Library*, Issue 4, 2003.
99. Bucher HC, Griffith LE, Guyatt GH, *et al.* Isoniazid prophylaxis for tuberculosis in HIV infection: a meta-analysis of randomized controlled trials. *AIDS* 1999;**13**:501–7.
100. Halsey NA, Coberly JS, Desormeaux J, *et al.* Randomized trial of isoniazid versus rifampicin and pyrazinamide for prevention of tuberculosis in HIV-1 infection.s. *Lancet* 1998;**351**:786–92.
101. Gordin FM, Chaisson RE, Matts JP, *et al.* Rifampin and pyrazinamide vs. isoniazid for prevention of tuberculosis in HIV-infected persons: an international randomized trial. *JAMA* 2000;**283**:1445–50.
102. Jasmer RM, Saukkonen JJ, Blumberg HM, *et al.* Short-course rifampin and pyrazinamide for latent tuberculosis infection: a multicenter clinical trial. *Ann Intern Med* 2002;**137**:640–7.
103. Update: fatal and severe liver injuries associated with rifampin and pyrazinamide for latent tuberculosis infection, and revisions in American Thoracic Society/CDC recommendations – United States, 2001. *MMWR* 2001;**50**:733–5.
104. From the Centers for Disease Control and Prevention. Update: fatal and severe liver injuries associated with rifampin and pyrazinamide treatment for latent tuberculosis infection. *JAMA* 2002;**288**:2967.
105. Papastavros T, Dolovich LR, Holbrook A, Whitehead L, Loeb M. Adverse events associated with pyrazinamide and levofloxacin in the treatment of latent multidrug-resistant tuberculosis. *CMAJ* 2002;**167**:131–6.

8 Diarrhea

Guy de Bruyn, Alain Bouckenooghe

Case presentation 1

A 52-year-old previously healthy woman is brought to the emergency room with symptoms of vomiting, severe abdominal cramps, and bloody diarrhea. About 3 days prior she developed abdominal pain and diarrhea, that was watery at the time of onset and for which she was given amoxicillin by her family healthcare provider. She got sicker with abdominal cramping and the stools became bloody over the 24 hours preceding admission. Earlier she had twice had spontaneous nose bleeding with loss of only small amounts of blood. No other family members are currently ill, but several coworkers who had eaten lunch with the patient at a local fast food restaurant developed diarrhea around the same time. She has not travelled outside of her city of residence in the last 6 months.

On physical examination, she appears ill. She complains of severe abdominal pain. Her vital signs indicate she is afebrile and has a mild tachycardia with normal blood pressure. There is pallor of the conjunctiva. Her abdomen is mildly tender to palpation. Laboratory analysis is as follows: hemoglobin 84 g/liter (8·4 mg/dL), hematocrit 24%, platelets 70×10^9/liter, lactate dehydrogenase 855 U/liter, liver function tests normal, urea 52·8 mmol/liter (148 mg/dL), creatinine 548 micromol/liter (6·2 mg/dL), reticulocyte count 5·2%, The Coombs test was negative and coagulation tests were normal with the exception of slightly elevated fibrin degradation products.

Infectious diarrhea

Diagnosis

Epidemiology

Diarrhea is a syndrome that is readily recognized. Definitions for diarrhea typically use duration as an organising principle (see Box 8.1), although pathophysiological or anatomic definitions are also common. In general, the clinical concern is discerning infectious from non-infectious causes, as well as likely pathogens that may be encountered in infectious cases.

Globally, infectious diarrhea is a major cause of morbidity and mortality, accounting for an

Box 8.1 Definitions used in published Infectious Diseases Society of America guidelines

- *Acute diarrhea*. Diarrhea episode lasting less than fourteen days
- *Chronic diarrhea*. Diarrheal episode lasting more than thirty days
- *Diarrhea*. Alteration of normal bowel movement, associated with increase in stool volume or water content or frequency. Also decreased stool consistency (unformed or liquid stools)
- *Infectious diarrhea*. Diarrheal episode from infection with an enteropathogenic organism
- *Persistent diarrhea*. Diarrheal episode lasting more than fourteen days

Table 8.1 Population-based estimates of diarrheal disease incidence

Location, period	Cohort	Incidence [cases/100 person years] (95% CI)	Reference
Cleveland, US 1948–57	Community	150	2
Tecumseh, US 1965–71	Community	100	
Brazil (urban), 1978–80	Community	143	3
Egypt (rural), 1980–1	Community	100	4
United Kingdom, 1993–6	Community	19·4 (18·1–20·8)	5
	General practice	3·3 (2·9–3·8)	
Netherlands, 1998–9	Community	28·3 (25·2–31·5)	6
	General practice	0·8	

estimated 99·6 million disability-adjusted life years (DALYs) lost.[1] Estimates of incidence of acute infectious diarrhea vary between 0·8 and 100 cases per 100 person-years (Table 8.1). Studies based in general practice settings tend to have lower incidence estimates, reflecting the large number of symptomatic persons who do not seek medical care as well as under-ascertainment of cases. For every person attending their primary care provider, a further five to six[5] or more symptomatic cases may not seek care.[6] Incidence rates also vary by age, with a bimodal distribution. Infants have the highest rates, with lowest rates in the late teens, which rise slightly in early adulthood. Although recent data are scarce, prior reports indicate very high peak age-specific rates of disease in developing countries of 9·7 cases per person year.[7] Healthcare-seeking behaviour is modified by age, symptom severity, and duration, and the presence of particular alarm symptoms such as fever or blood in the stool. One study found that only age, fever, and abdominal cramps were independently associated with seeking medical consultation.[6]

Globally, poor water, sanitation, and hygiene are the greatest risk factors for diarrheal disease.[1] Aside from age, other personal characteristics such as underlying medical conditions (HIV infection, prior gastric surgery, intake of medications that lower gastric acidity) are associated with elevated risk of acquiring diarrhea,[8,9] as are other factors including sexual preference.[8]

In travellers to tropical or subtropical destinations, diarrhea is amongst the commonest of acute ailments encountered. The attack rate of travellers' diarrhea varies by location, season of travel, consumption of high risk food or beverages (for example, tap water, ice cubes, ice cream, food from street vendors, salads, raw or uncooked shellfish), and other factors.[10–14] Rates in expatriates from developed nations may approach that for children under 5 years of age in these locations.[13]

Clinical findings

Inquiry regarding certain physical symptoms may assist in defining patients in whom stool cultures are more likely to yield pathogenic organisms. Clinicians should ask about duration of symptoms; characteristics of stool (consistency, frequency, volume, presence of blood or mucus); symptoms of hypovolemia, abdominal cramps, or fever; travel history; recent medications; and ingestion of raw or undercooked meat, unpasteurized dairy products, or raw seafood.

Physical examination should identify hypovolemia. However, the clinical diagnosis of hypovolemia in adults has best been validated in acute blood loss, and remains unproved in volume loss from diarrhea.[15] Therefore, physical findings such as postural vital signs, dry tongue, dry axillae, decreased skin turgor, or prolonged capillary refill time may need to be supplemented by measurement of serum electrolytes, urea, and creatinine to confirm the diagnosis.

Laboratory findings

A meta-analysis of 25 studies of the diagnostic use of fecal screening tests as a predictor of a stool culture positive for a known invasive enteropathogen reported the superior performance of fecal lactoferrin over fecal leukocytes or stool occult blood.[16] However, joint maximum sensitivity and specificity, as estimated from summary receiver operating characteristic (ROC) curves were only 86%, 63%, and 68%, respectively. Subsequent studies have indicated that lactoferrin has a sensitivity of 85–93% with a corresponding likelihood ratio positive (LR+) of 3·97–5·47[17,18] and fecal leukocytes a sensitivity of 57% with LR+ of 5·0 (95% CI 2·9, 8·8) among outpatients.[19] These studies do not highlight the operational issues in using these tests in the clinical setting, including need for an experienced microscopist (in the case of fecal leukocytes), need for a fresh specimen (for fecal leukocytes), and integration into clinical care.

Initial work up should therefore include a fecal lactoferrin measurement or, if microscopy can be performed on a fresh stool sample, presence of fecal leukocytes. If this is positive, a stool culture is indicated as the probability of finding an invasive pathogen is increased and this information is relevant towards further therapy of the patient and is also important from a public health standpoint.

Stool culture

Culture of fresh stool specimens remains the standard for determining an etiological diagnosis. The rationale for continued use of stool culture includes directed antimicrobial therapy, and assistance with public health goals, such as disease surveillance, identification of outbreaks, further evaluation in cases of suspected inflammatory enteritis, and protection from secondary transmission from sick food service workers.[20–22] The yield of stool cultures in the evaluation of diarrhea in recent travellers is typically below 50% and, in the case of community-acquired diarrhea in developed regions, this is significantly less (1·5–6%), because of relative increased importance of viral pathogens. Because acute diarrheal disease is often self-limited, and because of the delay in receiving culture results, the contribution of culture results to therapeutic decision-making is often limited. This must be balanced with the need for identification of invasive pathogens and pathogens of public health importance, and also with the need to minimize empiric therapy, which may be inappropriate. Most societal guidelines advise obtaining stool cultures selectively when the patient is moderately or severely ill, in cases with clinical signs of fever, mucus or blood visible in the stool, tenesmus, severe abdominal cramping, or treatment failure.[23–25] For public health reasons, stool cultures should also be tested for specific subpopulations: food handlers, day care attendees, day care employees, and any time an outbreak is suspected.

Treatment

Fluid management

Although the goal of fluid management is to reduce morbidity and mortality, most trials of these interventions have assessed other endpoints, such as stool output or need for intravenous rehydration. A direct comparison of intravenous versus oral rehydration has been reported in one small randomized controlled trial (RCT) among 20 adults with cholera and severe dehydration, which compared enteral rehydration through a nasogastric tube versus intravenous rehydration.[26] Both groups received initial intravenous fluids. The RCT found no significant difference in the total duration of diarrhea (44 hours with i.v. fluids *v* 37 hours with nasogastric fluids; difference +7 hours, 95% CI – 6 to + 20 hours), total volume of stool passed (8·2 liters *v* 11 liters; difference 2·8 liters, 95% CI – 8 to + 3 liters), or duration of *Vibrio cholerae* excretion (1·1 days *v* 1·4 days; difference 0·3 days, 95% CI 0 days to 1 day).

Many subsequent modifications to the formulation of oral rehydration solution (ORS) have been tested in prospective studies. These include amino acid ORS, bicarbonate-free ORS, citrate-containing ORS, reduced osmolarity ORS, and rice-based solutions.[27] Amino acid-containing ORS was found to reduce the total duration of diarrhea and the total volume of stool in two RCTs.[28,29] Replacing ORS bicarbonate with chloride was not beneficial in one small RCT, nor was any significant effect of replacing ORS bicarbonate with citrate found in three RCTs that have tested that modification. Reduced osmolarity ORS was associated with fewer unscheduled intravenous infusions in a systematic review of trials in children.[30] Fewer trials have examined the efficacy in adults, and among available trials, no consistent effect has been demonstrated. The risk of asymptomatic hyponatremia is higher among those receiving reduced osmolarity ORS (OR 2·1, 95% CI 1·1–4·1).[31] Despite the uncertainty of the data in adults, the World Health Organization recently changed the formulation of standard oral rehydration solution to a reduced osmolarity formulation.[32]

One systematic review (search date 1998, 22 RCTs conducted in Bangladesh, India, Indonesia, Pakistan, Egypt, Mexico, Chile, and Peru) in people with cholera and non-cholera diarrhea found that rice-based ORS significantly reduced the 24-hour stool volume compared to standard ORS (adults: four RCTs, WMD 51 mL/kg, 95% CI 66, 35 mL/kg; children: five RCTs, WMD 67 mL/kg, 95% CI 94, 41 mL/kg).[33] One RCT found that both rice-based ORS and low sodium rice-based ORS reduced stool output compared with standard ORS (4 liters for rice-based ORS *v* 5 liters for standard ORS, $P < 0{\cdot}02$; 3 liters for low sodium rice-based ORS *v* 5 liters for standard ORS, $P < 0{\cdot}05$).[34]

Antimicrobial therapy

The use of antibiotics for treatment of domestically-acquired diarrhea has been evaluated in at least 10 RCTs (1848 people) comparing one or more antibiotics with placebo.[35–42] These trials have evaluated fluoroquinolones (N = 8), co-trimoxazole (N = 4), clioquinol (N = 1) (no longer widely used; this drug is not available in the United States but is available for otic and dermatological use in several countries), and nifuroxazide (N = 1). Six RCTs found that antibiotics reduced illness duration or decreased number of liquid stools at 48 hours, while three RCTs found no benefit in reducing illness duration. One RCT found reduced duration of diarrhea for ciprofloxacin but not for co-trimoxazole.

Antibiotics have been extensively investigated for the treatment of travellers' diarrhea. A systematic review[43] and one additional RCT[44] describing the effects of treatment have been reported. The review (search date 1999) compared empirical use of antibiotics versus placebo and found 12 RCTs, among 1474 people with travellers' diarrhea, including students, package tourists, military personnel, and volunteers. Antibiotics evaluated in these trials included aztreonam, bicozamycin, ciprofloxacin, co-trimoxazole (trimethoprim/sulfamethoxazole; TMP/SMX), fleroxacin, norfloxacin, ofloxacin, and trimethoprim. The duration of therapy varied from a single dose to 5 days. The review found that antibiotics significantly increased the cure rate at 72 hours (defined as cessation of unformed stools, or less than one unformed stool/24 hours without additional symptoms; OR 5·9, 95% CI 4·1, 8·6). The additional RCT (598 people, 70% of whom had travelled recently) compared norfloxacin versus placebo. It found that norfloxacin significantly increased the number of people cured after 6 days (34/46 [74%] with norfloxacin *v* 18/48 [38%] with placebo; RR 2·0, 95% CI 1·3–3·0).

The systematic review found that the rate of adverse effects varied with each antibiotic, ranging from 2% to 18%. Gastrointestinal, dermatological, and respiratory symptoms were most frequently reported. The emergence of resistance of the infecting organism to the agent was also documented in a number of the trials. Antimicrobial resistance is clearly of concern for public health. One small RCT included in the review found a significant association between taking ciprofloxacin and isolation of resistant bacteria at 48 hours from these patients' stool samples (ciprofloxacin *v* placebo; absolute risk increase [ARI] 50%, 95% CI 15–85%). Another RCT in the review (181 adults with acute diarrhea) reported three cases of continued excretion of *Shigella* in people taking co-trimoxazole versus one person taking placebo.[45] Two of these isolates selected for resistance towards the drug, although the participants were clinically well. The additional RCT found that people with salmonella infection treated with norfloxacin versus placebo had significantly prolonged excretion of *Salmonella* species (median time to clearance of *Salmonella* species from stool: 50 days with norfloxacin *v* 23 days with placebo; CI not provided). In addition, six of nine *Campylobacter* isolates obtained after treatment showed some degree of resistance to norfloxacin.

The continued evolution of antimicrobial resistance among enteropathogens has meant that agents previously found to be effective in clinical trials, such as trimethoprim–sulfamethoxazole or ampicillin, no longer show *in vitro* activity.[46,47] Further active-control trials, not mentioned above, have evaluated a number of additional candidates, which could be considered. These include aztreonam,[48] azithromycin,[49] and rifaximin.[50]

Antidiarrheals

A number of antidiarrheal compounds, drugs that generally act by prolonging intestinal transit time through an effect on bowel motility, have been evaluated in clinical trials. These agents include difenoxin, diphenoxylate–atropine,[51] lidamidine,[52,53] loperamide,[53–57] and loperamide-oxide.[55–59] These trials of patients with acute diarrhea have generally been conducted among general practice networks. Trials evaluating loperamide or loperamide oxide have generally used "time to first relief" and "time to complete relief" as endpoints, the latter indicating the time between taking the loading dose and the start of the 24-hour period in which no watery or loose stools were passed. The majority of these reports have indicated a benefit of antidiarrheals on symptoms. Some have reported the benefit being experienced in the early phase of the illness, with no impact on total duration of symptoms. The most common adverse effect of these medications was constipation. Two RCTs found that constipation was significantly more frequent in people taking loperamide versus placebo (25% *v* 7%; ARI 18%, 95% CI 8%–28%[53]; 22% *v* 10·3%; ARI 12%, 95% CI 5%–29%;[52]). Another RCT (230 people) found that symptom scores for tiredness and sleepiness were significantly higher in people taking loperamide oxide 1 mg compared with placebo.[58] Other feared complications such as toxic megacolon have not been reported in clinical trials.

Antisecretory agents

A number of compounds have been developed that modify intestinal fluid secretion and thereby produce a clinical benefit. These include racecadotril, an inhibitor of enkephalinase which prolongs the antisecretory effect of endogenous enkephalins, and octreotide. An overview including four trials of racecadotril compared with placebo or another active agent reported that racecadotril shortened the duration of diarrhea and decreased stool weight in the first 24 hours of illness.[60] The rate of constipation was lower compared with loperamide (8·1% for racecadotril 100 mg t.i.d. *v* 31·3% for loperamide 1·33 mg t.i.d.) in one of the included trials. Octreotide has been reported to shorten the duration of diarrhea due to *Vibrio cholerae* in one small study, although did not affect the purging rate.[61]

Other modalities

Probiotic agents, which are dietary supplements of living commensal micro-organisms of low or no pathogenicity, have been proposed as potential therapy for a number of clinical indications.[62] A few small trials of therapy in adults with acute enteric infections have been reported, although the results appear conflicting.

Dietary modification, although frequently recommended for patients with acute diarrheal illnesses, has not been evaluated in prospective studies.

Supplementation of certain micronutrients has been evaluated as adjunctive therapy in acute diarrhea. The use of zinc supplementation has been extensively evaluated in children although not in adults.

Prognosis

Duration of symptoms

Acute diarrhea in adults is typically self-limited. Among travellers, symptoms typically last 3–5 days, may persist for over a week in 8–15%, and 2% develop chronic diarrhea.[63]

Need for hospitalization

Based on hospital discharge data from the United States, approximately 452 000 persons per year were hospitalized with acute diarrhea between 1979 and 1995. This represents < 1% of all cases of diarrhea, and approximately 1·5% of all hospitalizations.[64]

Other serious adverse outcomes

One particular concern in those patients with diarrhea due to *Escherichia coli* O157:H7 (enterohemorrhagic *E. coli*, EHEC) and other shiga-toxin-producing *E. coli* strains is the development of hemolytic uremic syndrome (HUS), a disorder characterized by hemolytic anemia, thrombocytopenia, and acute renal failure.[65] A recent meta-analysis assessed the risk of HUS after antibiotic treatment of EHEC in nine studies.[66] No association between antibiotic use and HUS was demonstrated [Pooled OR 1·04, 95% CI 0·59–1·82]. However, the authors reported significant heterogeneity of effect among the studies included in the meta-analysis. As a result, the topic remains controversial, and the value of antibiotics in this setting remains unresolved, hence the use of antibiotics is not advised.[67]

Reactive arthritis and Reiter's syndrome are further serious potential complications of enteric infection. The risk of these complications has been documented in the setting of outbreaks of enteric infection with *Salmonella typhimurium* or *S. enteritidis*, *Shigella flexneri*, *Yersinia pseudotuberculosis*, and sporadic cases of *Campylobacter* spp. or enterotoxigenic *E. coli* (ETEC).[68–70] The prevalence of joint symptoms after infection has been reported to be as high as 37%, although most estimates are in the range of 1–15%. Reiter's syndrome usually affects less than 3%. The prevalence of certain high-risk HLA types (such as HLA-B27) in the affected population has generally not been reported, although is clearly relevant to the development of joint symptoms.

Death

Worldwide, death from acute diarrhea remains a major cause of mortality, particularly in children under 5 years. Mortality trends from diarrhea for the United States for the period 1979–1987 showed a significant decline in deaths among young children, but rates for those 75 years or older remain around 15 deaths per 100 000 persons. Mortality from dysentery in hospitalized patients in Rwanda in the setting of a nationwide outbreak during the civil war was associated with age less than 5 years or greater than 50 years, severe dehydration on admission (assessed clinically), edema of the legs, and prescription of nalidixic acid (resistance to this agent emerged rapidly during the outbreak).[71,72]

Case presentation 2

A 73-year-old woman with diabetes mellitus and community-acquired pneumonia was admitted to hospital and treated with a third generation cephalosporin, intravenous fluids, insulin, and supplemental oxygen. She gradually improved, with defervescence of her fever by day 5 and improvement in her cough and dyspnea. On day 8 she developed watery offensive diarrhea with severe abdominal cramping. She was anorexic and hypoglycemic. Her temperature increased to 38·5° C, her heart rate increased to 135 beats per minute, she became hypotensive, and on her peripheral blood smear she had 22·4 × 10^9 WBC/L with 15% bands. Given her worsening clinical picture, she was transferred to the intensive care unit.

Nosocomial diarrhea

Diagnosis

Epidemiology

Diarrhea occurring during hospitalization may be due to a number of infectious or non-infectious causes. The leading cause of infectious nosocomial diarrhea is cytotoxin-producing *Clostridium difficile*. Other infectious pathogens account for a smaller proportion of nosocomial diarrhea, but may be important in outbreak settings. The patient population and locally prevalent pathogens are additional influences on the spectrum of pathogenic organisms encountered. Antibiotic-associated diarrhea may be caused not only by disruption of normal intestinal flora, but also by overgrowth of pathogenic organisms like *C. difficile*. The effects of the antibiotic may be directly on the intestinal mucosa, gastrointestinal motility, or mediated through alteration of colonic metabolism induced through changes in the normal resident bacterial flora.[73]

The rates of nosocomial diarrhea vary, in part due to the definition of diarrhea; rates of over 30% of admissions have been reported.[74] Among a large cohort of antibiotic-treated hospitalized patients, diarrhea occurred in 12 %.[75] *C. difficile* accounts for approximately 25% of cases of antibiotic-associated diarrhea.[75,76]

Clinical findings

Clinical findings often start shortly after use of an antibiotic although a delayed onset of up to 8 weeks is possible. Most patients have foul smelling watery greenish diarrhea, the presence of mucus and blood in the stool, with signs of focal abdominal tenderness or tenesmus often present. However, milder presentations without diarrhea occur, and fulminant colitis is estimated to occur in 1–3% of cases.[76] Leukocytosis is common, and may even be markedly elevated.[77]

Stool culture

A widely used policy in microbiology laboratories is to reject stool specimens obtained more than 3 days after admission (the "3-day rule"). The rationale for this is illustrated by the difference in stool culture yield for specimens taken < 72 hours after admission compared with specimens taken 72 hours or more after admission: 3·3% versus 0·5%.[78] A recent prospective study to derive guidelines for stool culture of inpatients proposed a modification to the 3-day rule, suggesting that cultures be obtained in the case of nosocomial diarrhea (> 72 hours after admission) if at least one of the following criteria are met: age ≥ 65 years, HIV infection, neutropenia, or if a nosocomial outbreak was suspected. This would have resulted in only two missed positive cultures for enteropathogens (other than *C. difficile*) of 65 positive cultures from over 27 000 stool cultures obtained in three hospitals over a cumulative period of 14 years. The rule would have led to a reduction in workload for the microbiology laboratory of between 47% and 62% in these hospitals. The detection of nosocomial outbreaks may have been delayed in some instances, especially if cases were widely distributed across hospital wards.

Identification of *C. difficile* in a stool culture is not sufficient as strains that do not produce toxins are not pathogenic, and the presence of one or both of the toxins must be established. In addition, isolation of *C. difficile* may take 48–72 hours, which delays the diagnosis.

Special examinations

The use of stool biomarkers has been examined as an aid to identification of patients with a higher likelihood of positive tests for *C. difficile*. The odds of a positive stool cytotoxin assay in persons with positive tests for stool leukocytes have been reported to be increased, whether detection is by lactoferrin assay (OR 3·7, 95% CI 1·8–7·8) or by light microscopy (OR 2·4, 95% CI 1·1–5·4).[79] Both have imperfect sensitivity, although stool microscopy may be the less sensitive screening test.[19,80]

The gold standard test for diagnosing *C. difficile*-associated diarrhea is a cell culture-based cytotoxin assay, which takes 24–48 hours. The impetus for alternative diagnostic tests has been the diagnostic delay and requirement for a tissue culture facility. A variety of rapid assays have been developed to address these needs. Enzyme immunoassays (EIA) have been developed for toxin A and B, or the combination of both, with reduced sensitivity (72–94% compared with tissue culture), but results are available in a few hours.[81] If the initial test is negative and diarrhea persists, a second sample should be evaluated to compensate for limited sensitivity. The combined toxin A/B tests have superior sensitivity to EIAs that test for toxin A alone, possibly owing to the detection of toxin A–/B+ strains.[82] Polymerase chain reaction assays to detect toxigenic strains have been reported,[83–85] although use remains limited. The use of latex agglutination assays that detect glutamate dehydrogenase has been discouraged by the Society for Healthcare Epidemiology in America because of the low sensitivity of the test, despite the ease of performance of the test, low cost, and high specificity.[81]

Radiographic studies lack both sensitivity and specificity but toxic megacolon or thumbprinting can be suggestive of infection with *C. difficile*. Abdominal computed tomography scanning typically shows thickening of the mucosa, yet this is not a pathognomonic sign.[86,87]

When a diagnosis needs to be made more rapidly, flexible sigmoidoscopy should be considered. This is particularly useful in situations where ileus has developed and stool studies cannot be obtained. In severe cases, pseudomembranous colitis may be visualized on examination. The typical appearance is of yellow adherent plaques about 10 mm in diameter scattered over the colonic mucosa and separated by hyperemic areas. Biopsies of the area show plentiful neutrophils in a classic “volcano” exudate of fibrin. About 10% of the cases of pseudomembranous colitis are in the proximal parts of the colon and can be visualized by a full colonoscopy.

Treatment

Usual interventions that are applicable to the management of diarrhea in other settings, such as correction of volume deficits and electrolyte imbalance, are important. Beyond this, the first consideration in therapy is to stop the offending antibiotic, whenever possible. This will often be sufficient to resolve the symptoms promptly. If the antibiotic needs to be continued or if symptoms are more severe, antibiotic therapy can be considered. Several effective therapies are available including vancomycin, teicoplanin, fusidic acid, metronidazole, and bacitracin.[88–90] Even though the efficacy of several antibiotics is similar,[91,92] the drug of choice is metronidazole 500 mg orally t.i.d. for 10–14 days. It is recommended that vancomycin use be restricted where possible.[81] Sometimes longer therapy is required, particularly when the offending antibiotic is still given. When therapy is needed, patients usually improve within 72 hours of the first dose of metronidazole. Vancomycin given orally at a dose of 125 mg q.i.d. is also effective,[93] but, because of its higher cost and because of efforts to limit the spread of vancomycin-resistant organisms, metronidazole is preferred. Vancomycin can be considered for patients who have not responded to at least two courses of metronidazole, patients with allergies or intolerance to metronidazole, pregnant women, and children. If there is no adequate clinical response, the oral dose of vancomycin can be increased to 500 mg p.o. q.i.d. For patients who are toxic or unable to take oral medication and in absence of a feeding tube, intravenous metronidazole at a dose of 500–750 mg every 6 hours can be used, although intravenous therapy is inferior and parenteral vancomycin is ineffective. Alternatives are under further study. Linezolid shows *in vitro* sensitivity but needs further clinical testing. Antimotility agents (for example, loperamide, etc.) are contraindicated.

Relapses can occur in up to 20% despite appropriate therapy. Reinfection can also occur. A second course of metronidazole is usually sufficient but prolonged courses of vancomycin can be considered in the face of multiple relapses with clinical signs, for example, oral vancomycin courses followed by a slow taper over 6 weeks.[94] Use of probiotics such as *Saccharomyces boulardii* may be useful, although the evidence remains equivocal.[95,96] Historically, fecal enemas from healthy donors have been tried in an effort to restore normal healthy bowel flora in an effort to competitively displace enteric pathogens.[97]

Diarrhea in HIV patients

Case presentation 3

A 27-year-old man is seen in the outpatient department for symptoms of diarrhea over the last 3 months. He reports stools every 2–3 hours that are watery or consist of poorly digested food he had consumed over the previous day. Occasionally the stool has an oily consistency. He has noted no fever, blood in the stool, tenesmus, or other abdominal complaints. He is known to be HIV-positive, although had declined close monitoring of his immune and virological status, and has not been receiving antiretroviral therapy. He is taking no regular medications apart from multivitamins and a herbal supplement. He has not travelled recently, has not been sexually active for several months preceding the onset of symptoms, and has no pets.

On examination he is afebrile, with normal vital signs. His abdominal examination is unremarkable. His laboratory studies disclose: sodium 137 mmol/liter, potassium 3·6 mmol/liter, urea 3·6 mmol/liter (10 mg/dL), creatinine 70·7 micromol/liter (0·8 mg/dL), and CD4 lymphocyte count 27 per microliter.

Diagnosis

Epidemiology

Chronic diarrhea is a heterogeneous illness, encompassing symptoms caused by infections, inflammatory bowel disease, functional bowel syndromes, malabsorption, and other idiopathic syndromes. A consequence of this heterogeneity is a complex epidemiology, which remains relatively poorly defined. Methodological flaws in the criteria for assembly of study cohorts, definition of diarrhea, and definition of "chronic" may all be important. The age- and sex-adjusted prevalence of this symptom have been estimated at 6 cases per 100 persons (95% CI 4·4–7·7).[98–102]

Persons infected with the human immunodeficiency virus (HIV) are commonly affected by diarrhea. The incidence of chronic diarrhea among participants in the Swiss HIV Cohort study was 8.5 per 100 person years (95% CI 7·4–9·9) between July 1992 and June 1994, and 9·1 (95% CI 7·8–10·7) between July 1994 and March 1996.[103] Prior studies have demonstrated that the risk of chronic diarrhea is related to degree of immunosuppression and transmission category,[104,105] and more recently medication use has emerged as a risk factor.[103,106]

Clinical findings

Limited data are available regarding the use of physical findings for making an etiological diagnosis in patients presenting with chronic diarrhea. Among HIV-infected patients, the history and physical examination have been reported not to be helpful in determining whether or not an enteropathogen will be identified, with the exception that abdominal tenderness was commoner in patients with CMV.[107] The American Gastroenterological Association has recommended that complete evaluation of persons seeking care for chronic diarrhea include evaluation of fluid balance, nutritional status, presence of flushing or rashes, mouth ulcers, thyroid masses, wheezing, arthritis, cardiac murmurs, hepatomegaly, abdominal masses, ascites, and edema. Attention should be paid during anorectal examination to the anal sphincter tone and the presence of perianal fistula or abscess.[100]

Stool culture

The use of stool studies for detection of enteric pathogens is well documented for the evaluation of chronic diarrhea in HIV infection. The yield of stool studies (including culture for enteric bacteria and mycobacteria, and microscopy for parasite ova) varies depending on the patient characteristics of the study population and the intensity of the diagnostic evaluation (Table 8.2).

Recommendations regarding the most appropriate diagnostic strategy for patients infected with HIV have not been formally tested in prospective studies examining a broad range of outcomes, including quality of life. Strategies range from an intensive workup, including upper endoscopy and colonoscopy with mucosal biopsy, to a minimal evaluation involving only stool cultures. The American Gastroenterological Association guidelines, published in 1996, propose a stepwise approach, which may be modified according to the clinical judgment of the physician.[108] The initial step identifies enteric bacteria and parasites through stool studies. Three samples should be submitted initially.

Laboratory tests

The use of fecal biomarkers (the prototype being occult blood) as screening tools to detect gastrointestinal pathology have not been extensively evaluated in the setting of chronic diarrhea, particularly as a marker of intestinal inflammation in chronic diarrhea. When compared to another biomarker, the leukocyte-derived protein calprotectin, against a criterion standard of direct visualization at colonoscopy with biopsy among patients undergoing evaluation for chronic diarrhea of unknown cause or chronic colitis of unknown activity, fecal hemoglobin was of poor discriminatory value for the presence of intestinal inflammation (area under ROC curve [AUC] = 0·58 [95% CI 0·46–0·70]).[109] Fecal calprotectin levels were elevated and significantly associated with the

Table 8.2 Prevalence of enteric pathogens causing diarrhea in HIV-infected patients *

			Prevalence of pathogens		
Reference	N(%)†	Evaluation‡	Patients with diarrhea (%)	Patients without diarrhea (%)	Pathogens§
Dworkin[111]	22 (55)	Stools	75	10	MAC *Cryptosporidia*
Laughon[112]	77 (64)	Stools	50	11	*Cryptosporidia* *Campylobacter* spp.
Smith[113]	30 (67)	Stools, EGD, colonoscopy	85	10	CMV *Entamoeba histolytica*
Antony[114]	66 (100)	Stools	55	–	MAC CMV
Rene[115]	132 (52)	Stools, EGD, colonoscopy	59	28	*Cryptosporidia* CMV
Cotte[116]	81 (73)	Stools	64	15	*Cryptosporidia* CMV
Kotler[117]	194 (73)	Stools	83	2	*Microsporidia* *Cryptosporidia*
Blanshard[108]	155 (100)	Stools, EGD, sigmoidoscopy	83	–	*Cryptosporidia* *Microsporidia*
Prasad[118]	59 (44)	Stools	73‖	–	*Isospora* *Cryptosporidia*
Manatsathit[109]	45 (100)	Stools, EGD, colonoscopy	64		*Cryptosporidia* Tuberculosis

*Adapted from (108) and (110)

†Number of patients studied and proportion with diarrhea (%)

‡Endoscopic procedures listed only if performed in all patients

§Two most common organisms are listed

‖Prevalence of pathogens not reported separately for patients with and without diarrhea

presence of intestinal inflammation (AUC = 0·89 [95% CI 0·81–0·97]). Fecal lactoferrin, another leukocyte-derived protein, was reported to have sensitivity of 90%, specificity of 98%, PPV 82%, and NPV 99% for ulcerative colitis and Crohn's disease in patients being investigated for chronic diarrhea with biomarkers and "an extensive evaluation", which included endoscopy.[119]

Treatment

Antimicrobial therapy

Given the broad differential diagnosis, empiric antimicrobial therapy without initial evaluation is not recommended in this population. If no enteric pathogens are identified on stool studies, an empiric course of oral antibiotics may be considered. This may include a fluoroquinolone or a macrolide. Antiprotozoal therapy can also

Table 8.3 Special pathogens and therapy

Pathogens	Therapy
Cyclospora cayetanensis	Trimethoprim–sulfamethoxazole 800 mg/160 mg twice daily × 7 days
Isospora belli	Trimethoprim–sulfamethoxazole 800 mg/160 mg twice daily × 10 days
Cryptosporidium parvum	None (self-limited disease in immunocompetent host)
Giardia lamblia	Metronidazole 250 mg t.i.d. × 5 days
	Tinidazole 2000 mg/day × 1 day
	Quinacrine 100 mg t.i.d. × 7 days
	Furazolidone 100 mg q.i.d. × 7–10 days
	Albendazole 400 mg/day × 7 days
Entamoeba histolytica	Metronidazole 250 mg q.i.d. × 7 days
Mycobacterium avium complex (MAC)	Ethambutol and clarithromycin
Herpes simplex	Acyclovir
HIV	Antiretroviral combination therapy
Cytomegalovirus	Ganciclovir
	Valganciclovir

be considered such as empiric use of trimethoprim-sulfamethoxazole if *Cyclospora* or *Isospora* infections are suspected. Empiric use of metronidazole is indicated when the suspected pathogens include *Giardia lamblia* or *Entamoeba histolytica*, and would also be of benefit in cases of *Clostridium difficile* colitis. Directed therapy may be available against identified pathogens (Table 8.3).

Antidiarrheals

Non-specific treatment with antidiarrheals, such as loperamide, loperamide oxide, diphenoxylate–atropine, codeine, or tincture of opium, may be considered for empirical therapy. The situations in which such use is tenable include:

- as a temporizing measure prior to a planned diagnostic evaluation
- if diagnostic evaluation does not identify a specific etiology
- if a diagnosis is made for which no effective therapy is known or for which specific treatment fails.[101]

Antidiarrheals may also be considered in HIV-infected persons who have non-bloody diarrhea and a negative initial evaluation on stool testing, although these recommendations have not been evaluated in prospective studies.[108]

The somatostatin analog octreotide has been evaluated as a potential therapy for HIV-associated diarrhea, but has not been found to be superior to placebo.[120]

Other therapy

The evidence for the efficacy of probiotic agents in chronic diarrhea is limited. Dietary modifications, such as a diet based on medium chain triglycerides, have been evaluated as adjunctive therapy in HIV-infected patients with chronic diarrhea, and may be of value.[121]

Prognosis

Duration of symptoms

Remission rates of chronic diarrhea have been estimated to be 282 per 1000 person-years.[98]

Given a similar incidence rate, the overall prevalence of chronic diarrhea was stable in the survey.

Survival

Chronic diarrhea among HIV-infected persons in the Swiss HIV Cohort study was found to be an independent predictor of death (risk ratio 1·48, 95% CI 1·23, 1·80).[100]

References

1. Murray CJ, Lopez AD. Global mortality, disability, and the contribution of risk factors: Global Burden of Disease Study. *Lancet* 1997;**349**:1436–42.
2. Garthright WE, Archer DL, Kvenberg JE. Estimates of incidence and costs of intestinal infectious diseases in the United States. *Public Hlth Rep* 1988;**103**:107–15.
3. Guerrant RL, Kirchhoff LV, Shields DS, *et al.* Prospective study of diarrheal illnesses in northeastern Brazil: patterns of disease, nutritional impact, etiologies, and risk factors. *J Infect Dis* 1983;**148**:986–97.
4. el Alamy MA, Thacker SB, Arafat RR, Wright CE, Zaki AM. The incidence of diarrheal disease in a defined population of rural Egypt. *Am J Trop Med Hyg* 1986;**35**:1006–12.
5. Wheeler JG, Sethi D, Cowden JM, *et al.* Study of infectious intestinal disease in England: rates in the community, presenting to general practice, and reported to national surveillance. The Infectious Intestinal Disease Study Executive. *BMJ* 1999;**318**:1046–50.
6. De Wit MA, Kortbeek LM, Koopmans MP, *et al.* A comparison of gastroenteritis in a general practice-based study and a community-based study. *Epidemiol Infect* 2001;**127**:389–97.
7. Guerrant RL, Hughes JM, Lima NL, Crane J. Diarrhea in developed and developing countries: magnitude, special settings, and etiologies. *Rev Infect Dis* 1990;**12**(Suppl. 1): S41–50.
8. Baer JT, Vugia DJ, Reingold AL, *et al.* HIV infection as a risk factor for shigellosis. *Emerg Infect Dis* 1999;**5**:820–3.
9. Cobelens FG, Leentvaar-Kuijpers A, Kleijnen J, Coutinho RA. Incidence and risk factors of diarrhea in Dutch travellers: consequences for priorities in pre-travel health advice. *Trop Medicine Internat Hlth* 1998;**3**:896–903.
10. Kollaritsch H. Traveller's diarrhea among Austrian tourists in warm climate countries: I. Epidemiology. *Eur J Epidemiol* 1989;**5**:74–81.
11. von Sonnenburg F, Tornieporth N, Waiyaki P, *et al.* Risk and etiology of diarrhea at various tourist destinations. *Lancet* 2000;**356**:133–4.
12. Mattila L, Siitonen A, Kyronseppa H, *et al.* Seasonal variation in etiology of travelers' diarrhea. Finnish-Moroccan Study Group. *J Infect Dis* 1992;**165**:385–8.
13. Herwaldt BL, de Arroyave KR, Roberts JM, Juranek DD. A multiyear prospective study of the risk factors for and incidence of diarrheal illness in a cohort of Peace Corps volunteers in Guatemala. *Ann Intern Med* 2000;**132**: 982–8.
14. Steffen R, Collard F, Tornieporth N, *et al.* Epidemiology, etiology, and impact of traveler's diarrhea in Jamaica. *JAMA* 1999;**281**:811–7.
15. McGee S, Abernethy WB, 3rd, Simel DL. The rational clinical examination. Is this patient hypovolemic? *JAMA* 1999;**281**:1022–9.
16. Huicho L, Campos M, Rivera J, Guerrant RL. Fecal screening tests in the approach to acute infectious diarrhea: a scientific overview. *Pediatr Infect Dis J* 1996;**15**:486–94.
17. Choi SW, Park CH, Silva TM, Zaenker EI, Guerrant RL. To culture or not to culture: fecal lactoferrin screening for inflammatory bacterial diarrhea. *J Clin Microbiol* 1996;**34**:928–32.
18. Silletti RP, Lee G, Ailey E. Role of stool screening tests in diagnosis of inflammatory bacterial enteritis and in selection of specimens likely to yield invasive enteric pathogens. *J Clin Microbiol* 1996;**34**:1161–5.
19. Savola KL, Baron EJ, Tompkins LS, Passaro DJ. Fecal leukocyte stain has diagnostic value for outpatients but not inpatients. *J Clin Microbiol* 2001;**39**:266–9.
20. Slutsker L, Ries AA, Greene KD, *et al.* Escherichia coli O**157**:H7 diarrhea in the United States: clinical and epidemiologic features. *Ann Intern Med* 1997;**126**: 505–13.
21. Koplan JP, Fineberg HV, Ferraro MJ, Rosenberg ML. Value of stool cultures. *Lancet* 1980;**2**:413–6.
22. Feldman RA, Banatvala N. The frequency of culturing stools from adults with diarrhea in Great Britain. *Epidemiol Infect* 1994;**113**:41–4.

23. Guerrant RL, Van Gilder T, Steiner TS, *et al.* Practice guidelines for the management of infectious diarrhea. *Clin Infect Dis* 2001;**32**:331–51.
24. Manatsathit S, Dupont HL, Farthing M, *et al.* Guideline for the management of acute diarrhea in adults. *J Gastroenterol Hepatol* 2002;**17**(Suppl.):S54–71.
25. DuPont HL. Guidelines on acute infectious diarrhea in adults. The Practice Parameters Committee of the American College of Gastroenterology. *Am J Gastroenterol* 1997;**92**:1962–75.
26. Pierce NF, Sack RB, Mitra RC, *et al.* Replacement of water and electrolyte losses in cholera by an oral glucose-electrolyte solution. *Ann Intern Med* 1969;**70**:1173–81.
27. De Bruyn G. Diarrhea. *Clin Evid* 2002:627–35.
28. Nalin DR, Cash RA, Rahman M, Yunus M. Effect of glycine and glucose on sodium and water adsorption in patients with cholera. *Gut* 1970;**11**:768–72.
29. Patra FC, Sack DA, Islam A, Alam AN, Mazumder RN. Oral rehydration formula containing alanine and glucose for treatment of diarrhea: a controlled trial. *BMJ* 1989;**298**:1353–6.
30. Hahn S, Kim Y, Garner P. Reduced osmolarity oral rehydration solution for treating dehydration due to diarrhea in children: systematic review. *BMJ* 2001;**323**:81–5.
31. Alam NH, Majumder RN, Fuchs GJ. Efficacy and safety of oral rehydration solution with reduced osmolarity in adults with cholera: a randomized double-blind clinical trial. CHOICE study group. *Lancet* 1999;**354**:296–9.
32. Hirschhorn N, Nalin DR, Cash RA, Greenough WB, 3rd. Formulation of oral rehydration solution. *Lancet* 2002;**360**:340–1.
33. Fontaine C, Gore SM, Pierce NF. Rice-based oral rehydration solution for treating diarrhea. *Cochrane Database Syst Rev* 2000:CD001264.
34. Bhattacharya MK, Bhattacharya SK, Dutta D, *et al.* Efficacy of oral hyposmolar glucose-based and rice-based oral rehydration salt solutions in the treatment of cholera in adults. *Scand J Gastroenterol* 1998;**33**:159–63.
35. de la Cabada FJ, DuPont HL, Gyr K, Mathewson JJ. Antimicrobial therapy of bacterial diarrhea in adult residents of Mexico – lack of an effect. *Digestion* 1992;**53**:134–41.
36. Ellis-Pegler RB, Hyman LK, Ingram RJ, McCarthy M. A placebo controlled evaluation of lomefloxacin in the treatment of bacterial diarrhea in the community. *J Antimicrob Chemother* 1995;**36**:259–63.
37. Pichler HE, Diridl G, Stickler K, Wolf D. Clinical efficacy of ciprofloxacin compared with placebo in bacterial diarrhea. *Am J Med* 1987;**82**:329–32.
38. Goodman LJ, Trenholme GM, Kaplan RL, *et al.* Empiric antimicrobial therapy of domestically acquired acute diarrhea in urban adults. *Arch Intern Med* 1990;**150**:541–6.
39. Noguerado A, Garcia-Polo I, Isasia T, *et al.* Early single dose therapy with ofloxacin for empirical treatment of acute gastroenteritis: a randomized, placebo-controlled double-blind clinical trial. *J Antimicrob Chemother* 1995;**36**:665–72.
40. Dryden MS, Gabb RJ, Wright SK. Empirical treatment of severe acute community-acquired gastroenteritis with ciprofloxacin. *Clin Infect Dis* 1996;**22**:1019–25.
41. Butler T, Lolekha S, Rasidi C, *et al.* Treatment of acute bacterial diarrhea: a multicenter international trial comparing placebo with fleroxacin given as a single dose or once daily for 3 days. *Am J Med* 1993;**94**:187S–194S.
42. Lolekha S, Patanachareon S, Thanangkul B, Vibulbandhitkit S. Norfloxacin versus co-trimoxazole in the treatment of acute bacterial diarrhea: a placebo controlled study. *Scand J Infect Dis* 1988;**56**(Suppl.):35–45.
43. De Bruyn G, Hahn S, Borwick A. Antibiotic treatment for travellers' diarrhea. *Cochrane Database Syst Rev* 2000:CD002242.
44. Wistrom J, Jertborn M, Ekwall E, *et al.* Empiric treatment of acute diarrheal disease with norfloxacin. A randomized, placebo-controlled study. Swedish Study Group. *Ann Intern Med* 1992;**117**:202–8.
45. Ericsson CD, Johnson PC, Dupont HL, *et al.* Ciprofloxacin or trimethoprim-sulfamethoxazole as initial therapy for travelers' diarrhea. A placebo-controlled, randomized trial. *Ann Intern Med* 1987;**106**:216–20.
46. Isenbarger DW, Hoge CW, Srijan A, *et al.* Comparative antibiotic resistance of diarrheal pathogens from Vietnam and Thailand, 1996–1999. *Emerg Infect Dis* 2002;**8**:175–80.
47. Gomi H, Jiang ZD, Adachi JA, *et al.* In vitro antimicrobial susceptibility testing of bacterial enteropathogens causing traveler's diarrhea in four geographic regions. *Antimicrob Agents Chemother* 2001;**45**:212–6.

48. DuPont HL, Ericsson CD, Mathewson JJ, de la Cabada FJ, Conrad DA. Oral aztreonam, a poorly absorbed yet effective therapy for bacterial diarrhea in US travelers to Mexico. *JAMA* 1992;**267**:1932–5.
49. Kuschner RA, Trofa AF, Thomas RJ, *et al.* Use of azithromycin for the treatment of Campylobacter enteritis in travelers to Thailand, an area where ciprofloxacin resistance is prevalent. *Clin Infect Dis* 1995;**21**:536–41.
50. DuPont HL, Jiang ZD, Ericsson CD, *et al.* Rifaximin versus ciprofloxacin for the treatment of traveler's diarrhea: a randomized, double-blind clinical trial. *Clin Infect Dis* 2001;**33**:1807–15.
51. Lustman F, Walters EG, Shroff NE, Akbar FA. Diphenoxylate hydrochloride (Lomotil) in the treatment of acute diarrhea. *Br J Clin Pract* 1987;**41**:648–51.
52. Heredia Diaz JG, Alcantara I, Solis A. [Evaluation of the safety and effectiveness of WHR-1142A in the treatment of non-specific acute diarrhea]. *Rev Gastroenterol Mex* 1979;**44**:167–73.
53. Heredia Diaz JG, Kajeyama Escobar ML. [Double-blind evaluation of the effectiveness of lidamidine hydrochloride (WHR-1142A) vs loperamide vs. placebo in the treatment of acute diarrhea]. *Salud Publica Mex* 1981;**23**:483–91.
54. Van Loon FP, Bennish ML, Speelman P, Butler C. Double blind trial of loperamide for treating acute watery diarrhea in expatriates in Bangladesh. *Gut* 1989;**30**:492–5.
55. Van den Eynden B, Spaepen W. New approaches to the treatment of patients with acute, nonspecific diarrhea: a comparison of the effects of loperamide and loperamide oxide. *Curr Ther Res* 1995;**56**:1132–41.
56. Hughes IW. First-line treatment in acute non-dysenteric diarrhea: clinical comparison of loperamide oxide, loperamide and placebo. UK Janssen Research Group of General Practitioners. *Br J Clin Pract* 1995;**49**:181–5.
57. Cardon E, Van Elsen J, Frascio M, *et al.* Gut-selective opiates: the effect of loperamide oxide in acute diarrhea in adults. The Diarrhea Trialists Group. *Eur J Clin Res* 1995;**7**:135–44.
58. Dettmer A. Loperamide oxide in the treatment of acute diarrhea in adults. *Clin Ther* 1994;**16**:972–80.
59. Dreverman JW, Van der Poel AJ. Loperamide oxide in acute diarrhea: a double-blind, placebo-controlled trial. The Dutch Diarrhea Trialists Group. *Aliment Pharmacol Ther* 1995;**9**:441–6.
60. Lecomte JM. An overview of clinical studies with racecadotril in adults. *Int J Antimicrob Agents* 2000;**14**:81–7.
61. Abbas Z, Moid I, Khan AH, *et al.* Efficacy of octreotide in diarrhea due to *Vibrio cholerae*: a randomized, controlled trial. *Ann Trop Med Parasitol* 1996;**90**:507–13.
62. Alvarez-Olmos MI, Oberhelman RA. Probiotic agents and infectious diseases: a modern perspective on a traditional therapy. *Clin Infect Dis* 2001;**32**:1567–76.
63. Ericsson CD, DuPont HL. Travelers' diarrhea: approaches to prevention and treatment. *Clin Infect Dis* 1993;**16**:616–24.
64. Mounts AW, Holman RC, Clarke MJ, Bresee JS, Glass RI. Trends in hospitalizations associated with gastroenteritis among adults in the United States, 1979–1995. *Epidemiol Infect* 1999;**123**:1–8.
65. Gerber A, Karch H, Allerberger F, Verweyen HM, Zimmerhackl LB. Clinical course and the role of shiga toxin-producing *Escherichia coli* infection in the hemolytic-uremic syndrome in pediatric patients, 1997–2000, in Germany and Austria: a prospective study. *J Infect Dis* 2002;**186**:493–500.
66. Safdar N, Said A, Gangnon RE, Maki DG. Risk of hemolytic uremic syndrome after antibiotic treatment of *Escherichia coli* O**157**:H7 enteritis: a meta-analysis. *JAMA* 2002;**288**:996–1001.
67. Zimmerhackl LB. E. coli, antibiotics, and the hemolytic-uremic syndrome. *N Engl J Med* 2000;**342**:1990–1.
68. Locht H, Krogfelt KA. Comparison of rheumatological and gastrointestinal symptoms after infection with *Campylobacter jejuni/coli* and enterotoxigenic *Escherichia coli*. *Ann Rheum Dis* 2002;**61**:448–52.
69. Fendler C, Laitko S, Sorensen H, *et al.* Frequency of triggering bacteria in patients with reactive arthritis and undifferentiated oligoarthritis and the relative importance of the tests used for diagnosis. *Ann Rheum Dis* 2001;**60**:337–43.
70. Dworkin MS, Shoemaker PC, Goldoft MJ, Kobayashi JM. Reactive arthritis and Reiter's syndrome following an outbreak of gastroenteritis caused by Salmonella enteritidis. *Clin Infect Dis* 2001;**33**:1010–14.
71. Lew JF, Glass RI, Gangarosa RE, *et al.* Diarrheal deaths in the United States, 1979 through 1987. A special problem for the elderly. *JAMA* 1991;**265**:3280–4.
72. Legros D, Paquet C, Dorlencourt F, Saoult E. Risk factors for death in hospitalized dysentery patients in Rwanda. *Trop Med Int Hlth* 1999;**4**:428–32.

73. Hogenauer C, Hammer HF, Krejs GJ, Reisinger EC. Mechanisms and management of antibiotic-associated diarrhea. *Clin Infect Dis* 1998;**27**:702–10.
74. McFarland LV. Epidemiology of infectious and iatrogenic nosocomial diarrhea in a cohort of general medicine patients. *Am J Infect Control* 1995;**23**:295–305.
75. Wistrom J, Norrby SR, Myhre EB, *et al.* Frequency of antibiotic-associated diarrhea in 2462 antibiotic-treated hospitalized patients: a prospective study. *J Antimicrob Chemother* 2001;**47**:43–50.
76. Mylonakis E, Ryan ET, Calderwood SB. *Clostridium difficile*-associated diarrhea: A review. *Arch Intern Med* 2001;**161**:525–33.
77. Wanahita A, Goldsmith EA, Musher DM. Conditions associated with leukocytosis in a tertiary care hospital, with particular attention to the role of infection caused by *Clostridium difficile. Clin Infect Dis* 2002;**34**:1585–92.
78. Bauer TM, Lalvani A, Fehrenbach J, *et al.* Derivation and validation of guidelines for stool cultures for enteropathogenic bacteria other than *Clostridium difficile* in hospitalized adults. *JAMA* 2001;**285**:313–19.
79. Manabe YC, Vinetz JM, Moore RD, *et al. Clostridium difficile* colitis: an efficient clinical approach to diagnosis. *Ann Intern Med* 1995;**123**:835–40.
80. Schleupner MA, Garner DC, Sosnowski KM, *et al.* Concurrence of *Clostridium difficile* toxin A enzyme-linked immunosorbent assay, fecal lactoferrin assay, and clinical criteria with *C. difficile* cytotoxin titer in two patient cohorts. *J Clin Microbiol* 1995;**33**:1755–9.
81. Gerding DN, Johnson S, Peterson LR, Mulligan ME, Silva J, Jr. *Clostridium difficile*-associated diarrhea and colitis. *Infect Control Hosp Epidemiol* 1995;**16**:459–77.
82. Lyerly DM, Barroso LA, Wilkins TD, Depitre C, Corthier G. Characterization of a toxin A-negative, toxin B-positive strain of *Clostridium difficile. Infect Immun* 1992;**60**:4633–9.
83. Guilbault C, Labbe AC, Poirier L, *et al.* Development and evaluation of a PCR method for detection of the *Clostridium difficile* toxin B gene in stool specimens. *J Clin Micrcbiol* 2002;**40**:2288–90.
84. Karasawa T, Nojiri T, Hayashi Y, *et al.* Laboratory diagnosis of toxigenic *Clostridium difficile* by polymerase chain reaction: presence of toxin genes and their stable expression in toxigenic isolates from Japanese individuals. *J Gastroenterol* 1999;**34**:41–5.
85. Arzese A, Trani G, Riul L, Botta GA. Rapid polymerase chain reaction method for specific detection of toxigenic *Clostridium difficile. Eur J Clin Microbiol Infect Dis* 1995;**14**:716–19.
86. Boland GW, Lee MJ, Cats AM, *et al.* Antibiotic-induced diarrhea: specificity of abdominal CT for the diagnosis of *Clostridium difficile* disease. *Radiology* 1994;**191**:103–6.
87. Kawamoto S, Horton KM, Fishman EK. Pseudomembranous colitis: spectrum of imaging findings with clinical and pathologic correlation. *Radiographics* 1999;**19**:887–97.
88. Wenisch C, Parschalk B, Hasenhundl M, Hirschl AM, Graninger W. Comparison of vancomycin, teicoplanin, metronidazole, and fusidic acid for the treatment of *Clostridium difficile*-associated diarrhea. *Clin Infect Dis* 1996;**22**:813–18.
89. The Swedish CDAD Study Group. Treatment of *Clostridium difficile* associated diarrhea and colitis with an oral preparation of teicoplanin; a dose finding study. The Swedish CDAD Study Group. Scand *J Infect Dis* 1994;**26**:309–16.
90. Dudley MN, McLaughlin JC, Carrington G, *et al.* Oral bacitracin vs vancomycin therapy for *Clostridium difficile*-induced diarrhea. A randomized double-blind trial. *Arch Intern Med* 1986;**146**:1101–4.
91. Teasley DG, Gerding DN, Olson MM, *et al.* Prospective randomized trial of metronidazole versus vancomycin for *Clostridium difficile*-associated diarrhea and colitis. *Lancet* 1983;**2**:1043–6.
92. de Lalla F, Nicolin R, Rinaldi E, *et al.* Prospective study of oral teicoplanin versus oral vancomycin for therapy of pseudomembranous colitis and *Clostridium difficile*-associated diarrhea. *Antimicrob Agents Chemother* 1992;**36**:2192–6.
93. Fekety R, Silva J, Kauffman C, Buggy B, Deery HG. Treatment of antibiotic-associated *Clostridium difficile* colitis with oral vancomycin: comparison of two dosage regimens. *Am J Med* 1989;**86**:15–19.
94. Fekety R, McFarland LV, Surawicz CM, *et al.* Recurrent *Clostridium difficile* diarrhea: characteristics of and risk factors for patients enrolled in a prospective, randomized, double-blinded trial. *Clin Infect Dis* 1997;**24**:324–33.
95. Lewis SJ, Potts LF, Barry RE. The lack of therapeutic effect of *Saccharomyces boulardii* in the prevention of antibiotic-related diarrhea in elderly patients. *J Infect* 1998;**36**:171–4.

96. Surawicz CM, McFarland LV, Greenberg RN, *et al.* The search for a better treatment for recurrent *Clostridium difficile* disease: use of high-dose vancomycin combined with *Saccharomyces boulardii*. *Clin Infect Dis* 2000;**31**:1012–17.
97. Gustafsson A, Berstad A, Lund-Tonnesen S, Midtvedt T, Norin E. The effect of faecal enema on five microflora-associated characteristics in patients with antibiotic-associated diarrhea. *Scand J Gastroenterol* 1999;**34**: 580–6.
98. Talley NJ, Weaver AL, Zinsmeister AR, Melton LJ, 3rd. Onset and disappearance of gastrointestinal symptoms and functional gastrointestinal disorders. *Am J Epidemiol* 1992;**136**:165–77.
99. American Gastroenterological Association medical position statement: guidelines for the management of malnutrition and cachexia, chronic diarrhea, and hepatobiliary disease in patients with human immunodeficiency virus infection. *Gastroenterology* 1996;**111**: 1722–3.
100. American Gastroenterological Association medical position statement: guidelines for the evaluation and management of chronic diarrhea. *Gastroenterology* 1999;**116**:1461–3.
101. Fine KD, Schiller LR. AGA technical review on the evaluation and management of chronic diarrhea. *Gastroenterology* 1999;**116**:1464–86.
102. Huttly SR, Hoque BA, Aziz KM, *et al.* Persistent diarrhea in a rural area of Bangladesh: a community-based longitudinal study. *Int J Epidemiol* 1989;**18**: 964–9.
103. Weber R, Ledergerber B, Zbinden R, *et al.* Enteric infections and diarrhea in human immunodeficiency virus-infected persons: prospective community-based cohort study. Swiss HIV Cohort Study. *Arch Intern Med* 1999;**159**:1473–80.
104. Rabeneck L, Crane MM, Risser JM, Lacke CE, Wray NP. Effect of HIV transmission category and CD4 count on the occurrence of diarrhea in HIV-infected patients. *Am J Gastroenterol* 1993;**88**:1720–3.
105. Kaslow RA, Phair JP, Friedman HB, *et al.* Infection with the human immunodeficiency virus: clinical manifestations and their relationship to immune deficiency. A report from the Multicenter AIDS Cohort Study. *Ann Intern Med* 1987;**107**:474–80.
106. Eisenberg JN, Wade TJ, Charles S, *et al.* Risk factors in HIV-associated diarrheal disease: the role of drinking water, medication and immune status. *Epidemiol Infect* 2002;**128**:73–81.
107. Blanshard C, Francis N, Gazzard BG. Investigation of chronic diarrhea in acquired immunodeficiency syndrome. A prospective study of 155 patients. *Gut* 1996;**39**:824–32.
108. Wilcox CM, Rabeneck L, Friedman S. AGA technical review: malnutrition and cachexia, chronic diarrhea, and hepatobiliary disease in patients with human immunodeficiency virus infection. *Gastroenterology* 1996;**111**:1724–52.
109. Limburg PJ, Ahlquist DA, Sandborn WJ, *et al.* Fecal calprotectin levels predict colorectal inflammation among patients with chronic diarrhea referred for colonoscopy. *Am J Gastroenterol* 2000;**95**:2831–7.
110. Manatsathit S, Tansupasawasdikul S, Wanachiwanawin D, *et al.* Causes of chronic diarrhea in patients with AIDS in Thailand: a prospective clinical and microbiological study. *J Gastroenterol* 1996;**31**:533–7.
111. Dworkin B, Wormser GP, Rosenthal WS, *et al.* Gastrointestinal manifestations of the acquired immunodeficiency syndrome: a review of 22 cases. *Am J Gastroenterol* 1985;**80**:774–8.
112. Laughon BE, Druckman DA, Vernon A, *et al.* Prevalence of enteric pathogens in homosexual men with and without acquired immunodeficiency syndrome. *Gastroenterology* 1988;**94**:984–93.
113. Smith PD, Lane HC, Gill VJ, *et al.* Intestinal infections in patients with the acquired immunodeficiency syndrome (AIDS). Etiology and response to therapy. *Ann Intern Med* 1988;**108**:328–33.
114. Antony MA, Brandt LJ, Klein RS, Bernstein LH. Infectious diarrhea in patients with AIDS. *Dig Dis Sci* 1988;**33**:1141–6.
115. Rene E, Marche C, Regnier B, *et al.* Intestinal infections in patients with acquired immunodeficiency syndrome. A prospective study in 132 patients. *Dig Dis Sci* 1989;**34**:773–80.
116. Cotte L, Rabodonirina M, Piens MA, *et al.* M, Trepo C. Prevalence of intestinal protozoans in French patients infected with HIV. *J Acquir Immune Defic Syndr* 1993;**6**:1024–9.

117. Kotler DP, Orenstein JM. Prevalence of intestinal microsporidiosis in HIV-infected individuals referred for gastroenterological evaluation. *Am J Gastroenterol* 1994;**89**:1998–2002.

118. Prasad KN, Nag VL, Dhole TN, Ayyagari A. Identification of enteric pathogens in HIV-positive patients with diarrhea in northern India. *J Hlth Popul Nutr* 2000;**18**:23–6.

119. Fine KD, Ogunji F, George J, Niehaus MD, Guerrant RL. Utility of a rapid fecal latex agglutination test detecting the neutrophil protein, lactoferrin, for diagnosing inflammatory causes of chronic diarrhea. *Am J Gastroenterol* 1998;**93**:1300–5.

120. Simon DM, Cello JP, Valenzuela J, *et al.* Multicenter trial of octreotide in patients with refractory acquired immunodeficiency syndrome-associated diarrhea. *Gastroenterology* 1995;**108**:1753–60.

121. Wanke CA, Pleskow D, Degirolami PC, *et al.* A medium chain triglyceride-based diet in patients with HIV and chronic diarrhea reduces diarrhea and malabsorption: a prospective, controlled trial. *Nutrition* 1996;**12**:766–71.

9

Urinary tract infections

Thomas Fekete

Case presentation 1

A 35-year-old woman is seen in the outpatient clinic for a 2-day history of worsening urinary burning and frequency. She is a healthy woman with no medical problems. She has two children at home and is currently using oral contraceptives. She recalls a possible urinary tract infection (UTI) while she was in college but remembers only that she "took a bunch of pills all at once" and had no sequelae of UTI afterwards. On examination she looks mildly uncomfortable but otherwise in no distress. She is afebrile and has normal vital signs. There is no costovertebral angle tenderness. There is slight discomfort with deep palpation over the pubis, but the bladder is not enlarged. The patient refuses a pelvic examination since she has just seen her gynecologist 2 weeks earlier for a routine checkup and was told everything was normal.

UTIs are a common medical problem, with costs estimated at more than US $1·6 billion in 1995 in the United States.[1] While many people with serious underlying illnesses develop UTIs in healthcare facilities as a consequence of bladder dysfunction and catheterization, women are especially vulnerable to getting UTIs even in the absence of underlying illness. About 40% of adult women report having had a previous UTI.[2] In young, sexually active women the rate of UTIs has been reported to be as high as 0·5 episodes per woman-year.[3] Moreover, in a random telephone dialing survey, nearly 11% of women reported at least one UTI in the past 12 months.[1]

Case presentation 1 (continued)

Urine dipstick testing is done in the office. It is strongly positive for leukocyte esterase and nitrites but negative for blood, protein and glucose. Is there sufficient evidence to make a clinical diagnosis of UTI in this patient?

Diagnosis

In the case presentation, this woman has a short history of dysuria and frequency with no prior known urinary pathology. A systematic review assessing the accuracy of history-taking and physical examination for diagnosing acute uncomplicated UTI in women reveals that dysuria and frequency without vaginal discharge or irritation raises the probability of UTI from about 48% to more than 90%.[4] While a positive urine dipstick can raise this probability even higher, a negative result will still leave a high post-test probability of UTI. The clinical elements in our patient (dysuria, frequency) along with history of hematuria, back pain, and costovertebral angle tenderness all tend to increase the likelihood that the woman has a UTI, as do the *lack* of vaginal complaints (discharge, irritation), dysuria, or back pain. Since the pretest possibility of UTI in an otherwise healthy woman coming to the clinic with a suspicion of

Table 9.1 Likelihood ratios (LR) for some important UTI clinical features

Clinical features	Positive LR	Negative LR
Dysuria	1·5	0·5
Frequency	1·8	
Hematuria	2·0	
Vaginal discharge	0·3	
Vaginal irritation	0·2	
Back pain	1·6	0·8
Vaginal discharge on examination	0·7	
Costovertebral angle tenderness	1·7	

UTI is so high (48%), it would be a fair question to ask how low a probability would militate against the initiation of therapy. The study made a formal evaluation of clinical features of UTI by a systematic review of the literature (464 articles) and focusing on nine that met rigorous inclusion criteria. These individual studies were chosen because they allowed an assessment of individual features such as dysuria or vaginal irritation so that each one could be given a likelihood ratio for the presence of a UTI. This likelihood ratio could be applied to a prior probability of UTI (as determined by the patient or the physician) so that a reasonable clinical diagnosis could be made. The likelihood ratios for some of the most important clinical features (where the 95% CI did not include 1·0 or −1·0) are in the Table 9.1.

The two most common tests used on the commercial dipstick to assess possible UTI are the nitrite (nitrate reductase) and the leukocyte esterase tests.[5] The nitrite test measures the presence of the enzyme nitrate reductase – a bacterial enzyme present in many though not all gram-negative bacteria. False positives are rare, but the rate of false negatives ranges from 10 to 30% and is especially high in infections caused by nitrite-negative organisms, when the urine has a low pH or a large amount of urobilinogen or ascorbic acid. Leukocyte esterase measures the presence of white blood cells in the urine. While other conditions can cause pyuria, the clinical setting is usually sufficiently clear to rule out these infections. False negative results can be found with low concentrations of urinary leukocytes, the presence of ascorbic acid, phenazopyridine, or large amounts of protein. Data on the usefulness of these screening tools in hospitalized patients are variable, but their rapidity makes them helpful in office practice. One of the problems of these rapid tests for UTI is that they are affected by spectrum bias.[6] What this means is that the sensitivity of the test is influenced by the underlying characteristics of the population being studied. In this example, the sensitivity of a positive dipstick test was 0·92 (95% CI 0·82–0·98) whereas, if the prior probability was low, the sensitivity would be reduced to 0·56 (0·03–0·79). When the presence of a positive urine culture is used as the reference standard of a UTI, the performance characteristics of various components of the urinalysis can be disappointing.[7]

In terms of non-invasive diagnostic tests that can be done in the ambulatory setting, there are two options: microscopic analysis of the urinary sediment and urine culture. Urine microscopy (determining in a semiquantitative manner the concentration of leukocytes in the urine) is done as a routine part of the urinalysis in many hospital laboratories, but the urine dipstick is almost as reliable in confirming UTI as the microscopic analysis[8] and is quicker and less expensive than microscopy. Both tests are imperfect but, in an Emergency Room study, each test had roughly the same number of false negatives and false positives when compared with the results of urine culture.[9] In pregnancy, the urine culture is the test of choice, since even a negative urinalysis does not ablate the need for culture. Less is known about the usefulness of dipstick testing in hospitalized patients, where there exists higher rates of pyuria and UTI than in ambulatory patients. Zaman and colleagues found high specificity using > 10 WBC/microliter and > 5 WBC (94% and 90%), but lower sensitivity with these values (57% and 84% respectively).[10] The positive predictive values were 91% and 77% and the negative predictive values were 68% and 93% respectively. Quantitative determination of pyuria in uncentrifuged urine (as contrasted with the usual semiquantitative assessment of WBC in centrifuged urine) can be a useful tool for research[8] to assure a consistent definition of UTI, but it is time-consuming and rarely done.

A management strategy that does not include any kind of urine testing might be appealing as a way of reducing costs and perhaps avoiding clinic visits. Unfortunately, this could result in considerable overtreatment. In a cohort of 231 Canadian women presenting with dysuria, about 80% thought that they had a UTI.[11] Physician diagnosis of a UTI occurred in 92% of cases; however, UTIs were documented in only 53%. As a result, unnecessary antibiotics were prescribed frequently. Combining clinical features and urine testing for pyuria and nitrates could have reduced the number of unnecessary treatment courses considerably. Unfortunately, it would have delayed the treatment of infection in a number of women with true cystitis (positive urine culture but negative dipstick test). The lesson from this set of observations is that, in the case of a very common problem like UTI, there can be diagnostic uncertainty comparable to that of other problems seen in the ambulatory setting. The careful clinician might interpret this as a choice between overtreatment and overdiagnosis. Luckily the consequences of either approach are modest both economically (since the drugs and the diagnostic tests are fairly inexpensive) and in toxicity (since the medications are well tolerated and a short delay in the treatment of UTI almost never leads to serious sequelae). The McIsaac paper algorithm led to a reduction in unnecessary antibiotic use from 40% of all drugs used to 27%, and a reduction in total urine cultures obtained from 87% to 40%; however, it also led to a reduction in the sensitivity for UTI from 92% to 81%. These guidelines would result in one delay of therapy in every 13 women with UTI.

Treatment guidelines for telephone-based prescription strategies might have the same problem of overtreatment. In a large study of women in the Group Health Cooperative in Washington state, who stated on the telephone that they had dysuria and met certain clinical criteria, the use of nurse prescribers of antibiotics resulted in very few clinic visits for UTI.[12]

By strict definition, a UTI should have $> 10^3$ colony forming units of microbe per milliliter of urine,[13] but urine cultures demand time for processing and growth (at least 18 hours) and further time for identification of the microbe and determination of antimicrobial susceptibility. A treatment delay while these results are awaited can increase the morbidity of UTI, and the culture itself increases the cost of diagnosis. However, there are no RCTs that have randomized patients with presenting UTI symptoms to urine culture versus no culture.

Obtaining urine cultures in patients who require hospitalization, who are allergic to first-line antibiotics, or who fail therapy is done in anticipation of possible changes in treatment based on resistance or drug intolerance. Severely ill patients may also benefit from a urine culture insofar as it might guide appropriate changes in treatment if there is a failure to respond to initial therapy. Withholding treatment until a culture report is available is reasonable only for those patients with a low suspicion of infection or significant drug allergy. The only benefit of obtaining a culture when there is a plan to initiate treatment is to help interpret treatment failure. In most studies of healthy ambulatory women, this is rare (< 5%).[14]

Other diagnostic testing

UTI can be defined as *simple* or *complicated* based on the respective absence or presence of documented or suspected structural or physiologic abnormalities of the urinary tract. There is no information in Case 1 to suggest abnormal urinary anatomy and physiology and thus no need for radiological localization of the infection.[15]

Case presentation 1 (continued)

After checking to make sure the patient had no drug allergies, the physician prescribed a 3-day course of trimethoprim-sulfamethoxazole (TMP-SMX) (160/800 mg p.o. twice a day). A phone call to the patient 2 days after the completion of therapy showed that her symptoms were totally resolved and that she had experienced only mild nausea on antimicrobial therapy.

Therapy for the ambulatory patient

The results of urine cultures in ambulatory patients with UTIs show a great preponderance for *Escherichia coli*. Although *E. coli* is a common commensal of the GI tract, the strains that cause UTIs are a subset of GI adapted strains that are also able to adhere to the periurethral area and to the cells lining the urinary tract. Similarly other gram-negative bacteria (such as *Klebsiella* spp., *Proteus* spp.) with uropathogenic attributes can also cause UTIs in otherwise healthy people. There are two important gram-positive uropathogens of ambulatory women. *Staphylococcus saprophyticus* (a coagulase-negative staphylococcus) is present in young women especially during the summer months, and *Enterococcus* is uncommon in ambulatory patients but sometimes causes infection in people who have received antibiotics previously. The concentration of these organisms in the urine has been the source of some disagreement in the past. While quantitative cultures usually show a large number of organisms present (> 10^5/mL), about 25% to 30% UTIs will have fewer organisms (> 10^3/mL).[16]

There are many choices of antimicrobials for the treatment of UTIs and a number of potential treatment durations. Although the patient in Case 1 had resolution of symptoms of her first UTI after taking single-dose therapy, the failure rate and early recurrence rate for single-dose treatment of UTI is considerably higher than that for short-course (usually 3-day) treatments.[17,18] A systematic review of the relative efficacy of single-dose versus 3-day or longer therapy shows better outcomes with the 3-day or longer therapy. Studies of single-dose therapy using β-lactams, TMP, TMP-SMX, and fluoroquinolones have essentially been halted, not only because the clinical outcomes are worse, but also because the total costs (including time off from work, repeated visits to health care providers, etc.) are magnified by relatively small differences in the recurrence rate.[19,20] The only drug still given in a single dose is fosfomycin which has a long half-life (5·7 hours) and high urinary levels (a single 3 g dose is given as a sachet dissolved in water).[21] The use of single-dose fosfomycin or longer courses of nitrofurantoin (7 days) gives a more reduced cure rate than TMP-SMX or fluoroquinolones.[19,22,23] Therefore these agents find their greatest use in salvage regimens or when patients have significant drug allergies or intolerance. Furthermore, fosfomycin (about US $25 in 1997) and nitrofurantoin (about US $20 in 1997) are expensive.[24]

Numerous studies have demonstrated the inferiority of β-lactams for UTI.[19,25] That is not to say that some patients do not respond well to inexpensive β-lactamss such as amoxicillin but that the overall rates of response and relapse are disappointing as compared with other drugs. This is true even if there is not a great amount of β-lactam resistance in uropathogens. However, it is important to note that β-lactams are recommended for pregnancy given the favorable safety profile.

It is important to interpret the results of clinical trials of antimicrobial agents for UTIs in the context of the local antimicrobial resistance patterns. Changing patterns of resistance of the infectious agents occur constantly.[26] Therefore, changes in strains and resistance patterns of bacteria causing UTI, as well differences in dosages of antimicrobials used make the interpretation of older studies challenging. An example is a large, well-designed study comparing the outcome of treatment with either ciprofloxacin, ofloxacin, or TMP-SMX in women with UTI.[14] Although a large number of women were in this study (866 were recruited and 688 were available for analysis), there were no significant differences among the three study drugs in terms of outcome or adverse reactions. The study was powered to show significance assuming a success rate of 93% for ciprofloxacin, 80% for TMP-SMX and 90% for ofloxacin. The actual clinical success rates were 93% for ciprofloxacin, 95% for TMP-SMX, and 96% for ofloxacin. Of note, the patient outcomes were as good as or better than expected (bacteriologic responses of 92–97% and clinical responses of 93–96%) even though the ciprofloxacin dose used in this study was the lowest recommended dose. Resistance to any of the drugs used was quite low; therefore the results may not apply in situations where resistance to one or more of the drugs is higher. In that situation, the outcome might be less good with the drug to which resistance has now emerged. Finally, the overall "better-than-expected" outcome might reflect especially mild disease in the patients enrolled in this study – thus true differences in outcome (or even adverse events) might be underestimated as compared with a sicker population with less capacity for spontaneous or aided recovery. A Cochrane review about fluoroquinolones for uncomplicated cystitis in women indicates that, although as a class fluoroquinolones have shown good clinical outcomes in the published literature, there might be clinically important differences in efficacy and tolerability within the class or compared with other agents.[27]

Prognosis

While withholding therapy from an otherwise healthy ambulatory woman with dysuria and a positive urine culture would be difficult for most clinicians, there are some data on the expected outcome. A randomized trial in Belgium studied the benefit of a 3-day course of nitrofurantoin (100 mg p.o. every 6 hours) with a similar schedule of placebo.[28] Although 166 women were screened, only 78 had pyuria and agreed to participate. Thirty-five women in each group were evaluable at the conclusion of therapy and 77% of the nitrofurantoin recipients were better as compared with 54% of the placebo recipients. Excluding women with negative urine cultures showed that 17/23 (74%) of the nitrofurantoin recipients versus 9/22 (41%) of the placebo recipients were better at the 7-day evaluation. While this confirms a considerable benefit of antimicrobials for UTI (NNT for various favorable outcomes ranged from 1·7 to 4·4), clinical and microbial success was fairly common without any active treatment. In one meta-analysis of six double-blind clinical trials (over 3000 patients), the following four factors were associated with better outcomes:

- not using a diaphragm
- treatment for > 3 days
- symptoms for < 2 days
- African-American race.[29]

Patients infected with bacteria categorized as *Klebsiella* or "other" had a worse prognosis.

In the case presented, a failure to choose the right treatment would have been apparent quite rapidly. In many regions, the susceptibility of uropathogens to commonly used first-line antimicrobials (TMP-SMX or a fluoroquinolone) is so high that it is not cost-effective to check routine cultures. There is even some clinical success in women with organisms that are reported to be resistant to the drug chosen for treatment. This might result from spontaneous cure or from achieving high enough a concentration of antimicrobial in the urine to result in cure despite apparent resistance. The largest study looking at treatment success with TMP-SMX in patients with resistant strains was published by a group in Israel in 2002.[30] Their patients received a 5-day course of TMP-SMX and, in the patients with strains that were susceptible, the success rate was 82% as compared with 42% in whom the organism was resistant. In areas where resistance is more frequent to usual first-line agents, the approach is to use a second-line agent such as fosfomycin or an alternative (but perhaps more expensive) first-line agent such as a fluoroquinolone. The same would be true for women who are allergic or cannot tolerate the usual medical interventions.

Case presentation 2

A 63-year-old woman is seen in the office for a 2-day history of dysuria. She had recently retired from her secretarial job because of complications of her diabetes (early cataracts and mild, painful neuropathy) that had made it difficult for her to travel to work. She had recently completed a course of cefadroxil for cellulitis of the left foot with clinical improvement. Her current voiding symptoms were moderately severe. She thought she might have had a fever and some mild sweats but at the time of the clinic visit she was afebrile. The remainder of the examination was unremarkable except for mild left costovertebral angle tenderness and diminished sensation in both feet. A pelvic examination was normal. A urine specimen was obtained: the dipstick test was positive for leukocyte esterase and glucose and negative for all other tests including nitrite.

Like the previous patient, this woman also has a short history of irritative voiding symptoms, but there are some important distinctions. In addition to being older, this patient has long-standing diabetes with complications. As a result, bladder dysfunction due to diabetic neuropathy is a possibility. This patient's previous course of antibiotics (cephalosporins) may have changed the specific potential uropathogens, and may specifically have selected a more antibiotic-resistant flora.[31] The presence of significant diabetic neuropathy might portend autonomic neuropathy and incomplete bladder emptying. Significant residual bladder urine increases the risk of upper tract infection and treatment failure as well as the intrinsic risk for cystitis.[32,33] There are two potential strategies with respect to obtaining urine cultures for this patient:

- obtain a culture before initiating antibiotics (early culture)
- obtain a culture only if there is a clinical failure of therapy (late culture).

Early culture is reasonable when urine can be obtained in the office and if culture reports are promptly and reliably available. On the other hand, a late culture strategy makes sense if cultures are difficult to obtain and if adherence with medication and follow up is likely to be excellent. These strategies have not been formally compared in clinical trials.

Case presentation 2 (continued)

Because of the patient's recent antibiotic course, a urine culture was requested. While culture results were awaited, the patient began a course of antibiotics with TMP-SMX (160/800 mg p.o. twice a day) with the intention of giving a 14-day course of treatment. The laboratory report on the culture showed that she had an *E. coli* that was resistant to ampicillin and tetracycline but susceptible to all the other agents tested. The patient responded clinically within 2 days of starting treatment. At the conclusion of her 14-day course of therapy, she was asymptomatic and, at the time of follow up clinic visit, had no symptoms or physical findings of UTI.

Follow up

Follow up for the woman with a symptomatic UTI is simple. If all symptoms have resolved, the treatment is considered successful and no further visit or diagnostic testing is needed. Both of the cases presented had good responses and would not need follow up. It would be sufficient to have telephone contact to assure that the treatment was successful. The success rate with TMP-SMX in the IDSA study[34] was 93%, and the majority of treatment failures were symptomatic. In a large primary care database (104 099 infections) in the UK, the failure rate (i.e., need for a second course of therapy) was 14% at 28 days of follow up after the diagnosis of UTI was first made.[31] This study included women treated in 1992–1999. Of all the drugs used, TMP-SMX was the least likely to fail with a hazard ratio (HR) for failure of 1·39 for amoxicillin and 1·23 for nitrofurantoin, although ciprofloxacin (HR for failure of 1·12; 95% CI 0·90–1·40) and cefadroxil (HR of 1·17; 95% CI 0·93–1·48) were of comparable efficacy but were used much less often than TMP-SMX. There are certainly limitations of this non-randomized study design, but the large number of women studied gives some indication of the likelihood of a successful outcome, even though treatment was assigned by physician preference and not controlled. Since this study did not look at the result of follow up cultures, but only at the need for another course of antimicrobials, it is difficult to know whether to look for early failure with scheduled culture before the recurrence of symptoms. Since failure requiring retreatment is expected in about one in seven patients, and these failures can occur within a few days of the conclusion of the original therapy to a month later, the usefulness of routine follow up cultures is questionable.

Asymptomatic bacteriuria

Asymptomatic bacteriuria refers to the presence of significant numbers of bacteria in the urine in the absence of symptoms such as urinary burning, frequency, or urgency. In young, healthy women, the prevalence of asymptomatic bacteriuria is 5–6%.[35] In this study, it was shown that, in the vast majority of cases of asymptomatic bacteriuria, the bacteriuria resolves spontaneously. However, the likelihood of developing cystitis within a week of the detection of asymptomatic bacteriuria is eight times higher than the risk within a week of having a sterile urine culture. Thus in this setting, asymptomatic bacteriuria is an uncommon but unalarming entity that has a small chance of progressing to symptomatic disease. Underlying conditions known to be associated with higher rates of asymptomatic bacteriuria are pregnancy, post-bladder catheter removal, advanced age (> 65 years) and diabetes mellitus. There is evidence favoring treatment of asymptomatic bacteriuria during pregnancy[36,37] and following bladder catheter removal.[38] A Cochrane review of bacteriuria in pregnancy showed substantial benefits of treatment for asymptomatic bacteriuria during pregnancy. The elimination of bacteriuria was much greater with antibiotics than with placebo or no treatment (OR 0·07; 95% CI 0·05–0·10), the reduction of pyelonephritis was impressive (OR 0·24; 95% CI 0·19–0·32), and the pregnancy outcome (fewer preterm or low birth weight babies) was enhanced (OR 0·60; 95% CI 0·45–0·80). A randomized controlled clinical trial demonstrated that bacteriuria resolved spontaneously within 14 days of bladder catheterization in 36% and after a single dose of antibiotics in 81%.[38] More importantly, of the women who received no treatment, seven of 42 developed symptomatic UTIs. In general, untreated women under the age of 65 did better at clearing their bacteriuria (74%) than older women (4%). In other settings such as diabetes and old age, attempted treatment of bacteriuria is unhelpful in preventing subsequent infections and exposes patients to the potential toxicity of antimicrobials and the cost of repeated clinic visits and urine tests.[39,40] A recent prospective, randomized trial of treatment of asymptomatic bacteriuria in diabetic women showed no net benefit for a 14-day course of antibiotics directed at the organism isolated.[41] There was no reduction in symptomatic UTI in a 3-year follow up, but there was a considerable excess in the use of antibiotics (5-fold increase) and in treatment-related adverse effects (3-fold increase). A minor side note: a 3-day course of antibiotics for the eradication of asymptomatic bacteriuria was ineffective in all six cases in which it was tried, so that regimen was dropped from the study.

Case presentation 2 (continued)

Three months later, the patient noted the onset of dysuria and urinary frequency over a period of 2 days. At the time of the office visit, she was uncomfortable but had no fever or constitutional symptoms. Her urinalysis again showed a positive leukocyte esterase on the dipstick and a large number of white blood cells on microscopic analysis. She was given another course of TMP-SMX after a urine culture was sent. This time, the culture showed > 100 000 colony-forming units of *Klebsiella pneumoniae*. This organism was resistant to ampicillin but susceptible to all other antibiotics tested.

In this situation, the patient had a new infection after cure of the previous UTI. Recurrence of UTI is a common problem with rates reported as high as 44% at one year.[42] Recurrent symptoms following apparent cure of a UTI can represent a *relapse* of the previous infection or a *reinfection*. In this case, the patient clearly had a reinfection since the organism isolated was a different species from that of the prior infection. To document a relapse, it is essential to demonstrate not only the same species of bacteria in both infections but also the same strain. This can be done using molecular typing.

Case presentation 2 (continued)

Although she felt completely well at the conclusion of her second course of antibiotics, the patient is frustrated and asks, "Why does this keep happening to me? Can't something be done to prevent another one of these infections?"

Prevention

The timing and frequency of recurrent UTI is unpredictable. Most of the known risk factors for UTI are difficult to control. Efforts to reduce the adhesion of uropathogenic bacteria to the genitourinary epithelium by the ingestion of cranberry juice have been mildly effective while the use of a lactobacillus GG beverage was not helpful in preventing UTI.[43] Women who were at risk of recurrent UTIs were randomized to receive a cranberry/lingonberry juice daily or lactobacillus GG for 5 days/week. The study was not blinded, although the investigators were not informed which treatment the women were getting. In a 6-month period, the women using the cranberry beverage had a 20% absolute reduction in the rate of UTIs (95% CI 3–36). There was a very slight increase in the absolute rate of UTIs in the group taking the lactobacillus beverage. Change in vaginal pH, in particular the use of spermicide (often accompanying diaphragms), has been associated with an increased risk of UTI in several studies.[3,44] Sexual activity can predispose to UTI[3] and this may be especially problematic with newer sex partners. In postmenopausal women, not taking estrogen replacement therapy is a risk factor for recurrent UTI.[32] Topical or systemic estrogens will reduce the rate of recurrent UTI in these women.[45] Clearly, the use of systemic estrogens should be informed by their risk/benefit for medical problems other than UTI.

The controversy over seeking an anatomical explanation for recurrent UTI is not fully resolved, but in adults it is rare to identify correctable lesions.[46] In this study, 104 adult women referred to Urology for UTI consultation were evaluated with excretory urography and 74 of them also had cystoscopy. These women had a heterogeneous history of UTI, but most had had two or more UTIs in the past year. The radiographic workup showed only 12 abnormalities of which perhaps five were related to (but not likely to be causal) UTI. The cystoscopies showed that 18% of the women had abnormalities (most of which were mucosal inflammation) and that only 4% had a potentially treatable problem (urethral diverticula). For our patient, bladder function could be abnormal if she also has an autonomic neuropathy from diabetes. Obstructions to urine flow, poor emptying of the bladder and ureters, reflux of urine from the bladder to the ureter, and anatomical variations of the urethra can be found as causes of recurrent infection. However, standard techniques (radiographic imaging, cystoscopy, etc.) have a low yield in identifying such lesions.[46] Relatively common problems such as incomplete bladder emptying because of neural injury or disease are often difficult or impossible to correct.

Evidence exists to support antimicrobial prevention of recurrent infections. Women with frequent, uncomplicated recurrences (usually two or more infections in a 6-month period) may benefit from one of three antibiotic use strategies:

- continuous low-dose prophylaxis[47,48]
- postcoital prophylaxis[49]
- pre-emptive short course treatment (without medical consultation) at first sign of infection.[50]

Each of these strategies reduces the frequency and morbidity of UTI, but there are no controlled trials comparing them. Postcoital prophylaxis trimethoprim-sulfamethoxazole (TMP-SMX) was studied in a randomized, placebo-controlled trial and shown to reduce UTIs by 12-fold (from 3·6 per patient-year to 0·3 per patient-year.)[49] However, the very small number of women studied (16 in the TMP-SMX group and 11 in the placebo group) limits precision. Self-directed therapy appeals to many women, and there is evidence that women who have experienced UTI can self-diagnose and treat with impressive accuracy and good outcomes.[51] In this study, 172 women were given the opportunity to initiate levofloxacin therapy at the first indication of a UTI. There was no control group since all women were eligible to initiate therapy after obtaining a urine specimen for analysis and culture. Roughly 50% of the women studied had one or more UTIs after enrolling in the study (on average, two per woman for those who had UTI), and the urinalysis and/or urine culture was positive in 95% of these episodes. Clinical and microbiologic cures were attained in 92% and 96% of cases respectively.

Whether prophylaxis is offered or not, there tends to be a slow trend towards cessation of recurrent infections in women without anatomic or physiologic reasons to have recurrent UTI. For women on continuing prophylaxis or postcoital prophylaxis, it might make sense to stop this treatment every year or so to see if the propensity to recurrent infections has faded. The patient in Case 2 will need to be aware of her urinary infection pattern and attend to her possible bladder dysfunction. This may entail consultation with a urologist who can assess her urodynamics and help determine the best way to maintain good voiding patterns. There has also been a Cochrane review of cranberry juice as a preventive measure for UTI.[52] While several studies purport to show an advantage to cranberry juice over placebo juice or water, the modest benefit is possibly outweighed by having only five studies with a large number of withdrawals. Furthermore, the failure to show a benefit in an intention-to-treat analysis makes this intervention less appealing.

The use of special silver-coated catheters in people who need short-term bladder catheterization has been studied and been shown to reduce the risk of UTI. A randomized crossover study in hospitalized patients showed that the relative risk of infection per 100 catheters used was 0·68 (95% CI 0·54–0·86).[53] A report prepared for the US Agency for Healthcare Research and Quality indicated that silver-coated catheters could prevent bacteriuria and complications of UTI such as bacteremia, although these benefits might be somewhat vitiated with a long duration of catheterization.[54] This paper describes a number of randomized controlled trials of various silver-coated catheters versus standard silicon urinary catheters. The range of benefits is broad from a 4-fold reduction (at most) to no meaningful reduction. This large variation is related in part to differences in the patient populations and in the duration of catheterization. The true extent of benefit (and the costs associated with the catheters and with subsequent infections) is not yet known.

The problem of UTI in people with spinal cord injury has also led to the study of preventive measures. The US Agency for Health Care Policy initiated a meta-analysis of the role of prophylactic antibiotics in adults and adolescents with neurogenic bladder secondary to spinal cord injury.[55] They showed a reduction in the number of episodes of asymptomatic bacteriuria but not in the number of symptomatic UTIs.

Urinary tract infections in men

Case presentation 3

A 40-year-old man presented to his physician with a 3-day history of dysuria. The pain was moderately severe but only present during voiding. He had no urethral discharge and he had no pelvic pain. He had not been sexually active for over 1 month prior to his dysuria. On examination, his temperature was 37·4°C and the general physical exam was normal. The rectal examination showed a mildly enlarged but non-tender prostate. Urine analysis showed pyuria and bacteriuria. Urine culture was obtained and he was given ciprofloxacin 750 mg every 12 hours pending culture results. The culture eventually showed 10^5 colony forming units per milliliter of *Escherichia coli* susceptible to ciprofloxacin.

Clinical presentation

The presentation in this case is comparable to UTIs that are seen in women. However, in men it is important to consider involvement of the prostate gland as well as the bladder, ureters, and kidneys. The literature on UTI in men is limited and groups together urinary infections, such as cystitis and pyelonephritis, with prostatitis. It is easy to "rule in" prostatitis with a variety of clinical features (prostate tenderness, post-prostate examination urethral discharge) because acute prostatitis is often defined as a

UTI in a man with additional features supporting prostate inflammation.[56] However, in men with features of UTI, it can be impossible to rule out some degree of prostatitis at the time of initial diagnosis since there may be only subtle or subclinical features of prostate involvement, which would only be revealed by prostate biopsy or culture of prostatic secretions. Thus the absence of prostate tenderness or post-prostate examination urethral discharge does not exclude the possibility of prostatitis in a man with dysuria and positive urine cultures.[56] Because of this overlap, acute prostatitis and UTI can be considered to form a continuum in men. Some older literature refers to this as "recurrent UTI in men" or chronic prostatitis because of the incomplete response to the short courses of antibiotics used at the time.[57]

Prostatitis

Prostatitis is a common condition and has protean manifestations. Several classification schemes have been devised to account for the variable characteristics that can be present. A recent NIH consensus classification has been developed to standardize prostatitis variants and permit more meaningful research.[58] This system creates four categories:

- acute bacterial prostatitis
- chronic bacterial prostatitis
- chronic prostatitis/pelvic pain syndrome (with inflammatory and non-inflammatory subtypes)
- asymptomatic inflammatory prostatitis.

Although having reproducible definitions for the advancement of clinical research is reasonable, this division is difficult to translate into everyday clinical practice. Acute and bacterial chronic prostatitis share similarities with UTI since all three are infections. However, it is much less clear what the relationship is between infection and the other two forms of prostate disease. The exact distinction between acute and chronic bacterial prostatitis in this working definition is imprecise and does not specify the number of days of symptoms needed to invoke a diagnosis of prostatitis. This difficulty is also reflected in clinical trials of bacterial prostatitis. Of interest, it is widely believed that the chronic bacterial and non-bacterial forms of prostatitis account for about 90% of cases of prostatitis. A large population-based study in Canada showed that nearly 10% of men (aged 20–74) had symptoms consistent with prostatitis other than acute bacterial prostatitis and there was a fairly smooth age distribution throughout the group.[59] A similar survey in Minnesota also showed that 9% of men (aged 40–70) had symptoms typical of prostatitis other than acute bacterial prostatitis.[60] However, among men with prior prostatitis (including acute bacterial prostatitis), there was a significant increase in the age-related risk of prostatitis (20% at age 40, 38% at age 60, and 50% at age 50), suggesting that the various chronic prostatitis syndromes can have a remitting/relapsing form that tends not to resolve completely irrespective of the intervention.

Diagnosis

The diagnosis of UTI in men is made in a similar fashion to that in women. Urine collection is less likely to be compromised by contamination from skin flora. Pyuria and bacteriuria are both highly predictive of significant positive cultures. The lower limit of a positive quantitative culture is 10^3 colony-forming units per ml.[61] The sensitivity and specificity of this cut-off were both 97%, and it was unimportant as to whether a clean-catch mid-stream specimen or an uncleansed first void specimen was used.

Other investigations

The evaluation of the cause of UTI in men differs from that in women since it is believed that there should be some diagnosable anatomic or physiologic factor to account for the UTI in men.[62] Recent studies in this area mostly come from referral centers and thus may suffer from referral bias. For example, a Scandinavian study of 83 men with UTI showed that 19 men had some upper tract finding and 35 men had lower tract problems.[63] There was a correctable defect in only one man with an upper tract lesion, but 41% of the men had a lower tract abnormality. Only 18% of the men were found to have previously unrecognized, correctable abnormalities with the multiple modalities used to study the lower tract: cysto-urethroscopy, uroflowmetry, digital rectal examination, and measurement of post-void residual by abdominal ultrasound. There is no mention of how many of these men actually underwent a corrective procedure. A study designed to compare intravenous urography (IVU) with ultrasound and plain film showed that half of the men studied had some abnormality (most of which were not correctable).[64] The most common problem found was bladder outflow obstruction that was actually diagnosed by urodynamics (which was not part of the formal study protocol but was available for many but not all of the patients). There was no mention of how many men received treatment for any abnormality found. A community-based study from Australia showed that of gay men with UTI (one-third of whom were HIV-positive), clinical management was satisfactory and, of the men who underwent further investigation, only 14% had detectable abnormalities and again there was no report on how many of these men underwent a corrective procedure.[65] One thing lacking in all these studies is a sense of the rate of baseline abnormalities in similar populations of men without UTIs. Given the high rate of prostate symptoms recorded in community-based surveys,[59,60] UTIs might simply coexist with some of the voiding problems and other prostate complaints seen in so many men. An additional issue that might be contributory is the referral bias of the studies performed by urologists.[63,64] If the primary care providers suspected some anatomical or physiological problem in these men, they might have referred them for evaluation more quickly than for men with UTIs who evinced no symptoms.

Treatment strategies for men

The organisms that cause urinary tract infections in men (including acute and chronic prostatitis) are essentially the same as those found in women. The same virulence factors (P fimbriae, adhesins, hemolysins) that make bacteria good uropathogens in women (particularly as a cause of pyelonephritis) also make them uropathogenic in men.[66–68] Thus, *E. coli*, *Klebsiella* spp., *Proteus* spp., *Enterococcus* spp., and various other gram-negative bacteria comprise the vast majority of uropathogens in men.

There are few studies comparing treatment strategies for male urinary tract infection or prostatitis in randomized controlled trials. There are no systematic reviews. Because of the possibility of concurrent prostatitis in men with UTI, the drugs selected for initial therapy are often those that penetrate into the prostate gland. These include TMP and the fluoroquinolones. Whilst other classes of drugs may be effective in the treatment of UTI in men, these drugs are active against most uropathogens. TMP is often given in a fixed combination with SMX. Clinical trials of TMP-SMX for UTI in males have, however, been disappointing. In an effort to compare a short course (10 days) to a long course (12 weeks) for recurrent UTI, the investigators of a multicenter US Veterans Administration study tried to recruit appropriate patients to randomize.[69] Of the 306 patients screened, only 38 were randomized and only 30 were available for analysis at the end of the study period. Of the men screened, 17% were excluded because of comorbidity, 28% for paramorbidity, 6% for comedication, 24% for lack of compliance, and 9% for miscellaneous reasons. This left 46 men to study. Four of them did not have meaningful outcome on localization tests (which would likely not be considered very important today, but were required for study entry). Of the 42 remaining men, four could not be randomized. Eight more were dropped from the study for a variety of protocol violations leaving a total of 30. Notably, fewer than half of the men studied were symptomatic from their UTI, and two did not even have pyuria. Of interest, the long course of therapy was superior – 60% success for 12 weeks and only 20% for 10 days (RR 3; 95% CI 1·01–8·95). Recurrent infections were from the same organism in the majority of cases. Another study of 42 men with recurrent UTI showed that a longer course of treatment (6 weeks *v* 2 weeks) had a lower failure rate at a 6-week post-treatment follow up visit (68% *v* 32%; RR = 2·2; 95% CI 1·05–4·49).[70]

In contrast to TMP-SMX, the clinical response to fluoroquinolones in men with UTI is much better. Fluoroquinolones have good prostate penetration in animal models, and agents studied appear comparable in the treatment of male UTI/prostatitis. When norfloxacin was compared with TMP-SMX in 109 men in a randomized controlled trial, the bacterial eradication rate of 93% with norfloxacin compared with 67% with TMP-SMX ($P < 0{\cdot}05$).[71]

Ofloxacin, a drug that has largely been replaced by its *l*-isomer, levofloxacin, was studied in an unblinded comparison to indanyl carbenicillin (an oral form of the drug that has an FDA indication for UTI/prostatitis) and to TMP-SMX.[72] The population included men and women in equal numbers; however, treatment arms were not stratified by gender, an important limitation. Treatment failure with carbenicillin was 25% compared with no treatment failures with ofloxacin (0%) ($P = 0{\cdot}048$). The comparison with TMP-SMX was done in a larger group (173 patients) and the outcomes were similar in both treatment arms, although the trend for clinical cure favored ofloxacin. Only 117 patients were evaluable for clinical cure: 93% of ofloxacin-treated patients were cured as compared with 85% of TMP-SMX-treated patients for an RR of 0·92 (95% CI 0·81–1·04).

In another study, ciprofloxacin was compared with TMP-SMX in men with UTI.[73] There was no significant difference in outcomes at late follow up (4–6 weeks), but the early bacterial eradication rate (days 5–9 following antibiotics) favored ciprofloxacin (82% *v* 52% $P = 0{\cdot}035$). The drug doses used in the study were low (ciprofloxacin 250 mg p.o. every 12 hours, and TMP-SMX 160/800 mg p.o. every 12 hours) and the duration was brief (mean of 7 days). An open label study of ciprofloxacin for chronic bacterial prostatitis showed a good outcome with a 4-week course.[74] The bacteriologic cure rate was 92% at 3 months after the end of therapy and 70% at 2 years post therapy.

How does this evidence apply to the example of the patient in Case 3 above? The treatment with ciprofloxacin is rational and should be of at least 2 week's duration. Assuming that he makes a good recovery and has no further symptoms, he does not need investigative studies, but incomplete resolution or relapse should occasion a workup. An ultrasound and plain abdominal radiograph can look for structural lesions such as kidney stones or hydronephrosis. A urologic evaluation could find problems with bladder emptying or structural disease of the lower urinary tract (including the prostate gland). While his prognosis is good, he may require a longer course of antibiotics for subsequent UTI.

Severe and complex urinary tract infections

Case presentation 4

A 59-year-old diabetic woman with no other prior medical problems was seen in the Emergency Department with a 36-hour history of fever, chills, and flank pain. She attempted to go to work that day, but after 2 hours at the office, her coworkers became alarmed when she nearly fainted on the way to the copier. In the ED, she was slightly confused and sweaty. Her oral temperature was 38·9°C, pulse 110, and respiratory rate 24. Her blood pressure was 92/60 mmHg. She had right flank tenderness on palpation. Urine obtained by bladder catheterization was cloudy and had numerous WBC and bacteria on microscopic exam. She had a WBC of 22 000 with 80% PMNs, 14% bands, and 6% lymphocytes. Her fingerstick blood glucose was 21 mmol/liter^{-1} and her creatinine was 100 micromol/liter^{-1}.

This patient has a severe urinary tract infection requiring hospital admission.[4] In addition to fever and flank tenderness, she has signs of possible sepsis with hypotension, rapid heart and respiratory rates, and mental clouding. Furthermore, her diabetes is out of control. Based on her clinical presentation, she has upper urinary tract disease (kidney, renal pelvis, or ureter) otherwise known as pyelonephritis.

Because this woman is diabetic, she is by definition presenting with a complicated UTI. This is defined as either a disruption of the normal anatomy or physiology (as in this patient) of the urinary tract. Obstructions to urine flow such as stones, tumors or strictures can lead to more clinically severe infections. Alterations to barriers that normally maintain the unidirectional flow of urine such as vesicoureteral reflux and external bladder catheters can also predispose to severe infections. The presence of stones or catheters can also contribute a surface for the growth of microbes as well as some protection from host defenses such as complement and phagocytosis. Physiologic problems such as incomplete bladder emptying with residual urine or poor ureteral muscular function can contribute to UTI complexity.

Diagnosis of severe urinary tract infections

The diagnosis of severe UTI starts with urine collection for urinalysis and culture. Quantitation of pyuria or bacteriuria cannot distinguish mild from severe UTI. A review of quantitative pyuria in 1983 showed a sensitivity of 97% and a specificity of 98% for the finding of concomitant bacteriuria.[75] Pyuria and UTI in the setting of an indwelling bladder catheter is still a topic of interest, but a recent study has shown that the high specificity of pyuria for bacteriuria (90%) is offset by a low sensitivity (37%).[76]

Blood cultures are commonly performed in patients with severe UTI. The rate of blood culture positivity varies, but is rarely in excess of 20–25%, even in the most severe hospitalized cases.[77] In almost all cases, positive blood cultures have the same organism that is found in the urine and thus may add little to the determination of the specific etiology of the UTI.[78] Whether positive blood cultures are systematically associated with worse outcomes, such as prolonged hospitalization, has not been determined.[79] There is some evidence from a retrospective chart review that young women with severe UTI and positive blood cultures do have higher rates of genitourinary abnormality, persistent fever, and abnormal heart rate than women without bacteremia.[80] A study of pregnant women with severe UTI showed that those who were bacteremic had a longer hospital stay than those who were not.[81]

Site of care

The initial management of severe UTI includes a decision about hospitalization, which is based generally on the need for intravenous fluids, pressors, close nursing care, and adherence to a medical regimen. The patient presented might be stabilized in the Emergency Department, but would likely require hospital admission for assessment of her hemodynamic stability.

For patients with uncomplicated severe UTI, the choice of hospital admission greatly increases the cost of treatment. It is difficult to ascertain whether it improves outcome, however. This topic has not been studied in a controlled fashion except to show that for patients who *can* be managed in the ambulatory environment with oral therapy, there is no advantage to parenteral medications.[82,83] A retrospective survey of women evaluated in an Emergency Department showed that patients who were admitted (28 out of a total of 111) were older, had higher degrees of fever, were more likely to be diabetic or to have some genitourinary abnormality, or to be vomiting than women who were managed as outpatients.[84] The presence of vomiting was highly associated with admission (OR 12). It is notable that 12% of the patients initially discharged from the Emergency Department returned.

Treatment

After obtaining cultures and other laboratory tests, antibiotics are given empirically until susceptibility results are available.

The organisms that cause serious UTI are quite similar to those that cause cystitis. There is a preponderance of *E. coli* and other gram-negative rods. These bacteria usually have the same adherence properties as the ones that cause lower tract infection but may have additional virulence attributes that permit ascent of the ureter and in some cases deeper invasion such as bacteremia. For the very ill patient in whom even a short delay in treatment could be significant, broad therapy is appropriate until culture results permit a narrowing.

Fluoroquinolones are appropriate for empiric therapy of severe UTI (although they should be used with caution if the patient has recently had a course of fluoroquinolone therapy). In many cases, fluoroquinolones will still be effective for treatment of UTIs, but prior exposure to fluoroquinolones is the most significant risk factor for the presence of a drug resistant flora. This is true for resistance in gram-positive[85] as well as gram-negative[86] bacteria and irrespective of the indication for the previous course of fluoroquinolones.

So long as there is no contraindication, such as vomiting or hypotension, oral antibiotics are effective. In one study, route of administration of ciprofloxacin was randomized to intravenous or p.o. therapy with about 70 patients per arm.[82] Over one-third of the patients were bacteremic. There was no discernable difference in any of the outcome measures between oral and intravenous therapy, although the study was not powered to show modest superiority of either regimen. Because of the excellent bioavailability of oral ciprofloxacin, this outcome was not surprising. The presence of enterococci required a change in regimen in both groups, although the patients were doing well clinically at the time of the change. Among specific fluoroquinolones, there is no clear evidence as to which is most effective. This is largely because the comparative clinical trials have been powered for equivalence. For example, gatifloxacin was shown to be as effective as ciprofloxacin in a randomized trial evaluating 372 adults with complicated UTI and/or pyelonephritis.[87] In a smaller study, levofloxacin and lomefloxacin (the latter is no longer available in the USA) were comparable to ciprofloxacin.[88] Both of these studies used oral therapy.

There is evidence to suggest that for severe UTI, fluoroquinolones are superior to TMP-SMX. A randomized controlled trial comparing a 7-day course of ciprofloxacin with a 14-day course of

TMP-SMX showed a better microbiological and clinical outcome for ciprofloxacin at early (4–11 days) and late (22–48 days) follow up.[89] The magnitude of the difference was roughly that for every 9–10 patients treated with ciprofloxacin there would be one less failure than if they were treated with TMP-SMX (NNT about 9–10). This was likely due to a fairly high rate of TMP-SMX resistance in the bacterial strains collected in this multicenter (25 centers) US study. While > 90% of bacteria were *E. coli* as would be expected, 16% of the patients in the TMP-SMX arm had *E. coli* that were TMP-SMX resistant. About half of these patients failed therapy (clinically and microbiologically) at the time of early follow up. Although TMP-SMX is a very inexpensive drug, the pharmaco-economic analysis showed that the cost of treatment failures (such as repeat courses of therapy and repeat laboratory tests) made the TMP-SMX arm more expensive than the ciprofloxacin arm. What remains to be seen is the rate at which uropathogens acquire fluoroquinolone resistance and the concomitant rise in treatment failures.

Aminoglycosides are another therapeutic option for severe UTIs. Almost all uropathogens from ambulatory patients are still susceptible to aminoglycosides (with the exception of *Enterococcus* spp.). However, careful monitoring is required because of the possibility for nephrotoxicity and ototoxicity.

Other classes of drugs have been studied in equivalence trials for the treatment of severe UTI. In one study, piperacillin/tazobactam and imipenem were equivalent for severe UTI with a microbiological success rate of about 50% for each.[90] In another study, patients were randomized to a single dose of intravenous ceftriaxone followed by oral cefixime versus daily intravenous ceftriaxone. Both groups of patients got a 10-day course of therapy and their outcomes were nearly identical. This cohort of patients was well enough to tolerate oral therapy after the first day and had a good outcome overall (about 75% bacteriologic and 90% clinical cure for each arm). Our patient in Case 4 might well be able to be discharged home after one or just a few doses of parenteral antibiotics.

Durability of response is a concern with severe UTI. In a comparison of hospitalized patients with severe UTI who got a short course of intravenous cefuroxime (for 2–3 days), patients who had follow up with norfloxacin (a fluoroquinolone) did better microbiologically than those who had ceftibuten (a cephalosporin).[91] The relative probability of bacterial eradication at 7–14-day follow up after the conclusion of therapy was 0·84 (95% CI 0·74–0·97) with ceftibuten being less effective. This seems to parallel the experience of β-lactams and fluoroquinolones for simple cystitis. This study did not explain why the responses were shorter lived for the cephalosporin, but it would be logical to assume that failure to eradicate the organism in other gastrointestinal and genital sites might have led to recurrence despite the 10-day course of therapy and the initial use of a parenteral cephalosporin. Of incidental note, the side effects of norfloxacin were milder than those of ceftibuten, although the study was under-powered to look at this and it did not achieve statistical significance.

As is the case with less severe UTIs the prospect of more resistance can influence choices of initial therapy and may limit alternatives in the face of drug allergy. There is clearly an increase in resistance to TMP-SMX that has been tracked recently in the USA. Between 1992 and 1996 there was a doubling in the prevalence of TMP-SMX resistance in the Seattle area.[92] In the international arena, there is considerable variability of resistance – even within the USA, the range of resistance varies by region of the country.[26] In this analysis of > 100 000 strains of uropathogens, 22% of the isolates from the western states (adjacent to the Pacific ocean) of the USA showed TMP-SMX resistance as compared with 10% from the northeast (Pennsylvania and states north and east of it). As alarming as these numbers are, the rates of resistance worldwide are even more variable and the source of concern. In a review of resistance rates in the 1990s outside the USA, percentage of *E. coli* isolates resistant to TMP-SMX varied from 12% in Holland to 60% in Bangladesh, and resistance to fluoroquinolones varied from 0% to 13% in Spain and 18% in Bangladesh.[93]

How quickly should a severe UTI respond to therapy?

This leads to a reasonable question of how quickly a woman with severe UTI should respond to therapy. Considering fever duration as an easily measured indicator of response, the answer is that there is a wide range of rates of improvement. A large retrospective survey of patients admitted with fever and UTI showed that the mean duration of fever ($T > 37{\cdot}5°C$ at some point during a 12-hour interval) was 39 hours with a median of 34 hours.[94] At 48 hours, about a quarter of the patients were still febrile. Elements associated with longer fever were increased serum creatinine, younger age, higher initial white blood cell counts, and the presence of *E. coli* as the causative agent. The interpretation of this data is difficult since the choice of hospital admission and initial antibiotics were completely uncontrolled. At the least it demonstrates that it is possible to see persistent temperature elevations in people who do well on therapy and have no underlying problems that predispose them to severe UTI. In fact the presence of persistent fever is a poor reason to initiate a more detailed workup for potentially complicated UTI, since fever was weakly correlated with abnormal results of imaging studies of the urinary tract that were done at the physician's request in some patients in this study.

References

1. Foxman B, Barlow R, D'Arcy H, Gillespie B, Sobel JD. Urinary tract infection: self-reported incidence and associated costs. *Ann Epidemiol* 2000;**10**:509–15.
2. Kunin CM. An overview of urinary infections. In: Kunin CM, ed, *Urinary Tract Infections: Detection, Prevention and Management, 5th edn*, Baltimore:Williams Wilkins, 1997.
3. Hooton TM, Scholes D, Hughes JP *et al.* A prospective study of risk factors for symptomatic urinary tract infection in young women. *N Engl J Med* 1996;**335**:468.
4. Bent S, Nallamothu BK, Simel DL, Fihn SD, Saint S. Does this woman have an acute uncomplicated urinary tract infection? *JAMA* 2002;**287**:2701–10.
5. Pezzlo M. Detection of urinary tract infections by rapid methods. *Clin Microbiol Rev* 1988;**1**:268–80.
6. Lachs MS, Nachamkin I, Edelstein PH, Goldman J, Feinstein AR, Schwartz JS. Spectrum bias in the evaluation of diagnostic tests: lessons from the rapid dipstick test for urinary tract infection. *Ann Intern Med* 1993;**117**:135–40.
7. Van Nostrand JD, Junkins AD, Bartholdi RK. Poor predictive ability of urinalysis and microscopic examination to detect urinary tract infection. *Am J Clin Pathol* 2000;**113**: 709–13.
8. Komaroff AL. Urinalysis and urine culture in women with dysuria. *Ann Intern Med* 1986;**104**:212–18.
9. Lammers RL, Gibson S, Kovacs D, Sears W, Strachan G. Comparison of test characteristics of urine dipstick and urinalysis at various test cutoff points. *Ann Emerg Med* 2001;**38**:505–12.
10. Zaman Z, Borremans A, Verhaegen J, Verbist L, Blanckaert N. Disappointing dipstick screening for urinary tract infection in hospital inpatients. *J Clin Pathol* 1998;**51**: 471–2.
11. McIsaac WJ, Low DE, Biringer A, Pimlott N, Evans M, Glazier R. The impact of empirical management of acute cystitis on unnecessary antibiotic use. *Arch Intern Med* 2002;**162**:600–5.
12. Saint S, Scholes D, Fihn SD *et al.* The effectiveness of a clinical practice guideline for the management of presumed uncomplicated urinary tract infection in women. *Am J Med* 1999;**106**:636–41.
13. Rubin RH, Shapiro ED, Andriole VT, Davis RJ, Stamm WE. Evaluation of new anti-infective drugs for the treatment of

urinary tract infection. *Clin Infect Dis* 1992;**15** (Suppl.): S216–27.

14. McCarty JM, Richard G, Huck W *et al.* A randomized trial of short course ciprofloxacin, ofloxacin or trimethoprim-sulfamethoxazole for the treatment of acute urinary tract infection in women. *Am J Med* 1999;**106**:292–9.
15. Sandler CM, Amis ES, Bigongiari LR *et al.* Imaging in acute pyelonephritis. American college of radiology. ACR appropriateness criteria. *Radiology* 2000;**215**(Suppl.1): 677–81.
16. Stamm WE. Quantitative urine cultures revisited (editorial). *Eur J Clin Microbiol Infect Dis* 1984;**3**:279–81.
17. Norrby SR. Short-term treatment of uncomplicated lower urinary tract infections in women. *Rev Infect Dis* 1990;**12**:458–67.
18. Leibovici L, Wysenbeek AJ. Single-dose antibiotic treatment for symptomatic urinary tract infections in women: a meta-analysis of randomized trials. *Q J Med* 1991;**78**:43–57.
19. Hooton TM, Winter C, Tiu F, Stamm WE. Randomized comparative trial and cost analysis of 3-day antimicrobial regimens for treatment of acute cystitis in women. *JAMA* 1995;**273**:41–5.
20. Fekete T. Review of three-day trimethoprim-sulfamethoxazole was best for acute cystitis. *ACP J Club*, 1995;**123**:15.
21. Patel SS, Balfour JA, Bryson HM. Fosfomycin tromethamine. A review of its antibacterial activity, pharmacokinetic properties and therapeutic efficacy as a single-dose oral treatment for acute uncomplicated lower urinary tract infections. *Drugs* 1997;**53**:637–56.
22. Huang ES, Stafford RS. National patterns in the treatment of urinary tract infections in women by ambulatory care physicians. *Arch Intern Med* 2002;**162**:41–7.
23. Iravani A, Klimberg I, Briefer C, Munera C, Kowalsky SF, Echols RM. A trial comparing low-dose, short-course ciprofloxacin and standard 7 day therapy with co-trimoxazole or nitrofurantoin in the treatment of uncomplicated urinary tract infection. *J Antimicrob Chemother* 1999; **43**(Suppl. A):67–75.
24. Fosfomycin for urinary tract infections. *Med Lett Drugs Ther* 1997;**39**:66–8.
25. Stamm WE, McKevitt M, Counts GW. Acute renal infection in women: treatment with trimethoprim-sulfamethoxazole or ampicillin for two or six weeks. *Ann Intern Med* 1987; **106**:341–5.
26. Gupta K, Sahm DF, Mayfield D, Stamm WE. Antimicrobial resistance among uropathogens that cause community-acquired urinary tract infections in women: a nationwide analysis. *Clin Infect Dis* 2001;**33**:89–94.
27. Rafalsky V, Andreeva I, Rjabkova E. Quinolones for uncomplicated acute cystitis in women. *Cochrane Database of Systematic Reviews*, 2002.
28. Christiaens TC, De Meyere M, Verschraegen G, Peersman W, Heytens S, De Maseneer JM. Randomized controlled trial of nitrofurantoin versus placebo in the treatment of uncomplicated urinary tract infection in adult women. *Br J Gen Pract* 2002;**52**:708–10.
29. Echols RM, Tosiello RL, Haverstock DC, Tice AD. Demographic, clinical and treatment parameters influencing the outcome of acute cystitis. *Clin Infect Dis* 1999;**29**:113–19.
30. Raz R, Chazan B, Kennes Y *et al.* Empiric use of trimethoprim-sulfamethoxazole (TMP-SMX) in the treatment of women with uncomplicated urinary tract infections in a geographical area with a high prevalence of TMP-SMX resistant uropathogens. *Clin Infect Dis* 2002;**34**:1165–9.
31. Lawrenson RA, Logie JW. Antibiotic failure in the treatment of urinary tract infections in young women. *J Antimicrob Chemother* 2001;**48**:895–901.
32. Stamm WE, Raz R. Factors contributing to susceptibility of postmenopausal women to recurrent urinary tract infections. *Clin Infect Dis* 1999;**28**:723–5.
33. Beylot M, Marion D, Noel G. Ultrasonographic determination of residual urine in diabetic subjects: relationship to neuropathy and urinary tract infection. *Diabetes Care* 1982;**5**:501–5.
34. Warren JW, Abrutyn E, Hebel JR *et al.* Guidelines for antimicrobial treatment of uncomplicated acute bacterial cystitis and acute pyelonephritis in women. *Clin Infect Dis* 1999;**29**:745–58.
35. Velasco M, Horcajada JP, Mensa J *et al.* Decreased invasive capacity of quinolone-resistant *Escherichia coli* in patients with urinary tract infections. *Clin Infect Dis* 2001;**33**:1682–6.
36. Smaill F. Antibiotics for asymptomatic bacteriuria in pregnancy. *Cochrane Database of Systematic Reviews*. Issue 1. Oxford: Update Software, 2002.
37. Gratacos E, Torres P-J, Vila J, Alonso PL, Cararach V. Screening and treatment of asymptomatic bacteriuria in

pregnancy prevent pyelonephritis. *J Infect* Dis 1994; **169**:1390–2.

38. Harding GKM, Nicolle LE, Ronald AR *et al.* How long should catheter acquired urinary tract infection in women be treated? *Ann Intern Med* 1991;**114**:713–19.
39. Forland M, Thomas VL. The treatment of urinary tract infections in women with diabetes mellitus. *Diab Care* 1985;**8**:499–506.
40. Abrutyn E, Berlin J, Mossey J, Pitsakis P, Levison M, Kaye D. Does treatment of asymptomatic bacteriuria in older ambulatory women reduce subsequent symptoms of urinary tract infections? *J Am Geriatr Soc* 1996;**44**:293–5.
41. Harding GKM, Zhanel GG, Nicolle LE, Cheang M. Antimicrobial treatment in diabetic women with asymptomatic bacteriuria. *N Engl J Med* 2002;**347**: 1576–83.
42. Ikaheimo R, Siitonen A, Heiskanen T *et al.* Recurrence of urinary tract infection in a primary care setting: analysis of a 1-year follow up of 179 women. *Clin Infect Dis.* 1996;**22**:91–9.
43. Kontiokari T, Sundqvist K, Nuutinen M *et al.* Randomized trial of cranberry–lingonberry juice and Lactobacillus GG drink for the prevention of urinary tract infection in women. *BMJ* 2001;**30**:1571.
44. Fihn SD, Boyko EJ, Normand EH *et al.* Association between use of spermicide coated condoms and Escherichia coli urinary tract infections in young women. *Am J Epidemiol* 1996;**144**:512.
45. Raz R, Stamm WE. A controlled trial of intravaginal estriol in postmenopausal women with recurrent urinary tract infection. *N Engl J Med* 1993;**329**:753–6.
46. Fowler JE, Pulaski ET. Excretory urography, cystography, and cystoscopy in the evaluation of women with urinary-tract infection. *N Engl J Med* 1981;**304**:462–5.
47. Nicolle LE. Prophylaxis: recurrent urinary tract infection in women. *Infection* 1992;**20**(Suppl. 3):S203–10.
48. Nicolle LE, Harding GKM, Thomson M, Kennedy J, Urias B, Ronald AR. Efficacy of five years of continuous low-dose trimethoprim-sulfamethoxazole prophylaxis for urinary tract infection. *J Infect Dis* 1988;**157**:1239–42.
49. Stapleton A, Latham RH, Johnson C, Stamm WE. Postcoital antimicrobial prophylaxis for recurrent urinary tract infection. A randomized, double-blind, placebo-controlled trial. *JAMA* 1990;**264**:703–6.
50. Chew LD, Fihn SD. Recurrent cystitis in nonpregnant women. *West J Med* 1999;**170**:274–7.
51. Gupta K, Hooton TM, Roberts PL, Stamm WE. Patient-initiated treatment of uncomplicated recurrent urinary tract infections in young women. *Ann Intern Med* 2001;**135**:9–16.
52. Jepson RG, Mihaljevic L, Craig J. Cranberries for preventing urinary tract infections. *Cochrane Database of Systematic Reviews*, 2002.
53. Karchmer TB, Gianetta ET, Muto CA, Strain BA, Farr BM. A randomized crossover study of silver coated urinary catheters in hospitalized patients. *Arch Int Med* 2000;**160**:3294–8.
54. Saint S. *Prevention of nosocomial urinary tract infections.* Agency for Healthcare Research and Quality, Contract No. 290–97–0013 (http://www.ahcpr.gov/clinic/ptsafety/pdf/chap15.pdf).
55. Vickrey BG, Shekelle P, Morton S, Clark K, Pathak M, Kamberg C. *Prevention and Management of Urinary Tract Infections in Paralyzed Persons. Evidence Report/Technology Assessment No. 6.* (Prepared by the Southern California Evidence-Based Practice Center/RAND under Contract No. 290–97–0001.) AHCPR Publication No. 99–E008. Rockville, MD: Agency for Health Care Policy and Research, February 1999.
56. Lipsky BA. Prostatitis and urinary tract infection in men: What's new?; what's true? *Am J Med* 1999;**106**:327–34.
57. Lipsky BA. Urinary tract infections in men: Epidemiology, pathophysiology, diagnosis and treatment. *Ann Intern Med* 1989;**110**:138–50.
58. Krieger JN, Nyberg L, Nickel JC. NIH consensus definition and classification of prostatitis. *JAMA* 1999; **282**:236–7.
59. Nickel JC, Downey J, Hunter D, Clark J. Prevalence of prostatitis-like symptoms in a population based study using the National Institutes of Health chronic prostatitis symptom index. *J Urol* 2001;**165**:842–5.
60. Roberts RO. Lieber MM. Rhodes T. Girman CJ. Bostwick DG. Jacobsen SJ. Prevalence of a physician-assigned diagnosis of prostatitis: the Olmsted County Study of Urinary Symptoms and Health Status Among Men. *Urology* 1998;**51**:578–84.
61. Lipsky BA, Ireton RC, Fihn SD, Hackett R, Berger RE. Diagnosis of bacteriuria in men: specimen collection and culture interpretation. *J Infect Dis* 1987;**155**:847–54.
62. Sobel JD, Kaye D. Urinary tract infections. In: Mandell GL, Bennett JE, Dolin R, eds. *Principles and Practice of*

Infectious Diseases, 5th edn. Philadelphia: Churchill Livingston, 2000.

63. Ulleryd P, Zackrisson B, Aus G, Bergdahl S, Hugosson J, Sandberg T. Selective urological evaluation in men with febrile urinary tract infection. *BJU Int*. 2001;**88**:15–20.
64. Andrews SJ, Brooks PT, Hanbury DC *et al*. Ultrasonography and abdominal radiography versus intravenous urography in investigation of urinary tract infection in men: prospective incident cohort study. *BMJ* 2002;**324**:454–6.
65. Russell DB, Roth NJ. Urinary tract infections in men in a primary care population. *Aust Fam Phys* 2001;**30**: 177–9.
66. Ulleryd P, Lincoln K, Scheutz F, Sandberg T. Virulence characteristics of *Escherichia coli* in relation to host response in men with symptomatic urinary tract infection. *Clin Infect Dis* 1994;**18**:579–84.
67. Mitsumori K, Terai A, Yamamoto S, Ishitoya S, Yoshida O. Virulence characteristics of *Escherichia coli* in acute bacterial prostatitis. *J Infect Dis* 1999;**180**:1378–81.
68. Andreu A, Stapleton AE, Fennell C. *et al*. Urovirulence determinants in *Escherichia coli* strains causing prostatitis. *J Infect Dis* 1997;**176**:464–9.
69. Smith JW, Jones SR, Reed WP, Tice AD, Deupress RH, Kaijser B. Recurrent urinary tract infections in men. *Ann Intern Med* 1979;**91**:544–8.
70. Gleckman R, Crowley M, Natsios GA. Therapy of recurrent invasive urinary-tract infections of men. *N Engl J Med* 1979;**301**:878–80.
71. Sabbaj J, Hoagland VL, Cook T. Norfloxacin versus co-trimoxazole in the treatment of recurring urinary tract infections in men. *Scand J Infect Dis* 1986;**48**:S48–S53.
72. Cox CE. Ofloxacin in the management of complicated urinary tract infections, including prostatitis. *Am J Med* 1989;**87**: 61S-68S.
73. Allais JM, Preheim LC, Cuevas TA, Roccaforte JS, Mellencamp MA, Bittner MJ. Randomized, double-blind comparison of ciprofloxacin and trimethoprim-sulfamethoxazole for complicated urinary tract infections. *Antimicrob Agents Chemother* 1988;**32**:1327–30.
74. Weidner W. Ludwig M. Brahler E. Schiefer HG. Outcome of antibiotic therapy with ciprofloxacin in chronic bacterial prostatitis. *Drugs* 1999;**58**(Suppl. 2):103–6.
75. Stamm WE. Measurement of pyuria and its relation to bacteriuria. *Am J Med* 1983;**75** (Suppl. 1B):53–8.
76. Tambyah PA, Maki DG. The relationship between pyuria and infection in patients with indwelling urinary catheters. *Arch Intern Med* 2000;**160**:673–7.
77. McMurry BR, Wrenn KD, Wright SW. Usefulness of blood cultures in pyelonephritis. *Am J Emerg Med* 1997;**15**: 137–40.
78. Thanassi M. Utility of urine and blood cultures in pyelonephritis. *Acad Emerg Med* 1997;**4**:797–800.
79. Grover SA, Komaroff AL, Weisberg M *et al*. The characteristics and hospital course of patients admitted for presumed acute pyelonephritis. *J Gen Intern Med* 1987;**2**:5–10.
80. Smith WR, McClish DK, Poses RM *et al*. Bacteremia in young urban women admitted with pyelonephritis. *Am J Med Sci*. 1997;**313**:50–7.
81. Wing DA, Park AS, Debuque L, Millar LK. Limited clinical utility of blood and urine cultures in the treatment of acute pyelonephritis during pregnancy. *Am J Obst Gynecol* 2000;**182**:1437–40.
82. Mombelli G, Pezzoli R, Pinoja-Lutz G. Monotti R, Marone C, Franciolli M. Oral *v* intravenous ciprofloxacin in the initial management of severe pyelonephritis or complicated urinary tract infections: a prospective randomized clinical trial. *Arch Intern Med* 1999;**159**:53–58.
83. Sanchez M, Collvinent B, Miro O *et al*. Short-term effectiveness of ceftriaxone single dose in the initial treatment of acute uncomplicated pyelonephritis in women. A randomized controlled trial. *Emerg Med J* 2002;**19**:19–22.
84. Pinson AG, Philbrick JT, Lindbeck GH, Schorling JB. ED management of acute pyelonephritis in women: a cohort study. *Am J Emerg Med* 1994;**12**:271–8.
85. Goldstein EJ, Garabedian-Ruffalo SM. Widespread use of fluoroquinolones versus emerging resistance in pneumococci. *Clin Infect Dis* 2002;**35**:1501–11.
86. Lautenbach E, Fishman NO, Bilker WB *et al*. Risk factors for fluoroquinolone resistance in nosocomial *Escherichia coli* and *Klebsiella pneumoniae* infections. *Arch Intern Med* 2002;**162**:2469–77.
87. Cox CE, Marbury TC, Pittman WG *et al*. A randomized, double-blind multicenter comparison of gatifloxacin versus ciprofloxacin in the treatment of complicated urinary tract infection and pyelonephritis. *Clin Ther* 2002;**24**:223–36.

88. Richard GA, Klimberg IN, Fowler CL, Callery-D'Amico S, Kim SS. Levofloxacin versus ciprofloxacin versus lomefloxacin in acute pyelonephritis. *Urology* 1998; **52**:51–5.
89. Talan DA, Stamm WE, Hooton TM *et al.* Comparison of ciprofloxacin (7 days) with trimethoprim-sulfamethoxazole (14 days) for acute uncomplicated pyelonephritis in women: a randomized trial. *JAMA* 2000;**283**:1583–90.
90. Naber KG, Savov O, Salmen HC. Piperacillin 2g/tazobactam 0·5g is as effective as imipenem 0·5g/cilastatin 0·5g for the treatment of acute uncomplicated pyelonephritis and complicated urinary tract infections. *Int J Antimicrob Agents* 2002;**19**:95–103.
91. Cronberg S, Banke S, Bergman B *et al.* Fewer bacterial relapses after oral treatment with norfloxacin than with ceftibuten in acute pyelonephritis initially treated with intravenous cefuroxime. *Scand J Infect Dis* 2001;**33**: 339–43.
92. Gupta K, Scholes D, Stamm WE. Increasing prevalence of antimicrobial resistance among uropathogens causing acute uncomplicated cystitis in women. *JAMA* 1999;**281**: 736–8.
93. Gupta K, Hooton TM, Stamm WE. Increasing antimicrobial resistance and the management of uncomplicated community-acquired urinary tract infections. *Ann Intern Med* 2001;**135**:41–50.
94. Behr MA, Drummond R, Libman M, Delaney S, Dylewski JS. Fever duration in hospitalized acute pyelonephritis patients. *Am J Med* 1996;**101**:277–80.

10
Sexually transmitted infections

David N Fisman

Case presentation

A 17-year-old girl presents to the city sexual health clinic with vaginal discharge. She has a new boyfriend and is 'on the pill'; she and her partner do not use condoms as their relationship "is monogamous". On examination, she has mild lower abdominal tenderness to palpation, cervicitis, and cervical discharge. There is cervical motion tenderness and left adnexal tenderness on bimanual examination. Her 17-year-old boyfriend has accompanied her to the clinic and is assessed separately; he reports a small amount of urethral discharge and mild dysuria. Examination reveals copious urethral discharge with meatal edema. A Gram stain of discharge reveals Gram-negative intracellular diplococci. You review the literature to determine the following.

- How accurate is the clinical diagnosis of sexually transmitted infections (STI)?
- Does information obtained from the laboratory tests change the range of diagnostic possibilities in an individual with a possible STI?
- How helpful are historical and clinical findings in the diagnosis of pelvic inflammatory disease?
- Do condoms reduce the likelihood of transmission of STI?

STI are caused by a large and heterogeneous group of pathogens. Many of these pathogens can be transmitted by non-sexual as well as sexual routes; for example, enteric pathogens can be transmitted through food and water as well as via sexual intercourse. This chapter will focus on those infectious agents that are principally or exclusively transmitted via sexual contact, although the general principles described below can be applied to the larger group of STI. This chapter will not focus on human immunodeficiency virus (HIV) infection, which is discussed in Chapter 11.

STI are distinguished from other infectious diseases by several clinical and epidemiological features. Perhaps most notable is the extremely high incidence of these infections; not withstanding likely underdiagnosis, *Chlamydia trachomatis* infection is the most common reportable infectious disease in the USA and Canada.[1,2] Herpes simplex virus type 2 (HSV-2) infection and human papillomavirus (HPV) infections are also extremely common: approximately 22% of adults in the USA have serological evidence of HSV-2 infection.[3] Transient HPV infection is acquired through sexual activity by 33–55% of young adults in the USA and Europe.[4–6] Worldwide, it is estimated that over 330 million cases of syphilis, gonorrhea, trichomoniasis, and genital chlamydia infection occur annually.[7] The high incidence and prevalence of infection results in a high burden of disease, as well as large economic costs.[8–11]

The burden of disease associated with these infections is further augmented by the synergistic relationship between non-HIV STI and HIV infection, owing to physical disruption of host mucosa, recruitment of immunologically active cells to the genital tract, and increases in HIV viral burden in genital secretions. A meta-analysis of

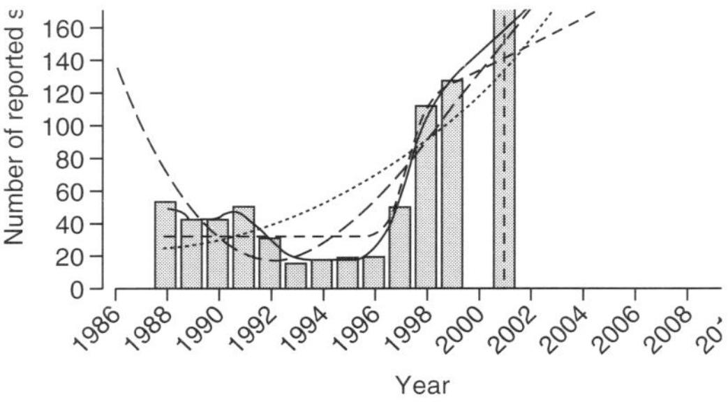

Figure 10.1 The impact of other sexually transmitted infections (STI) on risk of acquiring human immunodeficiency virus (HIV) infection. Forest plot showing the effect of other STI on HIV risk in individuals initially uninfected with HIV. Studies are listed on the vertical axis, with labels connoting author, year of publication, gender of initially uninfected partner, adjustment (a) or lack of adjustment (u) of effect estimate for other variables, and effect measure (OR, odds ratio; IRR, incidence rate ratio; RR, relative risk). Estimate of effect is plotted on the horizontal axis. The size of black boxes is proportional to study statistical precision, and horizontal lines represent 95% confidence intervals. The diamond represents the summary estimate of effect of sexually transmitted infection on HIV acquisition, and 95% confidence interval. Modified from Rottingen J, Cameron D, Garnett G. A systematic review of the epidemiological interactions between classic sexually transmitted diseases and HIV. *Sex Transm Dis* 2001;**28**(10):579–97 with permission of Lippincott Williams and Wilkins.

observational studies generated a summary estimate of the relative risk of HIV acquisition in the context of another sexually transmitted infection to be 3·7 (95% CI 2·7–5·0%) (Figure 10.1).[12]

However, STIs other than HIV infection may also result in chronic medical illness or long-term complications. Genital chlamydia infection is associated with tubal infertility,[13] ectopic pregnancies,[14,15] and chronic pelvic pain.[16,17] HPVs are strongly associated with cervical and anal cancers.[18,19] Infection of pregnant individuals with sexually transmitted pathogens may increase the risk of premature delivery, and may cause severe illness in the newborn.[20–25]

This chapter will review the evidence for the clinical and microbiological diagnosis of these infections, including evidence related to syndromic management (i.e. the use of more broadly targeted therapy in response to a clinical constellation of symptoms or signs). Evidence related to the interaction between contraceptive choice and STI is also reviewed. The second part of the chapter focuses on empiric and targeted management of STI, including some issues related to management in pregnancy. Finally, evidence of effectiveness for population-based STI prevention strategies is discussed.

Diagnosis of STI

Clinical and syndromic diagnosis

Sexually transmitted pathogens cause several common syndromes. Infection with *Neisseria gonorrhoea* or *Chlamydia trachomatis* frequently results in urethritis, cervicitis, or the constellation of symptoms and signs that suggest the presence of pelvic inflammatory disease. HSV, *Treponema pallidum*, and *Haemophilus ducreyi* are common agents of ulcerative genital disease, while vaginal discharge is commonly caused by infection with *Trichomonas vaginalis* or *Candida* spp. or by bacterial vaginosis.

The ability of clinicians to accurately diagnose infections caused by specific pathogens without the use of diagnostic tests appears poor. For example, a study involving a cohort of 446 men presenting to a New Orleans clinic found the clinical diagnosis of the causative agents of genital ulcer disease to be highly sensitive (94–98%), but non-specific (31–35%) when compared with culture, microscopy, and serologic diagnosis (Table 10.1).[26] Studies comparing clinical diagnosis of genital ulcer disease with the use of multiplex PCR have found similar limitations in clinician diagnostic accuracy.[27–29]

The accuracy of bedside diagnosis of vaginitis based on clinical features and simple bedside

Table 10.1 Sensitivity and specificity of ulcer appearance in identifying specific aeiologic agents of genital ulcer disease (modified from ref 26 with permission of the publisher)

Pathogen	Ulcer feature	Sensitivity (%)	Specificity (%)
Herpes simplex virus	3 or more lesions	63	64
	Shallow ulcer	60	88
	Moderate tenderness on examination	60	50
	All of the above features present	35	94
Haemophilus ducreyi	Undermined lesion border	85	68
	Moderate or severe tenderness on examination	57	52
	Purulent ulcer	64	75
	All of the above features present	34	94
Treponema pallidum	Indurated ulcer	47	95
	Non-purulent ulcer	82	53
	Ulcer painless or minimally painful	67	58
	All of the above features present	31	98

tests (i.e. pH testing, whiff test, microscopic evaluation of 'wet preps') also appears limited when compared with more comprehensive laboratory-based evaluations.[30] In a study performed in 153 women presenting to a clinic in Israel with vaginal discharge, only the finding of vaginal pH < 4·5 was associated with infection by a particular pathogen (yeast); the positive predictive value of low vaginal pH for vaginal candidiasis was 68%.

None the less, the limited availability of laboratory diagnostics in areas where STI are prevalent combined with concern that patients will not return for treatment has resulted in the development of the "syndromic" approach to diagnosis and treatment. In this approach, the presence of a given clinical history or constellation of physical exam findings results in the provision of broad-spectrum therapy targeting multiple treatable organisms.[31,32]

Relatively simple diagnostic algorithms exist for such syndromes as genital ulceration, lower abdominal discomfort, and genital discharge. The term "sensitivity" as applied to these algorithms indicates the proportion of individuals with infections diagnosed by laboratory methods who receive appropriate therapy as a result of algorithm use.

A recent review evaluated studies of syndromic diagnosis and management of STI; this review included no controlled trials comparing diagnostic approaches.[33] Rather, attempts were made to validate algorithms using more comprehensive laboratory testing as a gold standard. Algorithms used alone have been associated with high sensitivity for urethral discharge (91–97%) and in genital ulcer diseases from syphilis or chancroid (68–100%), and vaginal discharge syndromes. However, diagnostic sensitivity is achieved at a cost of low specificity (as low as 7% in diagnosis of urethral discharge) and low positive predictive values. Thus the decision to use algorithms in settings where diagnostic tests are unavailable needs to be based on the prevalence and health impact of a given infection in the local population, and balanced against the potential

Table 10.2 Use of urine leukocyte esterase for the diagnosis of gonorrhea or chlamydia in men

Population or specimen source	Prevalence	Study gold standard	Sensitivity (%)	Specificity (%)	Reference
55 male STD clinic patients, Mwanza Region, Tanzania	Gonorrhea: 40% Chlamydia: 7%	Gonorrhea detected by culture, chlamydia by EIA	96	38	334
1095 ambulatory emergency room patients, Atlanta, Georgia	Gonorrhea: 2·5% Chlamydia: 3·9%	Gonorrhea and chlamydia detected by culture	41	90	335
479 male college students, Songkla Province, Thailand	Gonorrhea: 0·2% Chlamydia: 4·0%	Gonorrhea and chlamydia detected by PCR	26	11	40

consequences and costs of unnecessary antibiotic treatment.

Basic laboratory testing for urethritis and cervicitis

Non-specific laboratory tests for the presence of gonorrheal and chlamydial cervicitis and urethritis include assessment of cervical, urethral and vaginal white blood cell counts, urine leukocyte esterase testing, and the use of Gram stains. Most of these modalities have proven disappointing. For example, a study evaluating the use of cervical or vaginal white blood cell counts for the identification of gonorrheal or chlamydial cervicitis found no white blood cell cut-off to be both sensitive and specific. The area under receiver operating curves created using a range of white blood cell cut-offs was ≤ 0·6 for the presence of either type of infection, suggesting that such tests provide little additional information (i.e. a random guess would have an area of 0·5).[34] Although specificity can be enhanced by the use of white blood cell cut-offs in concert with clinical findings of cervical erythema and mucopus, sensitivity of such testing remains poor, especially for chlamydia (sensitivity 41–52% for ≥ 10 polymorphonuclear cells/high powered field).[35,36]

In men, urine leukocyte esterase testing has had variable sensitivity and specificity in the diagnosis of urethritis (Table 10.2), while the evaluation of urethral Gram stain findings for leukocytes has low sensitivity (~67%) for the presence of chlamydia.[37]

In experienced hands, the use of urethral Gram stain for the identification of Gram-negative diplococci appears to be an extremely sensitive and specific tool for the identification of gonorrhea in men. An extremely high degree of correlation between Gram stain results and nucleic acid amplification-based testing was reported in more than 7000 specimens submitted to a sexually transmitted disease program in Houston ($\kappa = 0{\cdot}99$).[38] The ability to perform Gram stain evaluations on clinical specimens may markedly enhance the diagnostic usefulness of clinical algorithms, as described above. For example, in a study evaluating the diagnostic performance of an algorithm for urethritis, the addition of the Gram stain on urethral discharge markedly improved the specificity of algorithm diagnosis of gonorrhea (from 15% to 99%).[39]

The so-called "two glass test" (passage of ~50 mL of urine into the first glass, with the remainder passed into the second) has traditionally been used to distinguish infection in the anterior urethra from more proximal infection (anterior urethritis is thought to be present when only the first glass specimen has a cloudy appearance). The sensitivity and specificity of this test for the

Table 10.3 Estimated sensitivity of culture for *Neisseria gonorrhoea* relative to newer nucleic-acid based tests

Population	Culture source	Gonorrhea prevalence (%)	Sensitivity of culture (%) (95% CI)	Reference
Female commercial sex-trade workers in Benin, South Africa, and Thailand	Endocervical	5	70 (57–81)	44
Male STD clinic attendees, Baltimore, Maryland, USA	Urethral	22	77 (66–86)	45
Female STD clinic attendees, Baltimore, Maryland, USA	Endocervical	18	65 (46–80)	45
Female hospital emergency department attendees, Omaha, Nebraska, USA	Endocervical	7	89 (71–98)	46
Females using Duke University health system, North Carolina, USA	Endocervical	4	93 (76–99)	47

diagnosis of either gonococcal or chlamydial infection were 57% and 83% respectively in a cohort of Thai men.[40]

Identification of individual pathogens

Recent years have seen an explosion in the use of molecular diagnostic tests, particularly nucleic acid based methods such as the polymerase chain reaction (PCR), in the diagnosis of STI caused by fastidious pathogens. These newer testing methods may not only improve test sensitivity, but also permit the use of techniques that overcome traditional barriers to testing for sexually transmitted pathogens. For example, newer tests may yield satisfactory results when specimens are obtained via self-sampling, which may increase test acceptability.[41,42]

However, because newer tests may be more sensitive than the traditional "gold standards" (culture or microscopic visualization of an individual pathogen), calculation of sensitivity and specificity relative to a gold standard has become problematic. Furthermore, the use of additional tests to resolve discrepancies between negative culture tests and positive non-culture tests may introduce a form of verification bias, resulting in overestimation of sensitivity and specificity.[43] Such difficulties need to be taken into account in the interpretation of the data provided below.

Neisseria gonorhoea

Culture of *Neisseria gonorrhoea* from the genital tract is regarded as pathognomonic for infection. The sensitivity of *N. gonorrhoea* culture for genital tract specimens is relatively low when compared with newer nucleic acid amplification tests (Table 10.3).[44–47] Lack of sensitivity may be due in part to loss of viability associated with delays in transport; for example, a decline in sensitivity of culture testing from 89% to 78% was seen when on-site and off-site cultures were compared.[46] Specimen source also contributes to the sensitivity of culture, which is as low as 30–47% when specimens are obtained from the pharynx.[48,49] In a study in which 16 individuals had rectal gonorrhea identified by nucleic acid amplification, the organism was not identified by culture in any.[49]

More sensitive, non-culture methods for the diagnosis of gonococcal infection include enzyme immunoassay (EIA), nucleic acid hybridization ("probe") tests, and nucleic acid amplification tests. These tests have been the subject of a recent systematic review.[50] Nucleic acid amplification tests identified in this review were highly sensitive and specific in the diagnosis of gonococcal infections of the cervix (sensitivity 91–100%, specificity 97–100%), male urethra (sensitivity 98–100%, specificity 98–100%), and in urine testing (94–100%, specificity 98–100%). Studies of nucleic acid amplification tests not included in this review have reported similar test characteristics.[44,45,51–54]

Nucleic acid hybridization or "probe" tests were also highly sensitive and specific in the diagnosis of gonococcal infections of the cervix (sensitivity 91–100%, specificity 97–100%), male urethra (sensitivity 98–100%, specificity 98–100%), and in urine testing (94–100%, specificity 98–100%).[50] Although not approved for use on samples from non-genital sources, such as pharynx and rectum, probe tests and nucleic acid based tests appear to be sensitive and specific relative to culture testing, with sensitivity ranging from 86–94% and specificity 98–100% at these sites.[55,56]

A wide range of sensitivities (50–100%) have been reported for EIA for gonococcus, when performed on genital specimens, although these tests do appear specific (95–99%) for gonococcal infection when compared with culture.[57–62] Factors that may depress the sensitivity of gonococcal EIA include disturbances of normal vaginal flora associated with concommittant vaginitis in women,[62] and the degree of dilution of urinary sediment when these tests are used on urine.[58]

Chlamydia trachomatis

Sensitivity of culture for the recovery of *Chlamydia trachomatis* is more limited than is seen with gonococcus, as the former organism must be grown in cell culture, and recovery is influenced by the expertise of the testing laboratory, composition of the collection swab, and timely transport to the microbiology laboratory. The limited sensitivity of chlamydia culture for organism detection has resulted in substantial efforts being devoted to the development of non-culture methods for the diagnosis of chlamydial infection. Such methods include antigen detection methods such as direct fluorescent antigen assays (DFA), EIA, nucleic acid hybridization ("probe") tests, and nucleic acid amplification tests (including ligase chain reaction (LCR) and PCR).

A systematic review of the characteristics of non-culture tests for the identification of *C. trachomatis* in asymptomatic men and women aged 14–40 has been performed[63] The gold standard for diagnosis in this review was considered to be either culture of chlamydia or the identification of chlamydia by two different methods. All screening tests except the use of leukocyte esterase testing of urine (see above) were highly specific for the diagnosis of chlamydia (specificity 96–100%).

In this review, the sensitivity of non-culture tests for chlamydia was compared with the sensitivity of gold standard tests by calculation of odds ratios, expressed as the odds of a false-negative test with the non-culture test divided by the odds of a false-negative test with the gold standard assay. By these criteria, a test that is more sensitive than the gold standard will have an odds ratio <1, while a test that is inferior to the gold standard will have an odds ratio >1. The summary odds ratios for non-culture methods are presented in Figure 10.2. While this review did not include testing in individuals with symptomatic chlamydial infection, nucleic acid amplification tests appear to be equally sensitive and retain their high specificity in symptomatic individuals.[51,64,65]

Available evidence suggests that the sensitivity and specificity of nucleic acid amplification tests and probe testing for chlamydia on self-collected vaginal specimens or submitted tampons is similar to that seen with clinician-collected cervical specimens, and self-collection may have the advantage of greater acceptability or convenience in some circumstances.[66–69] The use

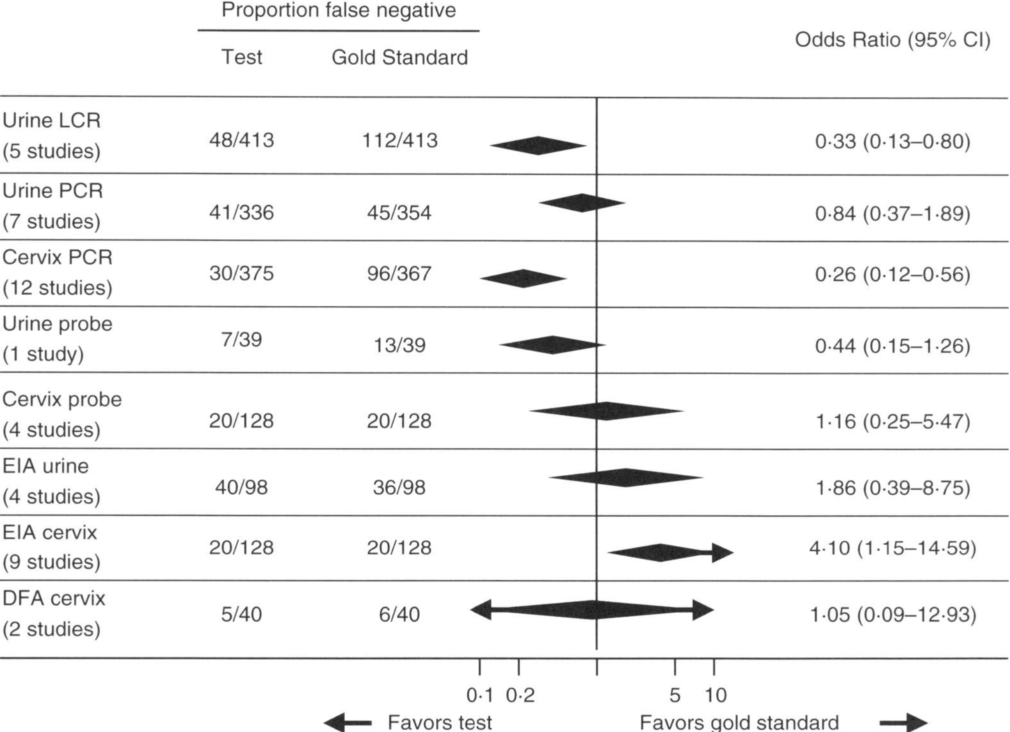

Figure 10.2 Pooled odds ratios for false negative results in screening tests for *Chlamydia trachomatis* infection. The authors of a meta-analysis of testing methods for asymptomatic chlamydial infection found most testing methods to be highly specific. Pooled sensitivity estimates were assessed by calculating the ratio of the odds of a false-negative result with each testing method (listed on the Y axis) and the odds of a false-negative result with gold standard tests. Odds ratios and 95% confidence limits are represented by black diamonds and listed on the right side of the figure; arrows indicate confidence limits that extend beyond the scale presented on the X axis. The sensitivity of PCR on cervical specimens and urine LCR were significantly better than those of gold standard assays, while the sensitivity of EIA on cervical specimens was significantly worse. Modified from *J Med Microbiol* 2000;**51**(12):1027, with permission from the Society for General Microbiology.

of self-collected specimens may open the way to approaches such as mail-in sampling for population-based screening. In a study performed in general practices in Denmark, testing of pooled self-collected mail-in specimens had a sensitivity and specificity comparable to that seen with testing of pooled physician-collected cervical and urethral swabs (sensitivity 96–100%, specificity of 93–100% with self-collected specimens; sensitivity 91%, specificity 100% with clinician-collected specimens).[70]

Pelvic inflammatory disease

Clinical assessment remains the mainstay of diagnosis of pelvic inflammatory disease (PID), a spectrum of pathological conditions including endometritis, salpingitis, tubo-ovarian abscess, and pelvic peritonitis. "Gold standard" tests (for example, endometrial biopsy, laparoscopy) are invasive and not readily available in many clinical settings. The triad of lower abdominal discomfort, cervical motion tenderness, and adnexal tenderness has been suggested to represent minimal diagnostic criteria for PID.[71]

Table 10.4 Sensitivity and specificity of ultrasonographic detection of fluid-filled fallopian tubes in the diagnosis of pelvic inflammatory diseases

Population	Type of sonography	Study gold standard	Sensitivity (%) (95% CI)	Specificity (%) (95% CI)	Reference
51 non-pregnant outpatients in Helsinki, Finland	Transvaginal	Plasma cell endometritis on biopsy	85 (55–98)	100 (91–100)	336
30 consecutive individuals hospitalized for suspected PID in Helsinki, Finland	Transvaginal	Presence of PID at laparoscopy	81 (58–95)	78 (40–97)	337
55 women with suspected PID in Providence, Rhode Island, USA	Transvaginal	Presence of PID at laparoscopy or histological endometritis on biopsy or culture of *N. gonorrhoea* or *C trachomatis* from upper genital tract specimen	32 (13–57)	97 (85–100)	338

A systematic review evaluated the sensitivity and specificity of historical, clinical, and laboratory findings for PID, when compared with laparoscopic diagnosis.[72] This review found no evidence that historical information (for example, history of irregular menses or history of intrauterine device use) can reliably identify the presence of PID in cohorts of women with abdominal pain and other signs of genital tract infection. The presence of individual clinical signs, such as purulent vaginal discharge or a palpable adnexal mass on examination in an individual with a complaint of abdominal tenderness, was both insensitive and non-specific.[72] In a study performed in Sweden in the 1960s, the presence of at least four clinical signs (such as pelvic tenderness, pelvic mass, fever, and abnormal vaginal discharge) was found to be specific (91%) for laparoscopically diagnosed PID but had a sensitivity of only 39%.[73]

The detection of gonorrhea or chlamydia may be helpful in the diagnosis of PID in individuals with compatible signs and symptoms. In a study performed in a cohort of women with abdominal pain and tenderness on bimanual examination, the isolation of one of these organisms from the lower genital tract had a sensitivity and specificity of 77% for the presence of PID.[74]

Two recent studies have used the presence of plasma cell endometritis, rather than laparoscopic evidence of PID, as the gold standard for the diagnosis of PID.[75,76] One study found the CDC "minimal diagnostic criteria" to be only 33% sensitive for the presence of plasma cell endometritis, but 88% specific,[75] while a second study found the CDC criteria to be more sensitive (83%) but less specific (22%).[76]

When available, ultrasonography may aid in the diagnosis of PID. The finding of fluid-filled fallopian tubes on ultrasound appears to be specific for the presence of PID, although the sensitivity of this finding has varied between studies (Table 10.4).

Trichomonas vaginalis

Trichomonas vaginalis is a unicellular flagellated organism that causes vaginitis in women and urethritis in men. The importance of diagnosis and treatment relates to the association between infection with this organism and adverse outcomes in pregnancy, as well as enhanced HIV transmission.[20,77] A meta-analysis of test characteristics associated with simple bedside tests, such as the use of 'wet mounts', and the use of Papanicolaou smear testing, found the sensitivity of these methods to be low (wet mount sensitivity 68% [95% CI 62–74]; Papanicolaou smear sensitivity 58%, [95% CI 43–73%]).[78]

Superior sensitivity is seen with other testing modalities, including culture using special media and PCR-based testing. A systematic review and meta-analysis found that culture using special media has a sensitivity of 90% (95% CI 77–93%), while PCR has a sensitivity of 95% (95% CI 91–99%) and specificity of 98% (95% CI 96–100%) relative to culture. Other non-culture tests, including DFA testing (sensitivity 85%, specificity 99%) and ELISA (sensitivity 82%, specificity 73%) also have good test performance, and are less expensive than culture methods.[79]

It has been noted that the high sensitivity of culture remains intact even with the use of standard transport media,[80] and despite delays in inoculation into special media.[81] This has led to the suggestion that a two-step process might be more efficient, with inexpensive and highly specific 'wet mount' testing used initially, and more expensive and sensitive tests reserved for specimens that test negative by wet mount.[82] However, it should be noted that such an approach would provide few advantages in settings where the prevalence of *T. vaginalis* infection is low.

Chancroid

Chancroid is an ulcerative genital disease caused by *Haemophilus ducreyi*. This organism has a distinct microscopic appearance, and direct Gram staining of purulent material from the ulcer base may reveal chains of short, Gram-negative bacilli. Such a finding had a sensitivity of 60% compared with culture in a cohort of individuals with genital ulcer disease attending a sexually transmitted diseases clinic in Nairobi.[83] Of 37 individuals who did not have *H. ducreyi* isolated by culture, 18 had Gram stain findings suggestive of *H. ducreyi*, suggesting either lack of sensitivity of culture or lack of specificity of Gram stain. When compared with the use of concurrent PCR assays for *H. ducreyi*-specific sequences, culture for *H. ducreyi* had a sensitivity ranging from 63% to 87%.[84–86]

Initial studies evaluating the use of PCR for the identification of *H. ducreyi* in clinical settings estimated sensitivity to be as low as 62% relative to culture.[87] However, subsequent technical improvements in specimen preparation have increased the sensitivity of PCR,[87] and more current estimates of the sensitivity of PCR for detection of *H. ducreyi* range from 79–98%, with specificity of 92–100% relative to culture.[85,86,88]

The use of PCR for the identification of *H. ducreyi* has provided important insights into the epidemiology of chancroid; for example, it has been observed that *H. ducreyi* may be present in ulcers co-infected with herpes viruses or *T. pallidum*.[27–29,86] Further, the phenomenon of asymptomatic carriage of *H. ducreyi* has been observed in 2% of commercial sex workers in The Gambia without signs or symptoms of chancroid.[89]

Other diagnostic modalities, including an indirect immunofluorescent assay, and an enzyme immunoassay, may also have value in the diagnosis of chancroid.[84]

Herpes simplex viruses

HSV are the most common agents of ulcerative genital disease in the developed world, and are increasingly recognized in the developing world as well.[90] The gold standard test for diagnosis of genital herpes has traditionally been culture of virus from genital lesions. If viral culture is not available, infection may be diagnosed by evaluating ulcer scrapings for the presence of multinucleated giant cells ("Tzank smear"). The sensitivity of Tzank smear relative to culture is

52–80% in anogenital lesions, with higher sensitivity in men than in women; the corresponding specificity is reported as 93%.[91] When used for orolabial herpes, the Tzanck smear has a reported sensitivity of 54% and a specificity of 100% relative to culture.[92]

Enzyme immunoassays provide a rapid and sensitive alternative to culture for identification of HSV. The sensitivity of these tests has been estimated to be 80–96%, while their specificity has been reported as 93–100%.[93–96] Direct immunofluorescent assays may also be useful for the diagnosis of HSV in the genital tract, and provide a more timely diagnosis than would be obtained with culture. Reported sensitivity is 74–80%, and specificity is 85–98% relative to culture.[97,98]

As has been noted, the quantification of the sensitivity and specificity of newer assays (for example, nucleic acid amplification-based assays) is difficult, since these assays are more sensitive than culture, the traditional gold standard. For example, in studies using PCR as the gold standard, viral culture has a sensitivity of 72–88%,[85,93,99,100] while EIA has a sensitivity of 65%.[93]

Older serologic assays for anti-herpes simplex antibody were unable to reliably distinguish between infection with HSV-1 and HSV-2.[101] More recent serologic assays, such as glycoprotein G-based Western blot, can differentiate the response to infection with these two viruses, and are more than 90% sensitive if performed 21 days or more after primary infection.[102] Based on individuals prospectively followed in the setting of randomized controlled trials, it can be estimated that approximately 40% of those who acquire HSV-2 infection (as evidenced by seroconversion) actually develop genital herpes.[103]

Newer ELISA-based assays for type-specific antibodies against HSV-1 and HSV-2 are sensitive and specific[104,105] when compared with Western blot assays, and are less expensive to perform. The role of antibody testing in the diagnosis of genital herpes remains poorly defined, but such tests might be used in counselling couples,[106] and in pregnancy-related screening.[107,108]

Syphilis

Primary and secondary syphilis may be diagnosed by visualization of spirochetes from ulcers, condylomata lata, and mucous patches using dark-field microscopy. Such diagnostic methods require both technical competence and experience; in the hands of an experienced microscopist, the sensitivity of dark-field microscopy has been estimated to range from 74 to 81% when compared with various reference standards.[85,109–111] The finding of motile spirochetes by dark-field microscopy in a sample from a genital lesion might be expected to be pathognomonic for syphilis, but other non-pathogenic genital tract spirochetes may lead to false positive test results.[112] Antibody-based assays and PCR may also be used to detect the presence of *T. pallidum* in lesions of primary or secondary syphilis, and may offer improved sensitivity in detection of treponemes (Table 10.5).

Serological testing is the mainstay of syphilis diagnosis in adults with non-primary disease; the characteristics of these tests have been reviewed in detail elsewhere.[112,113] Such tests can be classified as non-treponemal tests, which identify antibodies not directed against treponemes, and treponemal tests, which identify antibodies directed at treponemal components. Non-treponemal tests may be positive in the presence of a primary chancre, but are less than 90% sensitive in primary syphilis. Sensitivity is higher in secondary and early latent syphilis. By contrast, the fluorescent treponemal antibody absorbed assay (FTA-Abs), a treponemal test, is usually positive within a week of the development of a primary chancre (Figure 10.3).

Table 10.5 Diagnostic characteristics of commonly used tests for the detection of *Treponema pallidum* in early syphilis

Population or specimens source	Prevalence (%)	Comparator or study gold standard	Sensitivity (%)	Specificity (%)	Reference
		Darkfield microscopy			
128 individuals with anogenital lesions attending an STD clinic in Edmonton, Alberta, Canada	52	Positive darkfield evaluation or positive serologic test for syphilis	79	100	111
350 specimens taken from individuals with lesions suggestive of syphilis (>1 specimen per individual)	34	"Subsequent diagnosis of syphilis"	74	97	110
302 individuals with genital ulcer disease in Pune, India	14	Multiplex PCR	39	82	28
188 individuals with genital lesions attending STD clinics in Brooklyn, New York, and Seattle, Washington, USA	34	Direct fluorescent monoclonal antibody testing	85	96	122
295 men presenting to a New Orleans STD clinic with genital ulcer	25	Multiplex PCR	81	100	85
241 individuals assessed at county clinics in San Francisco and Los Angeles with lesions suggestive of primary syphilis	22	Direct fluorescent antibody testing	85	97	339
		Direct fluorescent antibody test			
241 individuals assessed at county clinics in San Francisco and Los Angeles with lesions suggestive of primary syphilis	18	Darkfield microscopy	86	93	339
156 individuals with genital ulcer disease from Malawi	17	PCR with dot-blot hybridization	85	97	340
128 individuals with anogenital lesions attending an STD clinic in Edmonton, Alberta, Canada	52	Positive darkfield evaluation or positive serologic test for syphilis	79	100	111
350 specimens taken from individuals with lesions suggestive of syphilis (>1 specimen per individual)	34	"Subsequent diagnosis of syphilis"	86	100	110

(Continued)

Table 10.5 Continued

Population or specimens source	Prevalence (%)	Comparator or study gold standard	Sensitivity (%)	Specificity (%)	Reference
188 individuals with genital lesions attending STD clinics in Brooklyn, New York, and Seattle, Washington, USA	34	Dark-field microscopy	91	93	109
		PCR			
295 men presenting to a New Orleans STD clinic with genital ulcer	22	Dark-field microscopy	100	99	85

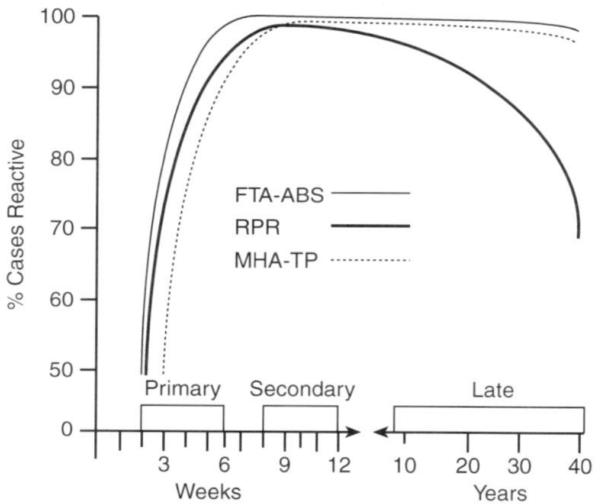

Figure 10.3 Timing of serological test positivity in syphilis. Comparison of timing of test positivity for a non-treponemal test (rapid plasma reagin or RPR), and two treponemal tests (fluorescent treponemal antibody absorbed (FTA-ABS) and microhemagglutination assay for *T. pallidum* (MHA-TP)). Both the RPR and FTA-ABS are positive in most individuals with a primary chancre, but FTA-ABS is more sensitive in primary syphilis. The two treponemal tests remain positive over time, while RPR will revert to negative in approximately one-third of untreated individuals. Reproduced from Larsen SA, Steiner BM, Rudolph AH. Laboratory diagnosis and interpretation of tests for syphilis. *Clin Microbiol Rev* 1995;**8**(1):1–21 with permission from the American Society for Microbiology.

A small proportion of individuals with syphilis have a negative non-treponemal test for syphilis due to "prozone" phenomena, which occur when extremely high titers of antibody disrupt the assay. This results in a false-negative test result, which becomes positive upon dilution.[114] Non-treponemal tests revert to negative over time in approximately 30% of untreated individuals;[115] treponemal tests may uncommonly revert to negative, a phenomenon that appears to be more common in individuals with HIV-associated immune dysfunction.[116]

The specificity of non-treponemal tests is problematic, and reports of falsely positive non-treponemal tests in the presence of other infectious diseases, rheumatologic diseases, and pregnancy are common.[117] The relative risk of a false-positive non-treponemal test in individuals with underlying HIV infection was 8·4 (95% CI 4·2–13·6%) in a Spanish cohort.[118] None the less, non-treponemal tests remain useful as screening tests because of their low cost, and because a reduction in titer following treatment is a useful indicator of microbiological cure.[119] Treponemal tests are more specific than non-treponemal tests, although false-positive test results are reported.[117] The characteristics of tests for the serologic diagnosis of syphilis are presented in further detail in Table 10.6.

The diagnosis of neurosyphilis is challenging. While VDRL testing of cerebrospinal fluid (CSF

Table 10.6 Ranges of sensitivity and specificity reported for serological tests for syphilis by stage

Test	Sensitivity				Specificity (%)	Reference
	Primary	Secondary	Latent	Late		
Non-treponemal tests						
VDRL	74–87	100	88–100	34–94	96–99	115,341,342
RPR	77–100	100	95–100	73	93–99	115,342
TRUST	77–86	100	95–100	—	98–99	115
USR	72–88	100	88–100	—	99	115
Treponemal tests						
FTA-Abs	70–100	100	99–100	96	84–100	115,341–343
MHA-TP	69–90	99–100	97–100	94	98–100	115,341–343
Non-standard tests						
ELISA	82–100	91–100	86–100	100	89–100	344–349
Western blot	78–100	98–100	83–100	100	97–100	350–352

Abbreviations: VDRL, Venereal Disease Research Laboratory; RPR, Rapid Plasma Reagin; TRUST, toluidine red unheated serum test; USR, unheated serum reagin; FTA-Abs, fluorescent treponemal antibody absorbed; MHA-TP, microhemagglutination assay for *T. pallidum*; ELISA, enzyme-linked immunosorbent assay. Modified with permission from Larsen SA, Pope V, Johnson RE, Kennedy EJ, eds. *A Manual of Tests for Syphilis, 9th ed.* 13–18. Copyright © 1998 by American Public Health Association.

VDRL) is often advocated, the sensitivity of this test is poor. A retrospective study was performed in 38 individuals with positive cerebrospinal fluid FTA-Abs (a test thought to be sensitive but non-specific for the diagnosis of neurosyphilis). Fifteen of 38 had likely neurosyphilis on the basis of a compatible clinical history and other CSF abnormalities (for example, leukocytosis or elevated protein), but only four of these 15 individuals had a positive CSF-VDRL (sensitivity 27%).[120]

The use of the "TPHA index" has been suggested as a more sensitive means of diagnosing neurosyphilis. This index is based on an antibody test (MHA-TP) that is more sensitive than CSF VDRL. False-positive test results are reduced by adjusting for CSF protein concentration, which in turn helps to control for blood contamination of the CSF sample.[121] However, a study in individuals co-infected with HIV and syphilis found high index values in only five of 40 individuals with possible neurosyphilis, and three of five individuals with positive CSF VDRL tests, suggesting that the TPHA index may also be relatively insensitive for active central nervous system infection.[122]

Existing evidence does not support the routine use of PCR for the diagnosis of neurosyphilis in adults, and published studies have yielded inconsistent results.[123,124] In a study conducted in infants born to mothers with untreated syphilis in Dallas, Texas, CSF PCR had a sensitivity of 65% when compared with a gold standard of rabbit infectivity testing; in this study PCR of blood or serum was more sensitive than CSF PCR for the presence of central nervous system disease (94%).[125]

Diagnosis of genital warts and human papillomavirus infection

The diagnosis of genital warts is usually made clinically, but rigorous studies of the sensitivity and specificity of clinical diagnosis are lacking. Although the intuition of experienced clinicians was more sensitive and specific than the use of a standardized diagnostic instrument in a small study of extragenital warts, the gold standard used in this study was the clinical judgment of one of the study investigators.[126]

Acetic acid (3–5%) has been used as an adjunct to the clinical diagnosis of genital warts, and whitening with acid application is said to signify the presence of underlying HPV infection. The application of acetic acid has also been advocated for the identification of subclinical warty lesions. However, whitening appears to be non-specific for the presence of HPV infection; in a cohort of Swedish army conscripts, HPV DNA was detected by PCR in only 17 of 39 biopsy specimens taken from aceto-white areas, and there was no difference in the detection of HPV DNA in urethral brushings from men with and without aceto-white lesions.[127] In another study HPV DNA was detected in only 55 of 91 aceto-white lesions detected by penoscopy, with other aceto-white biopsy specimens having histology suggestive of eczema.[128]

Furthermore, aceto-white lesions appear to be insensitive for the presence of HPV infection: in a cohort of Swedish women undergoing colposcopy, the finding of an aceto-white vulvar lesion had a sensitivity of 44% for the detection of HPV DNA by PCR.[129] Finally, many clinically typical genital warts do not turn white with the application of acetic acid. In a study of 202 men in Chandigarh, India, all hyperplastic warts turned white with the application of acetic acid, but only one of 12 typical verruca vulgaris-type lesions, and 15 of 59 flat warts did so.[130] Thus, the poor sensitivity and specificity of acetic acid testing for small or subclinical genital warts, combined with the lack of evidence to suggest that treatment of such lesions changes long-term outcome, makes it difficult to advocate the routine use of acetic acid testing for external genital warts.

Similarly, no evidence exists currently to support the use of HPV DNA testing in the clinical diagnosis of external genital warts. However, such testing may contribute substantially to cervical cancer screening programs. The presence of "high-risk" HPV DNA in genital tract specimens of women with atypical squamous cells of undetermined significance (ASCUS) on Papanicolaou smear is highly sensitive for the presence of underlying cervical neoplasia.[131–133] Mathematical models based on available screening data suggest that the incorporation of HPV DNA testing into screening practices would likely be cost-effective relative to current practices.[134–136] A more complete review of the relationship between human papillomavirus and cervical neoplasia is available elsewhere.[137]

Prevention of STI – condoms, other contraceptives

Evidence exists to support the effectiveness of latex male condoms in preventing transmission of several different STI. A prospective study of the impact of condom use on acquisition of either HIV or other STI in a community in Uganda found consistent condom use to be associated with a reduced risk of acquiring HIV infection (RR 0·4; 95% CI 0·2–0·9%), syphilis (OR 0·7; 95% CI 0·5–0·9%) and gonorrhea or chlamydia (OR 0·5; 95% CI 0·3–1·0%). These effects were seen despite the fact that condom users had riskier sexual practices than non-users.[138] No reduction in risk was associated with inconsistent condom use. Another prospective cohort study in a cohort of Kenyan sex trade workers found consistent condom use to be associated with a decreased risk of chlamydia (HR 0·6; 95% CI 0·4–0·9%); gonorrhea (HR 0·6; 95% CI 0·4–0·8%), genital ulcer disease (HR 0·5; 95% CI 0·3–0·9%), and PID (HR 0·6; 95% CI 0·4–0·9%), after adjustment for such covariates as place of work and number of sexual encounters per week.[139] A prospective study in American sailors suggested that consistent condom use reduced the risk of gonorrhea acquisition during shore leave from 10% to 0%, although this difference was not statistically significant, perhaps as a result of the small number of sailors who actually reported using condoms.[140]

The relationship between condom use and acquisition of genital herpes was studied in the context of a trial of a herpes vaccine in couples discordant for genital infection with HSV-2. Condom use by males during sexual intercourse in 25% of episodes or more was associated with a dramatic reduction in the hazard of acquisition of genital herpes by female partners (adjusted HR 0·09; 95% CI 0·01–0·7%). No effect was seen on female to male transmission but the study likely lacked statistical power to find such an effect.[141]

A systematic review and meta-analysis evaluated the relationship between condom use and acquisition of HPV infection, or HPV-associated disease (for example, genital warts or cervical intraepithelial neoplasia). The authors found no convincing evidence for a protective effect associated with condoms.[142]

Other contraceptive practices, including the use of spermicides, oral contraceptive pills, and intrauterine contraceptive devices (IUD) may affect the risk of STI. Despite the fact that it is bactericidal *in vitro*, there is no consistent evidence to suggest that the spermicide nonoxynol-9 reduces the risk of genital gonorrheal or chlamydia infection.[143–148] Further, nonoxynol-9 may increase the risk of ulcerative genital disease, which may enhance HIV transmission.[145,148]

A strong association between IUD and PID was noted in a multicenter case–control study conducted in the late 1970s,[149] but subsequent analyzes found the risk of PID to be most strongly associated with one particular type of IUD, the "Dalkon Shield" (OR 15·6; 95% CI 8·1–30·0%). The association of other types of IUD with PID is more controversial.[150–155]

Hormonal contraception, particularly oral contraceptive pills, may enhance the risk of acquisition of cervicitis, particularly due to *Chlamydia trachomatis*,[139] but a number of studies have found that symptomatic PID associated with *Chlamydia trachomatis* is less likely in women who use oral contraceptive pills.[156,157] This paradox may relate to the impact of oral contraceptive pills on recognition of PID: in a case–control study, individuals with asymptomatic PID were found to be 4·3 times as likely to use oral contraceptives as women with symptomatic disease (95% CI 1·6–11·7%).[158]

Management of sexually transmitted infections

Case presentation (continued)

The male adolescent described above is treated syndromically for urethritis with 1 g of oral azithromycin, and 400 mg of oral cefixime. Because of the presence of abdominal discomfort, adnexal tenderness, and cervical motion tenderness, his female partner is treated for PID. Despite some misgivings related to the question of compliance, the treating physician opts to manage her as an outpatient, with a 2-week course of oral metronidazole and levofloxacin. Subsequent laboratory testing shows both to be infected with *Chlamydia trachomatis* as well as gonorrhea. The female patient subsequently fails to return for scheduled follow up; when contacted by local public health personnel 2 weeks after presentation, she says that she took "all her medication", although she is still experiencing vaginal discharge and low abdominal discomfort. You wonder.

- How effective is syndromic management of STI?
- How effective is directed treatment of STI?
- Does treatment of sexual partners reduce the risk of relapse or reinfection?
- Are population-based interventions (including vaccination, screening, the use of mass antibiotic treatment) effective for control strategy for STI?
- Can behavioral interventions modify the future risk of sexually transmitted infection?

As discussed above, the syndromic diagnosis of STI is substantially less accurate than laboratory-based diagnosis. None the less, evidence exists to support management based on syndromic diagnoses, as this approach results in receipt of treatment by most infected individuals, and eliminates concerns related to non-treatment as a result of loss to follow up.

For example, despite the lack of accuracy of the clinical diagnosis of cervicitis, a study performed in female sex trade workers in Benin found that such a diagnosis was sufficient to warrant treatment for gonorrheal and chlamydial infections. The clinical diagnosis of cervicitis in this study was 48% sensitive and 75% specific for the presence of gonorrhea or chlamydia. This compared unfavorably to the 75% sensitivity and 100% specificity associated with laboratory diagnosis. However, the "effective sensitivity" of laboratory diagnosis, defined as the proportion of infected individuals detected by laboratory testing who actually returned to clinic within 30 days, was only 29%, worse than that seen with clinical diagnosis alone.[159]

A single non-randomized, controlled clinical trial has compared outcomes following the use of a diagnostic algorithm (with speculum examination) to a diagnostic approach incorporating basic microbiological testing in the evaluation of vaginal discharge. In this study, performed in a cohort of women in southern Thailand, the presence of gross cervical mucopus was a less sensitive indicator of cervical infection with gonorrhea and chlamydia than was the finding of microscopic mucopus on Gram stain (sensitivity 34% *v* 64%). However, no significant differences were seen between groups in the proportion of women with gonococcal or chlamydial infection at follow up, or in the proportion of women with persisting vaginal discharge 1–2 weeks after initial evaluation.[160] It should be noted that this study may have lacked statistical power to detect clinically significant differences in outcome.

Treatment of gonorrhea

A variety of drug regimens for the treatment of uncomplicated gonococcal urethritis and cervicitis have been assessed since the late 1960s via randomized controlled trials.[161–163] However, the relevance of early trials to current practice is limited, owing to the emergence of widespread antibiotic resistance in gonococcal isolates. Resistance to penicillins, tetracyclines, and macrolides have become commonplace throughout the world.[164,165] Although tetracycline and penicillin resistance have actually diminished in some areas in recent years, this probably reflects decreased selective pressure because of the non-use of these agents by treating clinicians.[134]

Prior to the emergence of widespread beta-lactam resistance, the use of a single 3 g oral dose of ampicillin or amoxicillin, combined with 1 g of probenecid, was highly effective for the treatment of uncomplicated gonorrhea.[162] However, a randomized controlled trial performed in an area of Ethiopia with high rates of penicillin resistance demonstrated that *in vitro* resistance to penicillin is associated with clinical treatment failure with such regimens; 19% of individuals treated with oral ampicillin and probenecid experienced clinical failure, while no failures were noted with a single 2 g intramuscular dose of spectinomycin.[166]

A subsequent randomized trial in Thailand showed single-dose therapy with third-generation cephalosporins to be equivalent in efficacy to single-dose spectinomycin therapy.[167] Treatment with either a single 400 mg dose of cefixime orally, or 250 mg of ceftriaxone intramuscularly reliably cured more than 95% of individuals with uncomplicated gonococcal urethritis or cervicitis in a randomized controlled trial performed in Nairobi, Kenya. Drug effectiveness was not diminished by gonococcal penicillinase production.[168] Single-dose cefixime and ceftriaxone have also been found to be highly effective and equivalent in a randomized controlled trial performed in the United States.[169]

Fluoroquinolones may be useful agents for single-dose therapy of uncomplicated gonococcal infections in areas where fluoroquinolone resistance is uncommon. A US trial completed in the 1980s found single dose ofloxacin (400 mg) to be equivalent to therapy with amoxicillin plus probenecid.[170] Comparison of a single 500 mg dose of ciprofloxacin with intramuscular ceftriaxone for urethritis treatment in an area of Zambia with a high prevalence of antibiotic-resistant gonococci found the two treatments to be equivalent.[171] However, resistance to fluoroquinolones has recently become widespread in Asia and in certain areas of the USA.[172,173] *In vitro* resistance to fluoroquinolones predicts clinical failure of fluoroquinolone therapy. A randomized controlled trial compared the efficacy of ceftriaxone to that of ciprofloxacin in *N. gonorrhoea*-infected sex-trade workers in the Philippines. The relative risk of clinical failure of therapy when individuals with a highly fluoroquinolone resistant organism (defined by ciprofloxacine MIC ≥ 0·4 micro g/mL), was 13·1 (95% CI 1·8–93·0%).[174]

A single 2 g dose of azithromycin may be an effective treatment for uncomplicated gonococcal infection. In a randomized trial both azithromycin and a single 250 mg intramuscular dose of ceftriaxone eradicated gonorrhea in more than 97% of participants; however, concomitant chlamydial infection was eradicated by azithromycin, but not by ceftriaxone.[175] The effectiveness of azithromycin outside the context of a clinical trial may be limited by the fact that over a third of individuals experience gastrointestinal discomfort with high-dose azithromycin, and by the emergence of azithromycin resistance in gonococcal solates.[176]

Although resistance to spectinomycin and third-generation cephalosporins remains uncommon, resistance to these agents has been reported, and has unfortunately become a significant problem in parts of China.[177]

Treatment of chlamydial infection and non-gonococcal urethritis or cervicitis

The past three decades have seen an evolution in the understanding of so-called non-gonococcal urethritis, post-gonococcal urethritis, and mucopurulent cervicitis, with increasing recognition that these syndromes are most commonly caused by *Chlamydia trachomatis*. As such, early data on the treatment of chlamydial infections are derived from studies that did not explicitly identify this pathogen, or which grouped chlamydial infections with those caused by other non-gonococcal organisms.

The efficacy of tetracyclines in the treatment of chlamydial infections has been demonstrated in several randomized controlled trials. An early trial compared spectinomycin to tetracycline for the treatment of gonorrhea, and found post-gonococcal urethritis to occur less frequently with tetracycline.[178] Tetracyclines were subsequently found to be superior to sulfa drugs combined with spectinomycin in a randomized trial in men with non-gonococcal urethritis.[179] Doxycycline was also significantly more efficacious than placebo in preventing post-gonococcal urethritis (RR 0·6; 95% CI 0·4–0·8%).[180]

Minocycline (100 mg twice daily), doxycycline (100 mg twice daily), and tetracycline (250 mg four times a day) had equal efficacy in the treatment of non-gonococcal urethritis and mucopurulent cervicitis in randomized trials.[181,182] A 2 g total daily dose of tetracycline may be more efficacious than a single gram total dose.[183]

Macrolide agents serve as a valuable alternative to the tetracyclines for the treatment of chlamydial infections. A week of therapy with 1 g per day of either erythromycin or tetracycline had equal efficacy in a randomized trial of treatment for men with chlamydial urethritis and their infected sex partners,[184] and newer macrolides such as clarithromycin (250 mg twice daily for 7 days) and roxithromycin (300 mg once a day for 10 days) also appear to be equivalent to doxycycline in the treatment of uncomplicated genital chlamydia infections and non-gonococcal urethritis and cervicitis.[185,186]

The development of azithromycin has had a dramatic impact on the treatment of chlamydial infections in the clinic setting, with a single 1 g dose of azithromycin proved equivalent to a 7 day course of doxycycline in the eradication of chlamydial infection, and in the resolution of cervicitis and urethritis. A systematic review and meta-analysis of 12 randomized controlled trials comparing azithromycin and doxycycline for the treatment of urethritis or cervicitis found no difference between these regimens in microbiological cure, or in the incidence of adverse drug events.[187]

Fluoroquinolones have had variable efficacy in the treatment of chlamydial infections. Two randomized trials comparing ciprofloxacin (750–1000 mg twice daily) to doxycyline found that elimination of chlamydia occurred in only 46–62% of those treated with ciprofloxacin, in contrast to 75–100% of those treated with doxycycline.[188,189] In contrast, one week of ofloxacin at a dose of 300–400 mg twice daily appears to be equivalent in efficacy to doxycycline dosed at 100 mg twice daily, with both drugs reported to eradicate chlamydial infections in 97–100% of individuals with urethritis or cervicitis.[190–192] Newer quinolones, such as sparfloxacin, grepafloxacin, and trovafloxacin, have been proven efficacious for the treatment of uncomplicated chlamydial infections of the genital tract, but their use has been limited by severe adverse drug effects, including cardiac arrhythmias and hepatotoxicity.[193–195]

Untreated lower genital tract chlamydial infection appears to be associated with adverse pregnancy outcomes including prematurity, low birth weight, stillbirth, post-partum endometritis, and pneumonitis and conjunctivitis in the newborn.[196–204] A retrospective cohort study found lower perinatal mortality associated with erythromycin treatment versus no treatment in pregnancies with a positive chlamydial culture.[205] A second retrospective cohort study found that women with successfully treated chlamydial cervicitis had lower frequencies of premature rupture of membranes and small-for-gestational-age infants compared with unsuccessfully treated women.[22] A randomized placebo-controlled trial evaluating chlamydia screening and erythromycin treatment in pregnancy found no differences between study arms, but this absence of effect may have occurred as a result of high rates of ancillary antibiotic use in the placebo arm.[206]

Subsequently, randomized controlled trials have compared amoxicillin (500 mg three times a day for 7 days) to non-estolate preparations of erythromycin for the treatment of uncomplicated chlamydial infection in pregnant women. A meta-analysis of trials comparing amoxicillin and erythromycin found the two drugs to be similar in efficacy, although amoxicillin is associated with a lower incidence of adverse effects, especially nausea.[207] With increasing comfort related to the use of azithromycin in pregnancy, randomized trials have been performed comparing this agent to amoxicillin; the two agents appear to have equivalent efficacy.[208,209]

Treatment of pelvic inflammatory disease

The agents of urethritis and cervicitis are strongly associated with the development of PID, a syndrome characterized clinically by the presence of lower abdominal pain, cervical motion tenderness, and uterine adnexal tenderness. However, while either *N. gonorrhoea* or *C. trachomatis* or both organisms are identifiable in cervical culture specimens of 70% of individuals with clinically diagnosed PID, this infection is typically polymicrobial, and therapeutic regimens include agents that are effective against these organisms, as well as Gram-negative bacilli and anaerobes. A systematic review of 34 trials and case series found most available drug regimens to be associated with probabilities of cure between 80–100%, although the pooled probability of cure was less than 80% when doxycycline and metronidazole were used without other agents.[210]

A key clinical branch point in the management of PID involves the question of whether individuals need to be admitted to hospital for therapy. A single randomized controlled trial (the "PEACH" trial) evaluated the question of inpatient versus outpatient therapy for women with moderate PID diagnosed clinically: 831 women received inpatient treatment with intravenous cefoxitin and doxycycline, or outpatient treatment with a single intramuscular injection of cefoxitin and oral doxycycline. No significant differences were seen in short-term cure rates, or in the development of longer term sequelae, including infertility, pelvic pain, and ectopic pregnancy in the 808 women available for long term follow up. The average follow-up time in these women was 35 months.[211]

Treatment of syphilis

Benzathine penicillin and aqueous penicillin G are the mainstays of therapy for syphilis, and are believed to be highly effective despite a lack of randomized controlled trials. Evidence supporting the use of tetracyclines as an alternative to penicillin for syphilis treatment is similarly based on descriptions of case series.[212,213] Recent randomized controlled trials of therapy for syphilis have compared alternative treatments to penicillin-based regimens.

Intramuscular ceftriaxone is commonly used as an alternative to benzathine penicillin for syphilis not affecting the central nervous system; however, there is little in the clinical trials literature to support this practice. A small randomized controlled trial compared a 15-day course of intramuscular penicillin to 1 g of intramuscular ceftriaxone given every other day for 7 days (i.e. four doses in total) in 28 patients with early syphilis. This study found an adequate serologic and clinical response in all participants.[214] A small randomized controlled trial comparing a single 2·4 million unit dose of benzathine penicillin to a single 3 g intramuscular dose of ceftriaxone and to 2 g of ceftriaxone given intramuscularly for 5 days found either clinical cure or sustained clinical response in 16 of 17 participants available for follow up. Although the single failure of treatment occurred with single-dose ceftriaxone, this study was too small to permit comparisons between treatment regimens.[215]

A promising alternative to benzathine penicillin in the treatment of early syphilis is azithromycin, which was compared with benzathine penicillin in an open-label pilot study[216]: 74 patients were randomized to receive standard dose benzathine penicillin, a single 2 g dose of azithromycin, or two 2 g doses of azithromycin one week apart. Of the 46 individuals available for evaluation a year after therapy, only three had experienced serological evidence of relapse or failure of response (defined as a < 2-fold reduction in RPR titers from pretreatment levels). While a larger study is needed to establish the efficacy of azithromycin in the treatment of early syphilis, these early data are promising.

Case reports and series suggesting that HIV-infected individuals are more prone to relapse after treatment of syphilis with standard drug regimens[217,218] prompted investigators to initiate two randomized controlled trials comparing usual therapy with penicillin to alternate therapies. The first of these trials[219] compared a standard regimen of 2·4 million units of benzathine penicillin G intramuscularly with standard therapy plus a 10-day course of amoxicillin and probenicid in 541 individuals with primary, secondary, or early latent syphilis: 101 participants were HIV-infected, with one-third of these having very low CD4 cell counts. No differences were seen between groups in clinical outcomes, regardless of HIV status or treatment regimens. A second trial compared 10 days of intramuscular ceftriaxone (2 g per day) to aqueous penicillin G (24 million units per day) in 36 individuals with neurosyphilis and HIV coinfection.[220] No difference was seen in the proportion of individuals with improvement in CSF VDRL titers, white blood cell counts, or protein concentrations at 14–26 weeks after therapy, although ceftriaxone was associated with a greater decline in serum RPR titers.

Preventive therapy is usually recommended for sex contacts of individuals found to have infectious syphilis. A randomized, open-label trial compared azithromycin to benzathine penicillin for the prevention of syphilis in individuals with an infectious sex partner. None of the 96 participants was documented to have developed syphilis during follow up, although fully one-third of participants were lost to follow up before completing 3 months of post-treatment surveillance.[221] Syphilis incidence also appears to be reduced in cohorts treated for gonorrhea with tetracyclines or erythromycin, suggesting that these agents are also effective against incubating syphilis.[222]

Intravenous penicillin G or intramuscular procaine penicillin have been recommended for the treatment of infants with clinical illness related to congenital syphilis.[223] However, a randomized controlled trial comparing a single dose of benzathine penicillin to a 10-day course of intramuscular procaine penicillin in 169 infants with asymptomatic congenital syphilis found no differences in efficacy between the two drug regimens. All 152 infants available for follow up at 2–3 months had a 4-fold decrease in RPR titers, while 149 became RPR non-reactive.[224] A small clinical trial performed in South Africa randomized asymptomatic infants of mothers with untreated syphilis and high serum reagin titers to single-dose benzathine penicillin or no therapy. While this study raises ethical concerns, it clearly demonstrated that non-treatment of such infants places them at high risk for the development of congenital syphilis. Congenital syphilis developed in four of eight infants randomized to no treatment, and none of the 11 infants who received penicillin ($P = 0{\cdot}04$).[225]

Treatment of genital herpes

Genital herpes may have a broad spectrum of clinical manifestations. First episodes of genital herpes may be primary (no previous infection with HSV-1 or HSV-2), or non-primary, with primary episodes often being more severe.[226–228] Among individuals with primary genital herpes infection, intravenous acyclovir at a dose of 5 mg/kg every 8 hours was shown to be superior to placebo in time to healing of genital ulcers and in speed of elimination of viral shedding.[229] Subsequently, oral acylovir at a dose of 200 mg five times per day was shown to be superior to placebo in individuals with first episodes of genital herpes, both primary and non-primary.[230,231] Further increasing the dose of antiviral drug does not result in improved outcomes; a randomized trial comparing a total of 4 g of acyclovir per day with 1 g per day found no differences between treatment groups.[232]

Treatment of recurrent genital herpes episodes with oral acyclovir at doses of 200 mg five times a day or 800 mg twice a day has been shown to be superior to placebo in the elimination of symptoms and viral shedding.[233–235] The related

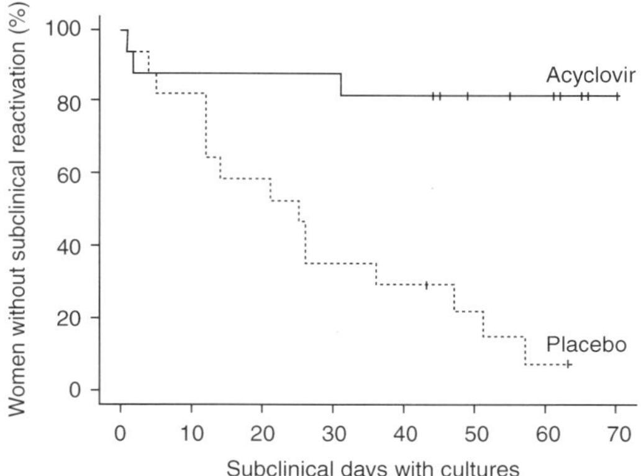

Figure 10.4 Impact of acyclovir on viral shedding in women with genital herpes. Thirty-four women with HSV-type 2 infection were randomized to receive acyclovir 400 mg b.i.d. or placebo. Viral cultures were performed on genital swab specimens collected daily. Rates of subclinical shedding of HSV-2 were significantly lower in women receiving acyclovir than in women receiving placebo ($P < 0.001$). Reproduced from Wald A, *et al.* Suppression of subclinical shedding of herpes simplex virus type 2 with acyclovir. *Ann Interm Med* 1996;**124**:8–15, with permission from the American College of Physicians.

drugs famciclovir (125 mg orally twice a day) and valacyclovir (500 mg orally twice a day), are superior to placebo,[236,237] and equivalent to acyclovir in efficacy.[238,239] Because many individuals with recurrent genital herpes recognize prodromal symptoms such as itching or tingling prior to experiencing an outbreak, patient-initiated therapy on the basis of such symptoms is often advocated, and appears effective in reducing outbreak duration and in aborting outbreaks.[236,237,239] More recently, evidence has emerged that traditional 5-day courses of therapy with antiviral drugs can be shortened. A 3-day course of valacyclovir appears equivalent in efficacy to a 5-day course,[240], while a 2-day course of oral acyclovir (800 mg three times per day) is superior to placebo in the reduction of duration of lesions and viral shedding.[241]

Individuals who experience frequent recurrences may prefer to use suppressive chronic therapy with antiviral drugs. The use of acyclovir at a dose of 400 mg twice a day is superior to placebo,[242–244] and to lower doses of acyclovir,[245] in the reduction of outbreak frequency. Treatment with daily acyclovir for as long as 6 years appears to be safe and well-tolerated by patients, and the emergence of viral resistance does not appear to be a problem in immunocompetent hosts.[246–248] Famciclovir (125 or 250 mg p.o. twice daily) and valacyclovir (250 mg twice daily, 500 mg once daily, or 1 g once daily) are also superior to placebo for the prevention of recurrences.[247,249–251]

Suppressive antiviral therapy appears to markedly reduce the frequency of asymptomatic viral shedding between recurrences as well (Figure 10.4);[252] this effect could theoretically reduce the transmission of genital herpes infections by asymptomatic individuals, but clear clinical evidence to support this idea is still lacking. Suppressive antiviral therapy in individuals with frequent recurrences does appear to significantly improve health-related quality of life, and also reduces anxiety and depression scores on standardized instruments.[253,254]

The epidemiology of maternal-fetal HSV transmission is complex. Available epidemiological evidence from a large cohort of women in Washington State suggests that the highest risk of maternal-fetal HSV transmission occurs with maternal acquisition of genital HSV infection in the third trimester of pregnancy (adjusted OR 59·3; 95% CI 6·7–525%).[25,255]

No randomized controlled trials exist to support the recommendation that women undergo cesarean section if herpetic lesions are present at the time of delivery.[256] However, among women in the Washington cohort with detectable HSV at delivery, a trend towards reduced transmission was seen in those who underwent cesarean delivery (adjusted OR 0·14; 95% CI 0·02–1·26%). Randomized controlled trials have found that suppressive antiviral drugs in pregnancy reduce the risk of cesarean section, by reducing the likelihood that active herpetic lesions are present at delivery[257–259] (Mantel–Haenszel pooled RR of cesarean section 0·49; 95% CI 0·33–0·74%). However, the question of whether antiviral drugs in pregnancy can actually reduce peripartum HSV transmission remains unresolved.

Treatment of chancroid

A variety of drug regimens have been proven efficacious in the treatment of chancroid in randomized controlled trials. However, the development of drug resistance in *H. ducreyi* has made some treatment options obsolete in certain geographic areas. Traditional agents of choice for the treatment of chancroid included tetracyclines and sulfonamides, but resistance to these agents is now extremely common, and macrolides, fluoroquinolones, and third-generation cephalosporins are now preferred for the treatment of chancroid.[260–265] The results of randomized controlled trials evaluating the efficacy of these agents are presented in Table 10.7.

Of note, single dose therapies with ciprofloxacin (500 mg) or azithromycin (1 g) have been proven equivalent to multiple dose antibiotic regimens, while ceftriaxone (250 mg intramuscularly) appears equivalent to single-dose azithromycin.[86,266–268]

Other antibiotic classes, including penicillins and aminoglycosides, may be useful in the treatment of chancroid. Although resistance to ampicillin by *H. ducreyi* is well described, resistance is mediated by beta-lactamase production, and chancroid can be effectively treated with the addition of a beta-lactamase inhibitor.[269] A single 2 g dose of spectinomycin is a useful alternative therapy for the treatment of chancroid. A trial comparing spectinomycin to trimethoprim-sulfamethoxazole in Thailand found spectinomycin to be more likely to result in cure (RR of cure with spectinomycin 2·0; 95% CI 1·7–2·0%).[270] However, a randomized trial comparing erythromycin (500 mg p.o. three times a day for 5 days) to a single 2 g dose of spectinomycin found higher rates of cure with erythromycin (RR of cure with spectinomycin 0·9; 95% CI 0·8–1·0%).[271]

Chancroid may be complicated by the development of fluctuant inguinal buboes. A small randomized trial compared aspiration to incision and drainage for the management of buboes during an outbreak of chancroid in New Orleans. Both forms of management appeared to be efficacious and acceptable, although six of 15 individuals who underwent aspiration experienced re-accumulation of purulent material, and required re-aspiration ($P = 0·05$).[272]

Treatment of genital warts

A number of treatment modalities are available for the management of genital warts. These include topical agents, cryotherapy, surgical modalities (including scissors excision, laser ablation, and electrocautery), and interferon. While it is often suggested that genital warts involute spontaneously over time, it has been pointed out that there is little evidence to support this contention.[273,274] Important clinical outcomes in the study of genital wart treatment include reductions in wart area and rates of relapse, as well as rates of wart clearance.

Podophyllotoxin and imiquimod are both patient-applied topical therapies that have been proven efficacious in the treatment of genital warts in randomized, placebo-controlled trials (Table 10.8). A randomized trial comparing thrice-weekly application of 5% imiquimod cream with more frequent applications found no benefit with more frequent applications, and identified an increase in the incidence of adverse events.[275]

Cryotherapy is commonly used for the treatment of genital warts, but has not been evaluated in placebo-controlled trials. This modality was

Table 10.7 Randomized controlled trials evaluating macrolides, fluoroquinolones, and third-generation cephalosporins for the treatment of chancroid

Study population	Treatment arms	Primary outcome measure	Results	Comments	Reference
245 men and women attending an urban STD clinic in Nairobi, Kenya, with genital ulcer disease compatible with chancroids	Single 500 mg dose of ciprofloxacin *v* erythromycin 500 mg t.i.d. for 7 days	Ulcer healing or improvement among individuals proven to have chancroid by culture or PCR	No difference between treatment arms in healing or improvement (RR of cure with ciprofloxacin 1·0, 95% CI 0·8–1·2)	Double-blind, placebo controlled	86
46 Indian men with clinical diagnosis of chancroid presenting to an outpatient specialty clinic	Ciprofloxacin 500 mg b.i.d. for 3 days *v* erythromycin 500 mg q.i.d. for 7 days v trimethoprim-sulfamethoxazole 160/800 mg b.i.d. for 7 days	Complete healing of ulcer 21 days after initial presentation	Cure in 29 of 31 individuals randomized to either erythromycin or ciprofloxacin. Relative risk of failure with trimethoprim-sulfamethoxazole 1·7, 95% CI 1·1–2·8	Open label trial. *H ducreyi* isolates resistant to trimethoprim-sulfamethoxazole. Individuals who failed initial therapy cured with ciprofloxacin or erythromycin	264
98 HIV-seronegative men presenting to a Nairobi clinic with culture-positive chancroid and negative syphilis evaluation	Single 400 mg oral dose of fleroxacin or trimethoprim-sulfamethoxazole 160/800 mg b.i.d. for 3 days	Clinical cure, defined as complete re-epithelialization at 1–2 weeks	Trend towards improved outcome with fleroxacin (RR of cure with fleroxacin 1·4, 95% CI 0·9–2·3)	Study performed as trimethoprim-sulfamethoxazole resistance being recognized in East Africa	265
204 men presenting to a Nairobi clinic with purulent genital ulcers	Azithromycin 1 g orally *v* erythromycin 500 mg q.i.d. for 7 days	Complete cure, defined as re-epithelialization of the ulcer base, ≤ 21 days after initial treatment	No differences between treatment regimens in outcome (cure in 73/82 with azithromycin and 41/45 with erythromycin)	HIV seropositivity associated with increased risk of failed therapy (OR 4·5, 95% CI 1·4–14·7)	266
139 men presenting to a Nairobi clinic with culture-positive chancroid and negative syphilis evaluation	500 mg ciprofloxacin as a single dose *v* 500 mg ciprofloxacin or trimethoprim-sulfamethoxazole 160/800 mg b.i.d. for 3 days	Complete cure, defined as re-epithelialization of the ulcer base, ≤ 21 days after initial treatment, and resolution of buboes	No differences between treatment regimens (cure seen in 28/46 with trimethoprim-sulfamethoxazole, 28/46 with single-dose ciprofloxacin, and 27/43 with 3-day ciprofloxacin regimen)	Double-blind, placebo controlled	267
197 men and women presenting to clinics in 4 US cities with genital ulcer but without evidence for syphilis	Single 1 g oral dose of azithromycin *v* 250 mg ceftriaxone given intramuscularly	Complete healing of ulcer ≥ 18 days after treatment in individuals with culture-proven chancroid	High rates of cure in both groups (32/32 with azithromycin, 29/33 with ceftriaxone), but azithromycin more efficacious (RR of cure 1·1, 95% CI 1·0–1·3)	High rates of healing among individuals with ulcers of uncertain etiology in both arms	268
48 men presenting to a Nairobi clinic with negative syphilis evaluation	Cefotaxime (1 g intramuscularly) with 1 g of probenecid orally, single treatment *v* once-daily treatment for 3 days	Complete healing of ulcer at 28 days of follow up	Total dose of 3 g cefotaxime superior to 1 g (RR of healing 1·4, 95% CI 1·0–2·0 with 3 g dose)	Double-blind, placebo controlled	353

Table 10.8 Randomized placebo-controlled trials of selected therapeutic modalities for the treatment of genital warts

Study population	Intervention	Results	Reference
	Podophyllotoxin		
60 men with a clinical diagnosis of genital warts attending government-affiliated clinics in Punjab region of Pakistan	Subjects randomized to treatment with podophyllotoxin 0·5% cream, interferon-alpha cream, or placebo up to 9 times per week for up to 4 weeks	Podophyllotoxin cured more individuals at 4 weeks than placebo (RR of cure 3·0, 95% CI 1·2–7·7), but less efficacious than interferon-alpha (RR of cure 0·7, 95% CI 0·5–1·0)	283
60 men with a clinical diagnosis of genital warts attending government-affiliated clinics in Punjab region of Pakistan	Subjects randomized to treatment with podophyllotoxin 0·5% cream, interferon-alpha cream, or placebo up to 9 times per week for up to 4 weeks	Podophyllotoxin cured more individuals at 4 weeks than placebo (RR of cure 3·7, 95% CI 1·2–11·2), but less efficacious than interferon-alpha (RR of cure 0·6, 95% CI 0·4–0·9)	284
57 men and women at several US centers, with prior complete resolution of genital warts	Participants randomized to receive 0.5% podophyllotoxin or placebo once daily, 3 days per week, for 8 weeks	Reduction in recurrence with podophyllotoxin 8 weeks after enrolment (RR of recurrence 0·4, 95% CI 0·1–1·0)	291
57 Swedish men with previously untreated genital warts	Subjects randomly assigned to receive up to 2 courses of 0·25% or 0·5% podophyllotoxin, or placebo, twice daily for 3 days	No resolution seen in placebo arm. Warts cleared after 2 cycles of treatment in 13/18 patients receiving 0·25% and 13/16 patients receiving 0·5% podophyllotoxin	354
109 men at several US centers, with a clinical diagnosis of genital warts	Subjects randomly assigned to 0·5% podophyllotoxin or placebo for 3 consecutive days, followed by 4 days without treatment. Applications repeated for 2–4 weeks	25/56 podophyllotoxin treated men wart-free at some point during study; no individual was wart-free in placebo arm. Reduction in total wart area also seen with podophyllotoxin	355
72 women with a clinical diagnosis of exophytic vulvar condyloma	Subjects randomly assigned to 0·5% podophyllotoxin in either alcohol or cream formulation or placebo, two applications per day, three consecutive days per week, for up to 4 weeks	Trend towards greater efficacy with podophyllotoxin at 10 weeks (RR for clearance 2·1, 95% CI 0·9–4·7)	356
38 men with genital warts in Seattle, Washington	Subjects randomly assigned to 0·5% podophyllotoxin or placebo applied three consecutive days per week for up to 4 weeks	11/19 podophyllotoxin treated men wart-free at some point during study; no individual was wart-free in placebo arm. Reduction in total wart area also seen with podophyllotoxin	357

Table 10.8 Continued

Study population	Intervention	Results	Reference
	Imiquimod		
311 men and women with anogenital warts at multiple US centers	Subjects randomized to 5% or 1% imiquimod cream or placebo, three applications per week for up to 16 weeks	Higher rates of clearance of warts seen with 5% imiquimod (RR of clearance 4·5, 95% CI 2·5–8·1) and 1% imiquimod than with placebo. 5% imiquimod more efficacious than 1% imiquimod (RR of clearance 2·4, 95% CI 1·6–3·7)	358
279 men and women with 2 or more biopsy-proven external genital warts, at multiple centers in the USA	Subjects randomized to daily application of 5% or 1% imiquimod cream or placebo, for up to 16 weeks	Higher rates of clearance of warts seen with 5% imiquimod (RR of clearance 16·3, 95% CI 5·3–51·1) and 1% imiquimod than with placebo. 5% imiquimod more efficacious than 1% imiquimod (RR of clearance 3·6, 95% CI 2·1–6·2)	359
60 women with genital warts in Punjab region of Pakistan	Subjects randomly assigned to 2% imiquimod or placebo, up to 10 applications per week for 6 weeks	Higher rates of clearance seen with 2% imiquimod than placebo after 6 weeks (RR of clearance 25, 95% CI 3·6–172·6)	360
60 men with genital warts attending public health centers and municipal dispensaries in Punjab region of Pakistan	Subjects randomized to 2% imiquimod cream or placebo, three applications weekly for 4 weeks	Higher rates of clearance seen with 2% imiquimod (RR of clearance 7·0, 95% CI 2·3–21·0)	361
	Intralesional interferon		
296 men and women with a clinical diagnosis of genital warts attending multiple centers in the USA	Subjects randomized to three weekly intralesional injections of interferon-alpha-2b or placebo, into up to three warts per subject, for 3 weeks	Higher rates of clearance of treated warts with interferon than with placebo at 16 weeks (RR for clearance of treated lesions 2·5, 95% CI 1·5–4·1). Higher percentage	362

Table 10.8 Continued

Study population	Intervention	Results	Reference
	Imiquimod		
		of interferon-treated subjects had a 50% or greater reduction in total wart area ($P < 0{\cdot}001$)	
158 men and women with a clinical diagnosis of at least two genital warts, covering at least 10 mm^2 in area, treated at four US centers	Warts injected with interferon alpha or placebo twice weekly for up to eight weeks, or until disappearance of warts	Interferon-alpha more efficacious than placebo 3 months after last injection (RR of clearance with interferon 2·9, 95% CI 1·8–4·8)	363
76 men and women from multiple USA centers, with genital warts present despite the use of conventional therapy	A single wart from each patient was injected three times per week for 4 weeks with one of three interferon preparations or placebo	Significant difference between interferon preparations and placebo in resolution of injected warts over 16-week follow up period ($P = 0.02$). No difference in efficacy between interferon preparations. Interferon did not affect non-injected warts	288
114 men and women with genital warts treated at six centers in the USA	Single wart injected intralesionally with high dose interferon-alpha, low dose interferon-alpha, or placebo, three times weekly for 3 weeks	High dose interferon-alpha more efficacious than low dose interferon-alpha (RR of clearance 2·8, 95% CI 1·3–6·3), and placebo (RR of clearance 3·8, 95% CI 1·5–10·2) at 12 weeks. Low dose interferon-alpha no better than placebo (RR of clearance 1·4, 95% CI 0·4–4·3)	364
41 women and 1 man aged 16 to 65 treated at a clinic in North Carolina	Six to nine injections of interferon-alpha-2b or placebo over a period of up to 29 days	Trend towards greater efficacy with interferon than placebo after 1 month (RR of clearance 3·0, 95% CI 0·9–10·0).	365

superior to podophyllin in a randomized trial (RR of clearance 3·2; 95% CI 1·7–6·1%), although this trial had high rates of loss to follow up.[276] More prolonged application of liquid nitrogen (> 10 s) increased the probability of wart clearance, but was associated with an increased risk of pain during treatment in a randomized trial (RR of clearance 1·7; 95% CI 1·2–2·4, RR of pain 2·3; 95% CI 1·4–3·9%).[277]

Two randomized trials have compared the efficacy of cryotherapy to trichloroacetic acid (TCAA), with no significant difference seen in rates of clearance (pooled RR for wart clearance with cryotherapy 1·0; 95% CI 0·7–1·4%).[278,279] However, cryotherapy may also be less likely to cause genital ulceration than TCAA (OR of ulceration with cryotherapy 0; 95% CI 0–0·3%).[279]

No placebo-controlled trials of surgical modalities for genital wart treatment have been performed to date. Randomized trials comparing laser surgery with conventional scissors excision, and electrocautery with cryotherapy, have failed to find any difference between modalities in terms of efficacy.[280,281] However, scissors excision of perianal warts was superior to podophyllin application both in initial wart clearance and in subsequent recurrence rates (RR of recurrence after scissors excision 0·3; 95% CI 0·2–0·7%).[282]

Topical, intralesional and systemic interferon preparations have been evaluated for the treatment of genital warts. Both topical and intralesional interferon are more efficacious than placebo in the eradication of genital warts (Table 10.8). Topical interferon-alpha was more efficacious than podophyllotoxin in two randomized trials (pooled RR of clearance with interferon-alpha 1·6; 95% CI 1·2–2·1%).[283,284] A randomized trial comparing podophyllin plus intralesional interferon-alpha to podophyllin alone found a higher rate of wart clearance with interferon, but a high rate of relapse was seen in both treatment groups, and intralesional interferon was associated with adverse effects including fever, myalgia, gastrointestinal distress, and headache.[285] Although systemic interferons have been more efficacious than placebo in the clearance of genital warts, the addition of systemic interferon to such standard therapies as cryotherapy or podophyllin has been no more efficacious than standard therapies alone.[286–291] Further, the expense and potential toxicity of systemic interferon limits its practical value in most clinical situations.

Treatment of genital warts in immunocompromised individuals, including those with HIV infection, may be particularly challenging. A randomized trial comparing imiquimod 5% to placebo in individuals with HIV infection and CD4 counts > 100 cells/mL found no difference between the two arms in rates of wart clearance.[292] Cidofovir 1% gel may be a useful therapeutic option in HIV infected individuals; a small randomized trial found higher rates of clearance with cidofovir (9/19 individuals) than with placebo (0/9 individuals, $P = 0{\cdot}006$). A second randomized trial found the combination of cidofovir 1% gel and scissors excision to be more efficacious than either scissors excision or cidofovir gel alone in a population of individuals with HIV infection.[293]

Patient factors other than frank immunocompromise may influence clearance of genital warts. An observational study carried out on individuals with genital warts in Leeds, UK, found increasing wart numbers associated with decreased clearance in response to therapy (hazard ratio for every 2-fold increase in wart numbers 0·70; 95% CI 0·45–0·86%). Smoking was evaluated as a possible predictor of persistence in this study, and was not found to be predictive of wart persistence.[294]

Treatment of trichomoniasis

Metronidazole appears to be a highly effective agent for the treatment of vaginal trichomoniasis.

Double-blind randomized controlled trials have found no significant difference in efficacy between a single 2 g dose of metronidazole and 5–7 day courses of the drug dosed at 750–800 mg per day. Both regimens appear to result in parasitological cure in over 85% of individuals.[295,296] Single-dose metronidazole for the treatment of trichomoniasis appears less efficacious if the drug is given as a single 1 g dose, although a single 1·5 g dose may be equivalent to a 2 g dose.[297,298] A single 2 g dose of tinidazole is equivalent in efficacy to 2 g of metronidazole for the treatment of vaginal trichomoniasis.[299–301] Tinidazole appears to be efficacious in individuals with prior failure of therapy associated with metronidazole-resistant trichomonads, and eradicated infection in 22 of 24 women who had previously failed therapy with metronidazole for trichomonal vaginitis.[302]

Topical therapies for trichomoniasis have been disappointing to date. A multicenter, open-label randomized trial comparing single-dose oral metronidazole to intravaginal clotrimazole or sulfanilamide-allantoin-aminacrine hydrochloride suppositories found metronidazole to be curative in 34/45 of subjects, while suppositories were associated with microbiologic failure in over 80% of participants.[303] Intravaginal 0·75% metronidazole gel was significantly less efficacious than oral metronidazole in a small randomized trial (RR of cure with gel 0·4; 95% CI 0·3–0·8%).[304] Topical nonoxynol-9 was ineffective in the treatment of vaginal trichomoniasis.[305]

The association between asymptomatic carriage of *T. vaginalis* and preterm delivery led investigators to hypothesize that screening for and treating subclinical infections in pregnancy could reduce the risk of preterm delivery. However, in a randomized placebo-controlled trial, the incidence of preterm delivery was significantly higher in women treated with metronidazole than among those treated with placebo (RR 3·0; 95% CI 1·5–5·9%). Screening for trichomoniasis in asymptomatic pregnant women cannot be recommended at this time.[20]

Treatment of partners for prevention of reinfection

The importance of treating sex partners for the prevention of repeated infection has been demonstrated for several curable sexually transmitted infections, including trichomonal vaginitis, genital chlamydia, and gonorrheal infection in women. In a study in which partners of women with trichomoniasis were randomized to receive either tinidazole or placebo, reinfection was strongly associated with the receipt of placebo (RR 4·7; 95% CI 1·3–25·3%).[306] Additionally, analysis of data from a randomized controlled trial of a behavioural intervention in women with a baseline sexually transmitted infection found reinfection with gonorrhea or chlamydia to be strongly associated with sex with a partner who was not adequately treated (OR 5·6; 95% CI 3·0–10·5%).[307]

Patient delivery of medications to sex partners might help ensure partner treatment, and two non-randomized studies have found lower rates of reinfection with chlamydia in women who delivered medications to their partners.[308,309] However, a more recent randomized controlled trial found patient-delivered partner treatment to be ineffective in preventing reinfection with chlamydia (OR of reinfection 0·80; 95% CI 0·62–1·05%).[310]

Strategies for control of STI in the community: vaccination, mass antibiotic treatment, counselling and behavioral interventions

Vaccine prevention of STI

Vaccination as a strategy for the prevention of bacterial STI has been unsuccessful to date. Effective vaccines are available for hepatitis A and B virus infections, which may be sexually transmitted.[311–315] A single small randomized, placebo-controlled trial has evaluated the use of hepatitis B vaccine for the post-exposure prophylaxis of infection in sex partners of individuals with acute hepatitis B. No protective effect was seen in this study.[316]

A novel glycoprotein-conjugate vaccine may be efficacious for the prevention of genital herpes in women. In a randomized placebo-controlled trial of couples discordant for HSV-2 infection, vaccination of women without prior serologic evidence of either HSV-1 or HSV-2 infection was associated with a reduction in genital herpes risk of 74% (95% CI 9–93%), although no reduction in HSV-2 infection risk was seen. The vaccine appeared ineffective in men.[317]

A novel virus-like particle conjugate vaccine against HPV type 16 (HPV-16) appears to be extremely efficacious in the prevention of infection with this viral type in young women (RR of acquisition of infection with vaccine 0; 95% CI 0–0·09). This vaccine represents a potentially important new tool for the prevention of cervical cancer.[318]

Population-based screening programs

Screening and use of curative or suppressive antibacterial and antiviral agents may provide an effective means of disrupting disease transmission, particularly if infections are asymptomatic or unrecognized in the absence of therapy. In non-pregnant populations, limited evidence exists to guide policy related to population-based screening for most pathogens. An exception is *Chlamydia trachomatis*, which is likely to be markedly underdiagnosed if testing is limited to those with symptoms.[319,320] A randomized controlled trial of screening for genital chlamydia infection in women enrolled in a Washington State health maintenance organization found a significant reduction in the incidence of PID after 1 year of follow up among screened women (RR 0·44; 95% CI 0·20–0·90%).[321] Screening for chlamydia may be a cost-saving health intervention in high-prevalence populations.[322]

Mass antibiotics treatment in high-risk populations and outbreaks

Existing data do not support the routine use of mass antibiotic treatment as a control measure for STI, either in high-risk populations or in the outbreak setting. However, existing data do support the use of empiric antimicrobial therapy for pregnant women in settings with high rates of STI.

Mass antibiotic treatment of adults was evaluated in a cluster-randomized controlled trial in the Rakai district of Uganda, where community-level treatment (azithromycin, ciprofloxacin, and metronidazole) was provided in an effort to slow HIV transmission. No impact was seen on HIV infection, but this trial did document significant reductions in syphilis (RR 0·8; 95% CI 0·7–0·9%) and trichomoniasis (RR 0·6; 95% CI 0·4–0·9%) in communities that received mass antibiotic therapy. The modest effect of the intervention and the potential impact of such a strategy on local antimicrobial susceptibility patterns argue against the use of such a strategy for primary control of STI other than HIV.[323]

However, in a pregnant subgroup of the above trial, empiric antibiotic therapy (with a regimen modified for safety in pregnancy) was associated with a significant reduction in neonatal death (RR 0·83; 95% CI 0·71–0·97%). Reductions in low birth weight, ophthalmia neonatorum, and maternal carriage of *T. vaginalis*, gonococcus, and *C. trachomatis* were also seen.[324] Two other randomized, placebo-controlled trials performed in Kenya found empiric administration of third-generation cephalosporins at 28–32 weeks of gestation to be associated with a reduced incidence of low birth weight (pooled RR 0·54; 95% CI 0·36–0·81%) and postpartum endometritis (pooled RR 0·50; 95% CI 0·31–0·81%), although these trials found no difference between groups in the incidence of stillbirth (pooled RR 0·69; 95% CI 0·26–1·81%).[325,326]

Prior attempts have been made to control gonorrhea in sex trade workers via mass antibiotic therapy. Mass treatment of female sex trade workers in the Philippines, reported as contacts by US sailors with gonorrhea, transiently reduced the prevalence of gonococcal carriage in sex-trade workers. However, no change in the incidence of gonorrhea was seen in navy personnel, and prevalence in sex-trade workers returned to baseline when mass treatment ended.[327]

Mass antibiotic treatment has also been used as a primary outbreak control strategy for syphilis. In controlling an outbreak of syphilis in sex-trade workers and migrant farm workers in California, mass treatment was associated with a decline in syphilis in both groups 1 year later.[328] However, in a more recent syphilis outbreak in Vancouver, the transient decline in syphilis rates which occurred with mass treatment was followed by a rebound in rates beyond baseline levels (Figure 10.5).[329]

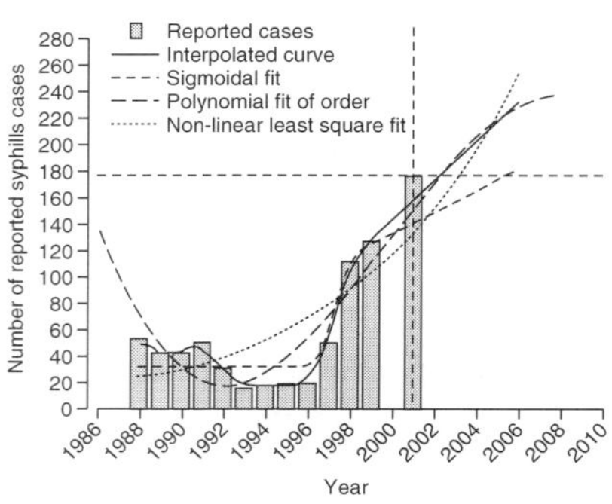

Figure 10.5 Failure of mass antibiotic treatment to control a syphilis outbreak in Vancouver. A mass antibiotic treatment effort was carried out in the year 2000 in an attempt to control a large urban syphilis outbreak. While a transient decrease in case numbers was seen, incidence rebounded sharply in 2002, possibly due to truncated immunity in individuals at highest risk of infection.[333] Curves fitted to these data using a variety of mathematical approaches were used to project a future increase case numbers. Rekart ML, Patrick DM, Chakraborty B, *et al.* Tangeted mass treatment for syphilis with oral azithromycin. *Lancet* 2003;**361**:313–4. Reproduced with permission.

Counselling and behavioural interventions

Several randomized controlled trials have evaluated behavioural interventions targeting groups perceived to be at increased risk of acquiring STI. A multicenter trial (Project RESPECT) conducted in publicly funded clinics in five US cities evaluated changes in behavior and incidence of infection in individuals receiving a brief didactic message, brief counseling, or extended counseling. Both brief and extended counseling reduced the risk of laboratory-confirmed sexually transmitted infection at 6 months (RR for brief intervention 0·7; 95% CI 0·6–0·9, RR for enhanced intervention 0·7; 95% CI 0·5–0·9%). A transient increase in condom use was also seen (Figure 10.6).[330] Other smaller clinic-based trials have failed to demonstrate similar changes in sexual behaviour or subsequent incidence of infection.[331,332]

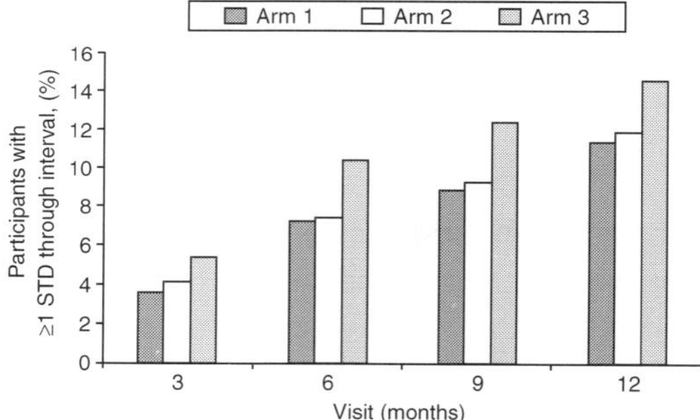

Figure 10.6 Effectiveness of clinic-based counselling interventions in the prevention of sexually transmitted infections. Clinic attendees enrolled in a multicenter trial were randomized to receive four interactive counseling sessions (Arm 1), two interactive counseling sessions (Arm 2), or didactic message on sexually transmitted infection risk-reduction (Arm 3). Reductions in sexually transmitted infection risk were seen with both counseling interventions, and persisted 12 months after initial counseling ($P = 0.008$). Reproduced from Kamb ML, *et al.* Efficacy of risk reduction counseling to prevent human immunodeficiency virus and sexually transmitted diseases: a randomized controlled trial. Project RESPECT Study Group. *JAMA* 1998;**280**(13):1165. Copyright © 1998, American Medical Association. All rights reserved.

References

1. 1998/1999 Canadian Sexually Transmitted Diseases (STD) Surveillance Report. *Can Commun Dis Rep* 2000;**26S6**.
2. *Centers for Disease Control and Prevention. Sexually Transmitted Disease Surveillance, 2000.* Atlanta, GA: US Department of Health and Human Services, 2001.
3. Fleming D, McQuillan G, Nahmias A, *et al.* Herpes simplex virus type 2 in the United States, 1976 to 1994. *N Engl J Med* 1997;**337**:1105–11.
4. Wikstrom A, Popescu C, Forslund O. Asymptomatic penile HPV infection: a prospective study. *Int J STD AIDS.* 2000;**11**:80–4.
5. Winer RL, Lee SK, Hughes JP, *et al.* Genital human papillomavirus infection: incidence and risk factors in a cohort of female university students. *Am J Epidemiol.* 2003;**157**:218–26.
6. Woodman CB, Collins S, Winter H, *et al.* Natural history of cervical human papillomavirus infection in young women: a longitudinal cohort study. *Lancet* 2001;**357**:1831–6.
7. Gerbase A, Rowley J, Heymann D, *et al.* Global prevalence and incidence estimates of selected curable STDs. *Sex Transm Infect.* 1998;**74**(Suppl.1):S12–16.
8. Szucs T, Berger K, Fisman D, Harbarth S. The estimated economic burden of genital herpes in the United States: an analysis using two costing approaches. *BMC Infect Dis.* 2001;**1**:5.
9. Washington A, Johnson R, Sanders L. *Chlamydia trachomatis* infections in the United States: what are they costing us? *JAMA* 1987;2**57**:2070–2.
10. Washington A, Katz P. Cost of and payment source for pelvic inflammatory disease: trends and projections, 1983 through 2000. *JAMA* 1991;**266**:2565–9.
11. Siegel J. The economic burden of sexually transmitted diseases in the United States. In: Holmes K, Sparling P, Mardh P et al, eds. *Sexually Transmitted Diseases.* New York: McGraw Hill, 1999:1367–79.
12. Rottingen J, Cameron D, Garnett G. A systematic review of the epidemiologic interactions between classic sexually transmitted diseases and HIV. *Sex Transm Dis* 2001;**28**:579–97.
13. World Health Organization Task Force on the Prevention and Management of Infertility. Tubal Infertility: serologic relationship to past chlamydial and gonococcal infection. *Sex Transmit Dis.* 1995;**22**:71–7.
14. Coste J, Laumon B, Bremond A, *et al.* Sexually transmitted diseases as major causes of ectopic pregnancy: results from a large case-control study in France. *Fertil Steril* 1994;**62**:289–95.
15. Ankum W, Mol B, Van der Veer F, Bossuyt P. Risk factors for ectopic pregnancy: a meta-analysis. *Fertil Steril* 1996;**65**:1093–9.
16. Stacey CM, Munday PE, Taylor-Robinson D, *et al.* A longitudinal study of pelvic inflammatory disease. *Br J Obstet Gynaecol* 1992;**99**:994–9.
17. Safrin S, Schachter J, Dahrouge D, Sweet RL. Long-term sequelae of acute pelvic inflammatory disease. A retrospective cohort study. *Am J Obstet Gynecol* 1992;**166**:1300–5.
18. Mitchell H, Drake M, Medley G. Prospective evaluation of risk of cervical cancer after cytological evidence of human papilloma virus infection. *Lancet* 1986; **1**:573–5.
19. Palefsky JM, Holly EA, Ralston ML, *et al.* Anal cytological abnormalities and anal HPV infection in men with Centers for Disease Control group IV HIV disease. *Genitourin Med* 1997;**73**:174–80.
20. Klebanoff MA, Carey JC, Hauth JC, *et al.* Failure of metronidazole to prevent preterm delivery among pregnant women with asymptomatic *Trichomonas vaginalis* infection. *N Engl J Med* 2001;**345**:487–93.
21. Sliverman N, Sullivan M, Hochman M, *et al.* A randomized, prospective trial comparing amoxicillin and erythromycin for the treatement of *Chlamydia trachomatis* in pregnancy. *Am J Obstet Gynecol* 1994;**170**:829–32.
22. Cohen I, Veille JC, Calkins BM. Improved pregnancy outcome following successful treatment of chlamydial infection. *JAMA* 1990;**263**:3160–3.
23. Temmerman M, Gichangi P, Fonck K, *et al.* Effect of a syphilis control program on pregnancy outcome in Nairobi, Kenya. *Sex Transm Infect* 2000;**76**:117–21.
24. Rotchford K, Lombard C, Zuma K, Wilkinson D. Impact on perinatal mortality of missed opportunities to treat maternal syphilis in rural South Africa: baseline results from a clinic randomized controlled trial. *Trop Med Int Health* 2000;**5**:800–4.
25. Brown ZA, Wald A, Morrow RA, *et al.* Effect of serologic status and cesarean delivery on transmission rates of herpes simplex virus from mother to infant. *JAMA* 2003;**289**:203–9.

26. DiCarlo R, Martin D. The clinical diagnosis of genital ulcer disease in men. *Clin Infect Dis* 1997;**25**:292–8.
27. Behets F, Andriamiadana J, Randrianasolo D, *et al.* Chancroid, primary syphilis, genital herpes and lymphogranuloma venereum in Antananarivo, Madagascar. *J Infect Dis* 1999;**180**:1382–5.
28. Risbud A, Chan-Tack K, Gadkari D, *et al.* The etiology of genital ulcer disease by multiplex polymerase chain reaction and relationship to HIV infection among patients attending sexually transmitted disease clinics in Pune, India. *Sex Transm Dis* 1998;**26**:55–62.
29. Behets F, Braitwaith A, Hylton-Kong T, *et al.* Genital ulcers: etiology, clinical diagnosis, and associated human immunodeficiency virus infection in Kingston, Jamaica. *Clin Infect Dis* 1999;**28**:1086–90.
30. Bornstein J, Lakovsky Y, Lavi I, *et al.* The classic approach to diagnosis of vulvovaginitis: a critical approach. *Infect Dis Obstet Gynecol* 2001;**9**:105–11.
31. World Health Organization. Report of a WHO Study Group: management of patients with sexually transmitted diseases. 810. 1991. Geneva, WHO. WHO Technical Reports Series.Ref Type: Report.
32. Dallabetta G, Gerbase A, Holmes K. Problems, solutions, and challenges in syndromic management of sexually transmitted diseases. *Sex Transm Infect* 1998;**74**(Suppl. 1):S1–S11.
33. Pettifor A, Walsh J, Wilkins V, Raghunathan P. How effective is syndromic management of STDs?: A review of current studies. *Sex Transm Dis* 2000;**27**:371–85.
34. Moore SG, Miller WC, Hoffman IF, *et al.* Clinical utility of measuring white blood cells on vaginal wet mount and endocervical gram stain for the prediction of chlamydial and gonococcal infections. *Sex Transm Dis* 2000;**27**: 530–8.
35. Myziuk L, Romanowski B, Brown M. Endocervical Gram stain smears and their usefulness in the diagnosis of *Chlamydia trachomatis*. *Sex Transm Infect* 2001;**77**:103–6.
36. Sellors J, Howard M, Pickard L, *et al.* Chlamydial cervicitis: testing the practice guidelines for presumptive diagnosis. *CMAJ* 1998;**158**:41–6.
37. Stamm W, Koutsky L, Benedetti J, *et al.* *Chlamydia trachomatis* urethral infections in men. Prevalence, risk factors, and clinical manifestations. *Ann Intern Med* 1984;**100**:47–51.
38. Juchau SV, Nackman R, Ruppart D. Comparison of Gram stain with DNA probe for detection of *Neisseria gonorrhoeae* in urethras of symptomatic males. *J Clin Microbiol* 1995;**33**:3068–9.
39. Moherdaui F, Vuylsteke B, Siqueira LF, *et al.* Validation of national algorithms for the diagnosis of sexually transmitted diseases in Brazil: results from a multicenter study. *Sex Transm Infect* 1998;**74**(Suppl.1):S38–S43.
40. Chandeying V, Skov S, Tabrizi SN, *et al.* Can a two-glass urine test or leucocyte esterase test of first-void urine improve syndromic management of male urethritis in southern Thailand. *Int J STD AIDS* 2000;**11**:235–40.
41. Wiesenfeld H, Lowry D, Heine R, *et al.* Self-collection of vaginal swabs for the detection of chlamydia, gonorrhea, and trichomoniasis. *Sex Transm Dis* 2001;**28**:321–5.
42. Sellors J, Lorincz A, Mahony J, *et al.* Comparison of self-collected vaginal, vulvar and urine samples with physician-collected cervical samples for human papillomavirus testing to detect high-grade squamous intraepithelial lesions. *CMAJ* 2000;**163**:513–8.
43. Hadgu A. Bias in the evaluation of DNA-amplification tests for detecting *Chlamydia trachomatis*. *Stat Med* 1997;**16**:1391–9.
44. Van Dyck E, Ieven M, Pattyn S, *et al.* Detection of *Chlamydia trachomatis* and *Neisseria gonorrhoeae* by enzyme immunoassay, culture, and three nucleic acid amplification tests. *J Clin Microbiol* 2001;**39**:1751–6.
45. Crotchfelt KA, Welsh LE, DeBonville D, *et al.* Detection of *Neisseria gonorrhoeae* and *Chlamydia trachomatis* in genitourinary specimens from men and women by a coamplification PCR assay. *J Clin Microbiol* 1997;**35**: 1536–40.
46. Iwen PC, Walker RA, Warren KL, *et al.* Effect of off-site transportation on detection of *Neisseria gonorrhoeae* in endocervical specimens. *Arch Pathol Lab Med* 1996;**120**:1019–22.
47. Livengood CH, III, Wrenn JW. Evaluation of COBAS AMPLICOR (Roche): accuracy in detection of *Chlamydia trachomatis* and *Neisseria gonorrhoeae* by coamplification of endocervical specimens. *J Clin Microbiol* 2001;**39**:2928–32.
48. Page-Shafer K, Graves A, Kent C, *et al.* Increased sensitivity of DNA amplification testing for the detection of pharyngeal gonorrhea in men who have sex with men. *Clin Infect Dis* 2002;**34**:173–6.

49. Stary A, Ching SF, Teodorowicz L, Lee H. Comparison of ligase chain reaction and culture for detection of *Neisseria gonorrhoeae* in genital and extragenital specimens. *J Clin Microbiol* 1997;**35**:239–42.
50. Koumans E, Johnson R, Knapp J, St Louis M. Laboratory testing for *Neisseria gonorrhoeae* by recently introduced non-culture tests: a performance review with clinical and public health considerations. *Clin Infect Dis* 1998;**27**:1171–80.
51. Van Der Pol B, Ferrero DV, Buck-Barrington L, *et al.* Multicenter evaluation of the BDProbeTec ET System for detection of *Chlamydia trachomatis* and *Neisseria gonorrhoeae* in urine specimens, female endocervical swabs, and male urethral swabs. *J Clin Microbiol* 2001;**39**:1008–16.
52. Mahony J, Luinstra KE, Tyndall M, *et al.* Multiplex PCR for detection of *Chlamydia trachomatis* and *Neisseria gonorrhoeae* in genitourinary specimens. *J Clin Microbiol* 1995;**33**:3049–53.
53. Martin DH, Cammarata C, Van Der Pol B, *et al.* Multicenter evaluation of AMPLICOR and automated COBAS AMPLICOR CT/NG tests for *Neisseria gonorrhoeae. J Clin Microbiol* 2000;**38**:3544–9.
54. Xu K, Glanton V, Johnson S, *et al.* Detection of *Neisseria gonorrhoeae* infection by ligase chain reaction testing of urine among adolescent women with and without *Chlamydia trachomatis* infection. *Sex Transm Dis* 1998;**25**:533–8.
55. Lewis JS, Fakile O, Foss E, *et al.* Direct DNA probe assay for *Neisseria gonorrhoeae* in pharyngeal and rectal specimens. *J Clin Microbiol* 1993;**31**:2783–5.
56. Young H, Anderson J, Moyes A, McMillan A. Non-cultural detection of rectal and pharyngeal gonorrhoea by the Gen-Probe PACE 2 assay. *Genitourin Med* 1997;**73**:59–62.
57. Thomas JG, Dul MJ, Badger S, *et al.* Multicenter clinical trial and laboratory utilization of an enzymatic detection method for gonococcal antigens. *Am J Clin Pathol* 1986;**86**:71–8.
58. Roongpisuthipong A, Lewis JS, Kraus SJ, Morse SA. Gonococcal urethritis diagnosed from enzyme immunoassay of urine sediment. *Sex Transm Dis* 1988; **15**:192–5.
59. Papasian CJ, Bartholomew WR, Amsterdam D. Modified enzyme immunoassay for detecting *Neisseria gonorrhoeae* antigens. *J Clin Microbiol* 1984;**20**:641–3.
60. Hossain A, Bakir TM, Siddiqui M, De Silva S. Enzyme immunoassay (EIA) in the rapid diagnosis of gonorrhoea. *J Hyg Epidemiol Microbiol Immunol* 1988;**32**:425–31.
61. Schachter J, McCormack WM, Smith RF, *et al.* Enzyme immunoassay for diagnosis of gonorrhea. *J Clin Microbiol* 1984;**19**:57–9.
62. Donders GG, van Gerven V, de Wet HG, van Stratem AM, de Boer F. Rapid antigen tests for *Neisseria gonorrhoeae* and *Chlamydia trachomatis* are not accurate for screening women with disturbed vaginal lactobacillary flora. *Scand J Infect Dis* 1996;**28**:559–62.
63. Watson EJ, Templeton A, Russell I, *et al.* The accuracy and efficacy of screening tests for *Chlamydia trachomatis*: a systematic review. *J Med Microbiol* 2002;**51**:1021–31.
64. Chernesky MA, Lee H, Schachter J, *et al.* Diagnosis of *Chlamydia trachomatis* urethral infection in symptomatic and asymptomatic men by testing first-void urine in a ligase chain reaction assay. *J Infect Dis* 1994;**170**:1308–11.
65. Mahony JB, Luinstra KE, Sellors JW, *et al.* Confirmatory polymerase chain reaction testing for *Chlamydia trachomatis* in first-void urine from asymptomatic and symptomatic men. *J Clin Microbiol* 1992;**30**:2241–5.
66. Gaydos C, Crotchfelt K, Shah N, *et al.* Evaluation of dry and wet transported intravaginal swabs in detection of *Chlamydia trachomatis* and *Neisseria gonorrhoeae* infections in female soldiers by PCR. *J Clin Microbiol* 2002;**40**:758–61.
67. Domeika M, Bassiri M, Butrimiene I, *et al.* Evaluation of vaginal introital sampling as an alternative approach for the detection of genital *Chlamydia trachomatis* infection in women. *Acta Obstet Gynecol Scand* 1999;**78**:131–6.
68. Knox J, Tabrizi SN, Miller P, *et al.* Evaluation of self-collected samples in contrast to practitioner-collected samples for detection of *Chlamydia trachomatis*, *Neisseria gonorrhoeae*, and *Trichomonas vaginalis* by polymerase chain reaction among women living in remote areas. *Sex Transmit Dis* 2002;**29**:647–54.
69. Quigley M, Munguti K, Grosskurth H, *et al.* Sexual behaviour patterns and other risk factors for HIV infection in rural Tanzania: a case-control study. *AIDS* 1997;**11**:237–48.
70. Ostergaard L, Moller J, Andersen B, Olesen F. Diagnosis of urogential *Chlamydia trachomatis* infection in women based on mailed samples obtained at home: multipractice comparative study. *BMJ* 1996;**313**:1186–9.

71. Centers for Disease Control and Prevention. 1998 Guidelines for treatment of Sexually Transmitted Diseases. *MMWR Morb Mortal Wkly Rep* 1998;**47**(RR-1):1–118.
72. Kahn J, Walker C, Washington A, *et al.* Diagnosing pelvic inflammatory disease: a comprehensive analysis and considerations for developing a new model. *JAMA* 1991;**266**:2594–604.
73. Jacobson L, Westrom L. Objectivized diagnosis of acute pelvic inflammatory disease: diagnostic and prognostic value of laparoscopy. *Am J Obstet Gynecol* 1969;**105**:1088–98.
74. Wasserheit J, Bell T, Kiviat N. Microbial causes of proven pelvic inflammatory disease and efficacy of clindamycin and tobramycin. *Ann Intern Med* 1986;**104**:187–93.
75. Korn AP, Hessol N, Padian N, *et al.* Commonly used diagnostic criteria for pelvic inflammatory disease have poor sensitivity for plasma cell endometritis. *Sex Transmit Dis* 1995;**22**:335–41.
76. Peipert JF, Ness RB, Blume J, *et al.* Clinical predictors of endometritis in women with symptoms and signs of pelvic inflammatory disease. *Am J Obstet Gynecol* 2001;**184**: 856–63.
77. Sorvillo F, Smith L, Kerndt P, Ash L. *Trichomonas vaginalis*, HIV, and African-Americans. *Emerg Infect Dis* 2001;**7**:927–32.
78. Wiese W, Patel SR, Patel SC, *et al.* A meta-analysis of the Papanicolaou smear and wet mount for the diagnosis of vaginal trichomoniasis. *Am J Med* 2000;**108**:301–8.
79. Patel SR, Wiese W, Patel SC, *et al.* Systematic review of diagnostic tests for vaginal trichomoniasis. *Infect Dis Obstet Gynecol* 2000;**8**:248–57.
80. Beverly A, Venglarik M, Cotton B, Schwebke JR. Viability of *Trichomonas vaginalis* in transport medium. *J Clin Microbiol* 1999;**37**:3749–50.
81. Schwebke JR, Venglarik M, Morgan S. Delayed versus immediate bedside inoculation of culture media for diagnosis of vaginal trichomoniasis. *J Clin Microbiol* 1999;**37**:2369–70.
82. Schwebke JR. Cost-effective screening for trichomoniasis. *Emerg Infect Dis* 2002;**8**:749–50.
83. Nsanze H, Fast M, D'Costa L, *et al.* Genital ulcers in Kenya: a clinical and laboratory study. *Br J Vener Dis* 1981;**59**:378–81.
84. Ahmed HJ, Borrelli S, Jonasson J, *et al.* Monoclonal antibodies against *Haemophilus ducreyi* lipooligosaccharide and their diagnostic usefulness. *Eur J Clin Microbiol Infect Dis* 1995;**14**:892–8.
85. Orle K, Gates C, Martin D, *et al.* Simultaneous PCR detection of *Haemophilus ducreyi*, *Treponema pallidum*, and herpes simplex virus types 1 and 2 from genital ulcers. *J Clin Microbiol* 1996;**34**:49–55.
86. Malonza I, Tyndall M, Ndinya-Achola J, *et al.* A randomized, double-blind, placebo-controlled trial of single-dose ciprofloxacin versus erythromycin for the treatment of chancroid in Nairobi, Kenya. *J Infect Dis* 1999;**180**:1886–93.
87. Johnson SR, Martin DH, Cammarata C, Morse SA. Development of a polymerase chain reaction assay for the detection of *Haemophilus ducreyi*. *Sex Transmit Dis* 1994;**21**:13–23.
88. Parsons LM, Waring AL, Otido J, Shayegani M. Laboratory diagnosis of chancroid using species-specific primers from *Haemophilus ducreyi* groEL and the polymerase chain reaction. *Diag Microbiol Infect Dis* 1995;**23**:89–98.
89. Hawkes S, West B, Wilson S, *et al.* Asymptomatic carriage of *Haemophilus ducreyi* confirmed by the polymerase chain reaction. *Genitourin Med* 1995;**71**:224–7.
90. Corey L, Handsfield HH. Genital herpes and public health: addressing a global problem. *JAMA* 2000;**283**:791–4.
91. Folkers E, Oranje AP, Duivenvoorden JN, *et al.* Tzanck smear in diagnosing genital herpes. *Genitourin Med* 1988;**64**:249–54.
92. Bagg J, Mannings A, Munro J, Walker DM. Rapid diagnosis of oral herpes simplex or zoster virus infections by immunofluorescence: comparison with Tzanck cell preparations and viral culture. *Br Dent J* 1989;**167**:235–8.
93. Slomka MJ, Emery L, Munday PE, *et al.* A comparison of PCR with virus isolation and direct antigen detection for diagnosis and typing of genital herpes. *J Med Virol* 1998;**55**:177–83.
94. Kudesia G, Van Hegan A, Wake S, *et al.* Comparison of cell culture with an amplified enzyme immunoassay for diagnosing genital herpes simplex infection. *J Clin Pathol* 1991;**44**:778–80.
95. Nerurkar LS, Namba M, Brashears G, *et al.* Rapid detection of herpes simplex virus in clinical specimens by use of a capture biotin-streptavidin enzyme-linked immunosorbent assay. *J Clin Microbiol* 1984;**20**:109–14.

96. Skar AG, Middeldorp J, Gundersen T, *et al.* Rapid diagnosis of genital herpes simplex infection by an indirect ELISA method. *NIPH Ann* 1988;**11**:59–65.
97. Chan EL, Brandt K, Horsman GB. Comparison of Chemicon SimulFluor direct fluorescent antibody staining with cell culture and shell vial direct immunoperoxidase staining for detection of herpes simplex virus and with cytospin direct immunofluorescence staining for detection of varicella-zoster virus. *Clin Diagn Lab Immunol* 2001;**8**:909–12.
98. Lafferty WE, Krofft S, Remington M, *et al.* Diagnosis of herpes simplex virus by direct immunofluorescence and viral isolation from samples of external genital lesions in a high-prevalence population. *J Clin Microbiol* 1987;**25**:323–6.
99. Scoular A, Gillespie G, Carman WF. Polymerase chain reaction for diagnosis of genital herpes in a genitourinary medicine clinic. *Sex Transm Infect* 2002;**78**:21–5.
100. Marshall DS, Linfert DR, Draghi A, *et al.* Identification of herpes simplex virus genital infection: comparison of a multiplex PCR assay and traditional viral isolation techniques. *Mod Pathol* 2001;**14**:152–6.
101. Ashley R, Cent A, Maggs V, *et al.* Inability of enzyme immunoassays to discriminate between infections with herpes simplex virus types 1 and 2. *Ann Intern Med* 1991;**115**:520–6.
102. Ashley RL, Militoni J, Lee F, *et al.* Comparison of Western blot (immunoblot) and glycoprotein G-specific immunodot enzyme assay for detecting antibodies to herpes simplex virus types 1 and 2 in human sera. *J Clin Microbiol* 1988;**26**:662–7.
103. Langenberg AG, Corey L, Ashley RL, *et al.* A prospective study of new infections with herpes simplex virus type 1 and type 2. Chiron HSV Vaccine Study Group. *N Engl J Med* 1999;**341**:1432–8.
104. Wald A, Ashley-Morrow R. Serological testing for herpes simplex virus (HSV)-1 and HSV-2 infection. *Clin Infect Dis* 2002;**35**(Suppl.2):S173–S182.
105. Scoular A. Using the evidence base on genital herpes: optimising the use of diagnostic tests and information provision. *Sex Transm Infect* 2002;**78**:160–5.
106. Fisman DN, Hook EW, III, Goldie SJ. Estimating the costs and benefits of screening monogamous, heterosexual couples for unrecognized infection with herpes simplex virus type 2. *Sex Transm Infect* 2003;**79**:45–52.
107. Lipsitch M, Davis G, Corey L. Potential benefits of a serodiagnostic test for herpes simplex virus type 1 (HSV-1) to prevent neonatal HSV-1 infection. *Sex Transm Dis* 2002;**29**:399–405.
108. Barnabas RV, Carabin H, Garnett GP. The potential role of suppressive therapy for sex partners in the prevention of neonatal herpes: a health economic analysis. *Sex Transm Infect* 2002;**78**:425–9.
109. Cummings MC, Lukehart SA, Marra C, *et al.* Comparison of methods for the detection of *Treponema pallidum* in lesions of early syphilis. *Sex Transmit Dis* 1996;**23**:366–9.
110. Daniels K, Ferneyhough H. Specific direct fluorescent antibody detection of *Treponema pallidum*. *Health Lab Sci.* 1977;**14**:164–71.
111. Romanowski B, Forsey E, Prasad E, *et al.* Detection of *Treponema pallidum* by a fluorescent monoclonal antibody test. *Sex Transmit Dis* 1987;**22**:156–9.
112. Larsen SA, Steiner BM, Rudolph AH. Laboratory diagnosis and interpretation of tests for syphilis. *Clin Microbiol Rev* 1995;**8**:1–21.
113. Hart G. Syphilis tests in diagnostic and therapeutic decision making. *Ann Intern Med* 1986;**104**:368–76.
114. Spangler A, Jackson J, Fiumara N, Warthin T. Syphilis with a negative blood test reaction. *JAMA* 1964;**189**:87–90.
115. Larsen S, Johnson R. Diagnostic tests. In: Larsen S, Pope V, Johnson R, Kennedy E, eds. *A Manual of Tests for Syphilis*. Washington, DC: American Public Health Association, 1998.
116. Haas JS, Bolan G, Larsen SA, *et al.* Sensitivity of treponemal tests for detecting prior treated syphilis during human immunodeficiency virus infection. *J Infect Dis* 1990;**162**:862–6.
117. Hook EW, III, Marra CM. Acquired syphilis in adults. *N Engl J Med* 1992;**326**:1060–9.
118. Joyanes P, Borborio M, Arquez J, Perea E. The association of false-positive rapid plasma reagin results and HIV infection. *Sex Transmit Dis* 1998;**25**:569–71.
119. Romanowski B, Sutherland R, Fick GH, *et al.* Serologic response to treatment of infectious syphilis. *Ann Intern Med* 1991;**114**:1005–9.
120. Davis LE, Schmitt JW. Clinical significance of cerebrospinal fluid tests for neurosyphilis. *Ann Neurol* 1989;**25**:50–5.

121. Luger A, Schmidt BL, Steyrer K, Schonwald E. Diagnosis of neurosyphilis by examination of the cerebrospinal fluid. *Br J Vener Dis* 1981;**57**:232–7.
122. Tomberlin MG, Holtom PD, Owens JL, Larsen RA. Evaluation of neurosyphilis in human immunodeficiency virus-infected individuals. *Clin Infect Dis* 1994;**18**:288–94.
123. Marra CM, Gary DW, Kuypers J, Jacobson MA. Diagnosis of neurosyphilis in patients infected with human immunodeficiency virus type 1. *J Infect Dis* 1996;**174**:219–21.
124. Noordhoek GT, Wolters EC, de Jonge ME, van Embden JD. Detection by polymerase chain reaction of *Treponema pallidum* DNA in cerebrospinal fluid from neurosyphilis patients before and after antibiotic treatment. *J Clin Microbiol* 1991;**29**:1976–84.
125. Michelow IC, Wendel GD, Jr, Norgard MV, *et al.* Central nervous system infection in congenital syphilis. *N Engl J Med* 2002;**346**:1792–8.
126. Young R, Jolley D, Marks R. Comparison of the use of standardized diagnostic criteria and intuitive clinical diagnosis in the diagnosis of common viral warts (verrucae vulgaris). *Arch Dermatol* 1998;**134**:1586–9.
127. Kataoka A, Claesson U, Hansson B, *et al.* Human papillomavirus infection of the male diagnosed by Southern-blot hybridization and polymerase chain reaction: comparison between urethral samples and penile biopsy samples. *J Med Virol* 1991;**33**:159–64.
128. Wikstrom A, Hedblad M, Johansson B, *et al.* The acetic acid test in evaluation of subclinical genital papillomavirus infection: a comparative study on penoscopy, histopathology, virology, and scanning electron microscopy findings. *Genitourin Med* 1992;**68**:90–9.
129. Jonsson M, Karlsson R, Evander M, *et al.* Acetowhitening of the cervix and vulva as a predictor of subclinical human papillomavirus infection: sensitivity and specificity in a population-based study. *Obstet Gynecol* 1997;**90**:744–7.
130. Kumar B, Gupta S. The acetowhite test in genital human papillomavirus infection in men: what does it add? *J Eur Acad Dermatol Venereol* 2001;**15**:27–9.
131. Manos MM, Kinney WK, Hurley LB, *et al.* Identifying women with cervical neoplasia: using human papillomavirus DNA testing for equivocal Papanicolaou results. *JAMA* 1999;**281**:1605–10.
132. Kuhn L, Denny L, Pollack A, *et al.* Human papillomavirus DNA testing for cervical cancer screening in low-resource settings. *J Natl Cancer Inst* 2000;**92**:818–25.
133. Ascus-LLIL Triage Study (ALTS) Group. Results of a randomized trial on the management of cytology interpretations of atypical squamous cells of undetermined significance. *Am J Obstet Gynecol* 2003;**188**:1383–92.
134. Kim J, Wright T, Goldie S. Cost-effectiveness of alternative triage strategies for atypical squamous cells of undetermined significance. *JAMA* 2002;**287**:2382–90.
135. Goldie SJ, Weinstein MC, Kuntz KM, Freedberg KA. The costs, clinical benefits, and cost-effectiveness of screening for cervical cancer in HIV-infected women. *Ann Intern Med* 1999;**130**:97–107.
136. Goldie SJ, Kuhn L, Denny L, *et al.* Policy analysis of cervical cancer screening strategies in low-resource settings: clinical benefits and cost-effectiveness. *JAMA* 2001;**285**:3107–15.
137. Burd EM. Human papillomavirus and cervical cancer. *Clin Microbiol Rev* 2003;**16**:1–17.
138. Ahmed S, Lutaloa T, Wawer M, *et al.* HIV incidence and sexually transmitted disease prevalence associated with condom use: a population study in Rakai, Uganda. *AIDS* 2002;**15**:2171–9.
139. Baeten J, Nyange P, Richardson B, *et al.* Hormonal contraception and risk of sexually transmitted disease acquisition: results from a prospective study. *Am J Obstet Gynecol* 2002;**185**:380–5.
140. Hooper R. Cohort study of venereal disease. I: The risk of gonorrhea transmission from infected women to men. *Am J Epidemiol* 1978;**108**:136–44.
141. Wald A, Langenberg A, Link K, *et al.* Effect of condoms on reducing the transmission of herpes simplex virus type 2 from men to women. *JAMA* 2001;**285**:3100–6.
142. Manhart LE, Koutsky LA. Do condoms prevent genital HPV infection, external genital warts, or cervical neoplasia? A meta-analysis. *Sex Transmit Dis* 2002;**29**:725–35.
143. Niruthisard S, Roddy R, Chutivongse S. Use of nonoxynol-9 and reduction in rate of gonococcal and chlamydial cervical infections. *Lancet* 1992;**339**:1371–5.
144. Louv W, Austin H, Alexander W, *et al.* A clinical trial of nonoxynol-9 for preventing gonococcal and chlamydial infections. *J Infect Dis* 1988;**158**:518–23.

145. Kreiss J, Ngugi E, Holmes K, *et al.* Efficacy of nonoxynol 9 contraceptive sponge use in preventing heterosexual acquisition of HIV in Nairobi prostitutes. *JAMA* 1992;**268**:477–82.

146. Richardson B, Lavreys L, Martin H, *et al.* Evaluation of a low-dose nonoxynol-9 gel for the prevention of sexually transmitted diseases. *Sex Transmit Dis* 2001;**28**:394–400.

147. Roddy R, Zekeng L, Ryan K, *et al.* Effect of nonoxynol-9 on urogenital gonorrhea and chlamydia infection: a randomized controlled trial. *JAMA* 2002;**287**:1117–22.

148. Roddy R, Zekeng L, Ryan K, *et al.* A controlled trial of nonoxynol 9 film to reduce male-to-female transmission of sexually transmitted diseases. *N Engl J Med* 1998;**339**:504–10.

149. Burkman RT. Association between intrauterine device and pelvic inflammatory disease. *Obstet Gynecol* 1981;**57**:269–6.

150. Grimes DA. Intrauterine device and upper-genital-tract infection. *Lancet* 2000;**356**:1013–19.

151. Lee NC, Rubin GL, Ory HW, Burkman RT. Type of intrauterine device and the risk of pelvic inflammatory disease. *Obstet Gynecol* 1983;**62**:1–6.

152. Farley T, Rosenberg M, Rowe P, *et al.* Intrauterine devices and pelvic inflammatory disease: an international perspective. *Lancet* 1992;**339**:785–8.

153. Kronmal RA, Whitney CW, Mumford SD. The intrauterine device and pelvic inflammatory disease: the Women's Health Study reanalyzed. *J Clin Epidemiol* 1991;**44**: 109–22.

154. Gareen IF, Greenland S, Morgenstern H. Intrauterine devices and pelvic inflammatory disease: meta-analyzes of published studies, 1974–1990. *Epidemiology* 2000;**11**:589–97.

155. Hubacher D, Lara-Ricalde R, Taylor DJ, *et al.* Use of copper intrauterine devices and the risk of tubal infertility among nulligravid women. *N Engl J Med* 2001;**345**:561–7.

156. Kimani J, Maclean IW, Bwayo JJ, *et al.* Risk factors for *Chlamydia trachomatis* pelvic inflammatory disease among sex workers in Nairobi, Kenya. *J Infect Dis* 1996;**173**:1437–44.

157. Wolner-Hanssen P, Eschenbach DA, Paavonen J, *et al.* Decreased risk of symptomatic chlamydial pelvic inflammatory disease associated with oral contraceptive use. *JAMA* 1990;**263**:54–9.

158. Ness RB, Keder LM, Soper DE, *et al.* Oral contraception and the recognition of endometritis. *Am J Obstet Gynecol* 1997;**176**:580–5.

159. Mukenge-Tshibaka L, Alary M, *et al.* Syndromic versus laboratory-based diagnosis of cervical infections among female sex workers in Benin: implications of nonattendance for return visits. *Sex Transm Dis* 2002;**29**:324–30.

160. Chandeying V, Skov S, Kemapunmanus M, *et al.* Evaluation of two clinical protocols for the management of women with vaginal discharge in southern Thailand. *Sex Transm Infect* 1998;**74**:194–201.

161. Waugh MA, Cooke EM, Nehaul BB, Brayson J. Comparison of minocycline and ampicillin in gonococcal urethritis. *Br J Vener Dis* 1979;**55**:411–14.

162. Brathwaite AR. Double-blind trial of amoxycillin and ampicillin plus probenecid in the treatment of gonorrhoea in men. *Br J Vener Dis* 1979;**55**:340–2.

163. Berry E. Treatment of gonorrheal urethritis evaluated in 230 men. *JAMA* 1967;**202**:657–9.

164. Nissinen A, Jarvinen H, Liimatainen O, *et al.* Antimicrobial resistance in *Neisseria gonorrhoeae* in Finland, 1976 to 1995. The Finnish Study Group For Antimicrobial Resistance. *Sex Transm Dis* 1997;**24**:576–81.

165. Rahman M, Sultan Z, Monira S, *et al.* Antimicrobial susceptibility of *Neisseria gonorrhoeae* isolated in Bangladesh (1997 to 1999): rapid shift to fluoroquinolone resistance. *J Clin Microbiol* 2002;**40**:2037–40.

166. Habte-Gabr E, Geyid A, Serdo D, *et al.* Single-dose treatment of uncomplicated acute gonococcal urethritis in Ethiopian men: comparison of rosoxacin, spectinomycin, penicillin, and ampicillin. *Sex Transmit Dis* 1987;**14**:153–5.

167. Panikabutra K, Ariyarit C, Chitwarakorn A, *et al.* Randomized comparative study of ceftriaxone and spectinomycin in gonorrhoea. *Genitourin Med* 1985;**61**: 106–8.

168. Plourde PJ, Tyndall M, Agoki E, *et al.* Single-dose cefixime versus single-dose ceftriaxone in the treatment of antimicrobial-resistant *Neisseria gonorrhoeae* infection. *J Infect Dis* 1992;**166**:919–22.

169. Handsfield HH, McCormack WM, Hook EW, III, *et al.* A comparison of single-dose cefixime with ceftriaxone as treatment for uncomplicated gonorrhea. The Gonorrhea Treatment Study Group. *N Engl J Med* 1991;**325**:1337–41.

170. Black JR, Long JM, Zwickl BE, *et al.* Multicenter randomized study of single-dose ofloxacin versus amoxicillin-probenecid for treatment of uncomplicated gonococcal infection. *Antimicrob Agents Chemother* 1989;**33**:167–70.

171. Bryan JP, Hira SK, Brady W, *et al.* Oral ciprofloxacin versus ceftriaxone for the treatment of urethritis from resistant *Neisseria gonorrhoeae* in Zambia. *Antimicrob Agents Chemother* 1990;**34**:819–22.

172. Kilmarx P, Knapp J, Xia M, *et al.* Intercity spread of gonococci with decreased susceptibility to fluoroquinolones: a unique focus in the United States. *J Infect Dis* 1998;**177**:677–82.

173. Trees D, Sandul A, Neal S, *et al.* Molecular epidemiology of *Neisseria gonorrhoeae* exhibiting decreased susceptibility and resistance to ciprofloxacin in Hawaii, 1991–1999. *Sex Transm Dis* 2001;(28):309–14.

174. Aplasca de los Reyes M, Pato-Mesola V, Klausner J, *et al.* A randomized trial of ciprofloxacin versus cefixime for treatment of gonorrhea after rapid emergence of gonococcal ciprofloxacin resistance in the Phillipines. *Clin Infect Dis* 2001;**32**:1313–8.

175. Handsfield HH, Dalu ZA, Martin DH, *et al.* Multicenter trial of single-dose azithromycin vs. ceftriaxone in the treatment of uncomplicated gonorrhea. Azithromycin Gonorrhea Study Group. *Sex Transmit Dis* 1994;**21**:107–11.

176. Zarantonelli L, Borthagaray G, Lee EH, *et al.* Decreased susceptibility to azithromycin and erythromycin mediated by a novel mtr(R) promoter mutation in *Neisseria gonorrhoeae*. *J Antimicrob Chemother* 2001;**47**:651–4.

177. Guoming L, Qun C, Shengchun W. Resistance of *Neisseria gonorrhoeae* epidemic strains to antibiotics: report of resistant isolates and surveillance in Zhanjiang, China: 1998 to 1999. *Sex Transm Dis* 2000;**27**:115–18.

178. Karney W, Pedersen A, Nelson M, *et al.* Spectinomycin versus tetracycline for the treatment of gonorrhea. *N Engl J Med* 1977;**296**:889–94.

179. Mahony J, McCann J, Harris J, *et al.* Oxytetracycline compared with single-dose therapy with sulfametopyrazine-streptomycin sulphate in nongonococcal urethritis in males. *Br J Clin Pract* 1974;**28**:179–81.

180. McLean K, Evans B, Lim J, Azadin B. Postgonococcal urethritis: a double-blind study of doxycycline vs placebo. *Genitourin Med* 1990;**66**:20–3.

181. Turnbull B, Stringer H, Meech R. Tetracycline and minocycline in the management of non-gonococcal urethritis: a comparison. *NZ Med J* 1982;**95**:460–2.

182. Romanowski B, Talbot H, Stadnyk M, *et al.* Minocycline compared with doxycycline in the treatment of non-gonococcal urethritis and mucopurulent cervicitis. *Ann Intern Med* 1993;**119**:16–22.

183. Bowie W, Yu J, Fawcett A, Jones H. Tetracycline in nongonococcal urethritis. Comparison of 2 g and 1 g daily for seven days. *Br J Vener Dis* 1980;**56**:332–6.

184. Scheibel J, Kristensen J, Hentzer B, *et al.* Treatment of chlamydial urethritis in men and *Chlamydia trachomatis*-positive female partners: comparison of erythromycin and tetracycline in treatment courses of one week. *Sex Transm Dis* 1982;**9**:128–31.

185. Lidbrink P, Bygdeman S, Emtestam L, *et al.* Roxithromycin compared with doxycycline in the treatment of genital chlamydial infection and non-specific urethritis. *Int J STD AIDS* 1993;**4**:110–13.

186. Stein GE, Mummaw NL, Havlichek DH. A preliminary study of clarithromycin versus doxycycline in the treatment of nongonococcal urethritis and mucopurulent cervicitis. *Pharmacotherapy* 1995;**15**:727–31.

187. Lau C, Qureshi A. Azithromycin versus doxycycline for genital chalmydial infections: a meta-analysis of randomized clinical trials. *Sex Transmit Dis* 2002;**29**:497–502.

188. Fong I, Linton W, Simbul M, *et al.* Treatment of nongonococcal urethritis with ciprofloxacin. *Am J Med* 1987;**82**:311–16.

189. Hooton T, Rogers M, Medina T, *et al.* Ciprofloxacin compared with doxycycline for nongonococcal urethritis. Ineffectiveness against *Chlamydia trachomatis* due to relapsing infection. *JAMA* 1990;**264**:1418–21.

190. Kitchen V, Donegan C, Ward H, *et al.* Comparison of ofloxacin with doxycycline in the treatment of non-gonococcal urethritis and cervical chlamydial infection. *J Antimicrob Chemother* 1990;**26**(Suppl.D):99–105.

191. Mogabgab WJ, Holmes B, Murray M, *et al.* Randomized comparison of ofloxacin and doxycyline for chlamydia and ureaplasma urethritis and cervicitis. *Chemotherapy* 1990;**36**:70–6.

192. Batteiger BE, Jones RB, White A. Efficacy and safety of ofloxacin in the treatment of nongonococcal sexually transmitted disease. *Am J Med* 1989;**87**(Suppl.6C): 75S–77S.
193. Phillips I, Dimian C, Barlow D, *et al.* A comparative study of two different regimens of sparfloxacin versus doxycycline in the treatment of non-gonococcal urethritis in men. *J Antimicrob Chemother* 1996;**37** (Suppl.A):123–34.
194. McCormack WM, Dalu ZA, Martin DH, *et al.* Double-blind comparison of trovafloxacin and doxycycline in the treatment of uncomplicated Chlamydial urethritis and cervicitis. Trovafloxacin Chlamydial Urethritis/Cervicitis Study Group. *Sex Transm Dis* 1999;**26**:531–6.
195. McCormack WM, Martin DH, Hook EW, III, Jones RB. Daily oral grepafloxacin vs. twice daily oral doxycycline in the treatment of *Chlamydia trachomatis* endocervical infection. *Infect Dis Obstet Gynecol* 1998;**6**:109–15.
196. Martin DH, Koutsky L, Eschenbach DA, *et al.* Prematurity and perinatal mortality in pregnancies complicated by maternal *Chlamydia trachomatis* infections. *JAMA* 1982;**247**:1585–8.
197. Rastogi S, Kapur S, Salhan S, Mittal A. *Chlamydia trachomatis* infection in pregnancy: risk factor for an adverse outcome. *Br J Biomed Sci* 1999;**56**:94–8.
198. Rastogi S, Salhan S, Mittal A. Detection of *Chlamydia trachomatis* antigen in spontaneous abortions. Is this organism a primary or secondary indicator of risk? *Br J Biomed Sci* 2000;**57**:126–9.
199. Claman P, Toye B, Peeling RW, *et al.* Serologic evidence of *Chlamydia trachomatis* infection and risk of preterm birth. *CMAJ* 1995;**153**:259–62.
200. Witkin SS, Ledger WJ. Antibodies to *Chlamydia trachomatis* in sera of women with recurrent spontaneous abortions. *Am J Obstet Gynecol* 1992;**167**:135–9.
201. Berman SM, Harrison HR, Boyce WT, *et al.* Low birth weight, prematurity, and postpartum endometritis. Association with prenatal cervical *Mycoplasma hominis* and *Chlamydia trachomatis* infections. *JAMA* 1987;**257**:1189–94.
202. Hammerschlag MR, Anderka M, Semine DZ, *et al.* Prospective study of maternal and infantile infection with *Chlamydia trachomatis*. *Pediatrics* 1979;**64**:142–8.
203. Schachter J, Lum L, Gooding CA, Ostler B. Pneumonitis following inclusion blennorrhea. *J Pediatr* 1975;**87**:779–80.
204. Wager GP, Martin DH, Koutsky L, *et al.* Puerperal infectious morbidity: relationship to route of delivery and to antepartum *Chlamydia trachomatis* infection. *Am J Obstet Gynecol* 1980;**138**:1028–33.
205. Ryan GM, Jr, Abdella TN, McNeeley SG, *et al.* *Chlamydia trachomatis* infection in pregnancy and effect of treatment on outcome. *Am J Obstet Gynecol* 1990;**162**:34–9.
206. Martin DH, Eschenbach DA, Cotch M, *et al.* Double-blind placebo-controlled treatment trial of *Chlamydia trachomatis* endocervical infections in pregnant women. *Infect Dis Obstet Gynecol* 1997;**5**:10–17.
207. Turrentine M, Newton E. Amoxicillin or erythromycin for the treatment of antenatal chlamydial infection: a meta-analysis. *Obstet Gynecol* 1995;**86**:1025.
208. Kacmar J, Cheh E, Montagno A, Peipert JF. A randomized trial of azithromycin versus amoxicillin for the treatment of *Chlamydia trachomatis* in pregnancy. *Infect Dis Obstet Gynecol* 2001;**9**:197–202.
209. Jacobson GF, Autry AM, Kirby RS, *et al.* A randomized controlled trial comparing amoxicillin and azithromycin for the treatment of *Chlamydia trachomatis* in pregnancy. *Am J Obstet Gynecol* 2001;**184**:1352–4.
210. Walker C, Kahn J, Washington A, *et al.* Pelvic inflammatory disease: meta-analysis of antimicrobial regimen efficacy. *J Infect Dis* 2002;**168**:969–78.
211. Ness R, Soper D, Peipert J, *et al.* Effectiveness of inpatient and outpatient treatment strategies for women with pelvic inflammatory disease: results from the Pelvic Inflammatory Disease Evaluation and Clinical Health (PEACH) Randomized Trial. *Am J Obstet Gynecol* 2002;**186**:929–37.
212. Fiumara NJ. Treatment of secondary syphilis: an evaluation of 204 patients. *Sex Transm Dis* 1977;**4**:96–9.
213. Fiumara NJ. Treatment of seropositive primary syphilis: an evaluation of 196 patients. *Sex Transm Dis* 1977;**4**:92–5.
214. Schofer H, Vogt HJ, Milbradt R. Ceftriaxone for the treatment of primary and secondary syphilis. *Chemotherapy* 1989;**35**:140–5.
215. Moorthy TT, Lee CT, Lim KB, Tan T. Ceftriaxone for treatment of primary syphilis in men: a preliminary study. *Sex Transmit Dis* 1987;**14**:116–18.
216. Hook E, Martin D, Stephens J, *et al.* A randomized, comparative pilot study of azithromycin versus

benzathine penicillin G for treatment of early syphilis. *Sex Transm Dis* 2002;**29**:486–90.

217. Gordon S, Eaton M, George R, *et al.* The response of sypmptomatic neurosyphilis to high-dose intravenous penicillin G in patients with human immunodeficiency virus infection. *N Engl J Med* 1994;**331**:1469–73.
218. Berry C, Hooton T, Collier A, Lukehart S. Neurologic relapse after benzathine penicillin therapy for secondary syphilis in a patient with HIV infection. *N Engl J Med* 1987;**316**:1587–9.
219. Rolfs R, Joesoef M, Hendershot E, *et al.* A randomized trial of enhanced therapy for early syphilis in patients with and without human immunodeficiency virus infection. *N Engl J Med* 1997;**337**:307–14.
220. Marra C, Boutin P, McArthur J, *et al.* A pilot study evaluating ceftriaxone and penicillin G as treatment agents for neurosyphilis in human immunodeficiency virus-infected individuals. *Clin Infect Dis* 2000;**30**: 540–4.
221. Hook E, Stephens J, Ennis D. Azithromycin compared with penicillin G benzathine for treatment of incubating syphilis. *Ann Intern Med* 1999;**131**:434–7.
222. Peterman T, Zaidi A, Lieb S, Wroten J. Incubating syphilis in patients treated for gonorrhea: a comparison of treatment regimens. *J Infect Dis* 1994;**170**:689–92.
223. Centers for Disease Control and Prevention. Sexually transmitted diseases treatment guidelines 2002. *MMWR Morb Mortal Wkly Rep* 2002;**51**(RR-6):26–8.
224. Paryani SG, Vaughn AJ, Crosby M, Lawrence S. Treatment of asymptomatic congenital syphilis: benzathine versus procaine penicillin G therapy. *J Pediatr* 1994;**125**:471–5.
225. Radcliffe M, Meyer M, Roditi D, Malan A. Single-dose benzathine penicillin in infants at risk of congenital syphilis–results of a randomized study. *S Afr Med J* 1997;**87**:62–5.
226. Benedetti JK, Zeh J, Selke S, Corey L. Frequency and reactivation of nongenital lesions among patients with genital herpes simplex virus. *Am J Med* 1995;**98**:237–42.
227. Reeves WC, Corey L, Adams HG, *et al.* Risk of recurrence after first episodes of genital herpes. Relation to HSV type and antibody response. *N Engl J Med* 1981;**305**:315–19.
228. Vontver LA, Reeves WC, Rattray M, *et al.* Clinical course and diagnosis of genital herpes simplex virus infection and evaluation of topical surfactant therapy. *Am J Obstet Gynecol* 1979;**133**:548–54.
229. Corey L, Fife K, Benedetti J, *et al.* Intravenous acyclovir for the treatment of primary genital herpes. *Ann Intern Med* 1983;**98**:914–21.
230. Bryson Y, Dillon M, Lovett M, *et al.* Treatment of first episodes of genital herpes simplex virus infection with oral acyclovir. A randomized double-blind controlled trial. *N Engl J Med* 1983;**308**:916–21.
231. Mertz G, Critchlow C, Benedetti J, *et al.* Double-blind placebo-controlled trial of oral acyclovir in first-episode genital herpes simplex virus infection. *JAMA* 1984;**252**:1147–51.
232. Wald A, Benedetti J, Davis G, *et al.* A randomized, double-blind, comparative trial comparing high- and standard-dose oral acyclovir for first-episode genital herpes infections. *Antimicrob Agents Chemother* 1994;**38**:174–6.
233. Ruhnek-Forsbeck M, Sandstrom E, Andersson B, *et al.* Treatment of recurrent genital herpes simplex virus infections with oral acyclovir. *J Antimicrob Chemother* 1985;**16**:621–8.
234. Reichman R, Badger G, Mertz G, *et al.* Treatment of recurrent genital herpes simplex infections with oral acyclovir. A controlled trial. *JAMA* 1984;**251**:2103–7.
235. Stone K, Whittington W. Treatment of genital herpes. Rev Infect *Dis* 1990;**12**(Suppl.6):610–19.
236. Spruance S, Tryring S, Degregorio B, *et al.* A large-scale, placebo-controlled, dose-ranging trial of peroral valacyclovir for episodic treatment of recurrent genital herpes. *Arch Intern Med* 1996;**156**:1729–35.
237. Sacks S, Aoki F, Diaz-Mitoma F, *et al.* Patient-initiated, twice-daily oral famciclovir for early recurrent genital herpes: a randomized, double-blind multicenter trial. *JAMA* 1996;**276**:44–9.
238. Chosidow O, Drouault Y, Leconte-Veyriac F, *et al.* Famciclovir vs. aciclovir in immunocompetent patients with recurrent gential herpes infections: a parallel groups, randomized, double-blind clinical trial. *Br J Dermatol.* 2001;**144**:818–24.
239. Bodsworth N, Crooks R, Borelli S, *et al.* Valaciclovir versus aciclovir in patient initiated treatment of

recurrent genital herpes: a randomized, double blind clinical trial. *Genitourin Med* 1997;**73**:110–16.

240. Leone P, Trottier S, Miller J. Valacyclovir for episodic treatment of genital herpes: a shorter 3-day treatment course compared with 5-day treatment. *Clin Infect Dis* 2002;**34**:958–62.

241. Wald A, Carrell D, Remington M, *et al.* Two-day regimen of acyclovir for treatment of recurrent genital herpes simplex virus type 2 infection. *Clin Infect Dis* 2002;**34**:944–8.

242. Mertz G, Jones C, Mills J, *et al.* Long-term acyclovir suppression of frequently recurring genital herpes simplex virus infection. A multicenter double-blind trial. *JAMA* 1988;**260**:201–6.

243. Kaplowitz L, Baker D, Gelb L, *et al.* Prolonged continuous acyclovir treatment of normal adults with frequently recurring genital herpes simplex virus infection. *JAMA* 1991;**265**:747–51.

244. Mattison H, Reichman R, Benedetti J, *et al.* Double-blind, placebo-controlled trial comparing long-term suppressive with short-term oral acyclovir therapy for management of recurrent genital herpes. *Am J Med* 1988;**85**:20–5.

245. Mindel A, Faherty A, Carney O, *et al.* Dosage and safety of long-term suppressive acyclovir therapy for recurrent genital herpes. *Lancet* 1988;**1**:926–8.

246. Goldberg L, Kaufman R, Kurtz T, *et al.* Long-term suppression of recurrent genital herpes with acyclovir: a 5-year benchmark study. *Arch Dermatol* 1993; **1993**:582–7.

247. Mertz G, Loveless M, Levin M, *et al.* Oral famciclovir for suppression of recurrent genital herpes simplex virus infection in women. A multicenter, double-blind, placebo-controlled trial. *Arch Intern Med* 1997;**157**:343–9.

248. Fife KH, Crumpacker CS, Mertz GJ, *et al.* Recurrence and resistance patterns of herpes simplex virus following cessation of > or =6 years of chronic suppression with acyclovir. Acyclovir Study Group. *J Infect Dis* 1994;**169**:1338–41.

249. Patel R, Bobsworth N, Woolley P, *et al.* Valaciclovir for the suppression of recurrent genital HSV infection: a placebo controlled study of once daily therapy. *Genitourin Med* 1997;**73**:105–9.

250. Reitano M, Tyring S, Lang W, *et al.* Valaciclovir for the suppression of recurrent genital herpes simplex virus infection: a large-scale dose range-finding study. *J Infect Dis* 1998;**178**:603–10.

251. Diaz-Mitoma F, Sibbald R, Shafran S, *et al.* Oral famciclovir for the suppression of recurrent genital herpes: a randomized controlled trial. *JAMA* 1998; **280**:887–92.

252. Wald A, Zeh J, Barnum G, *et al.* Suppression of subclinical shedding of herpes simplex virus type 2 with acyclovir. *Ann Intern Med* 1996;**124**:8–15.

253. Patel R, Tyring S, Strand A, *et al.* Impact of suppressive antiviral therapy on the health related quality of life of patients with recurrent genital herpes infection. *Sex Transm Infect* 1999;**75**:398–402.

254. Carney O, Ross E, Ikkos G, Mindel A. The effect of suppressive oral acyclovir on the psychological morbidity associated with recurrent genital herpes. *Genitourin Med* 1993;**69**:457–9.

255. Brown Z, Selke S, Zeh J, *et al.* The acquisition of herpes simplex virus during pregnancy. *N Engl J Med* 1997;**337**:515.

256. Prober CG, Corey L, Brown ZA, *et al.* The management of pregnancies complicated by genital infections with herpes simplex virus. *Clin Infect Dis* 1992;**15**:1031–8.

257. Watts DH, Brown ZA, Money D, *et al.* A double-blind, randomized, placebo-controlled trial of acyclovir in late pregnancy for the reduction of herpes simplex virus shedding and cesarean delivery. *Am J Obstet Gynecol* 2003;**188**:836–43.

258. Brocklehurst P, Kinghorn G, Carney O, *et al.* A randomized placebo controlled trial of suppressive acyclovir in late pregnancy in women with recurrent genital herpes infection. *Br J Obstet Gynaecol* 1998;**105**:275–80.

259. Stray-Pedersen B. Acyclovir in late pregnancy to prevent neonatal herpes simplex. *Lancet* 1990; **336**:756.

260. Hammond G, Slutchuk M, Lian C, *et al.* The treatment of chancroid: comparison of one week of sulfisoxazole with single dose doxycycline. *J Antimicrob Chemother* 1979;**5**:261–5.

261. Meheus A, Ursi J, Van Dyck E, Ballard R. Treatment of chancroid with single-dose doxycycline compared with a two-day course of co-trimoxazole. *Ann Soc Belg Med Trop.* 1981;**61**:119–24.

262. Rutanarugsa A, Vorachit M, Polnikorn N, Jayanetra P. Drug resistance of *Haemophilus ducreyi*. *SE Asian J Trop Med Publ Health* 1990;**21**:185–93.
263. Fast M, Nsanze H, D'Costa LJ, *et al*. Antimicrobial therapy of chancroid: an evaluation of five treatment regimens correlated with in vitro sensitivity. *Sex Transmit Dis* 1983;**10**:1–6.
264. D'Souza P, Pandhi RK, Khanna N, *et al*. A comparative study of therapeutic response of patients with clinical chancroid to ciprofloxacin, erythromycin, and cotrimoxazole. *Sex Transmit Dis* 1998;**25**:293–5.
265. Plourde PJ, D'Costa LJ, Agoki E, *et al*. A randomized, double-blind study of the efficacy of fleroxacin versus trimethoprim-sulfamethoxazole in men with culture-proven chancroid. *J Infect Dis* 1992;**165**:949–52.
266. Tyndall M, Agoki E, Plummer FA, *et al*. Single dose azithromycin for the treatment of chancroid: a randomized comparison of erythromycin. *Sex Transmit Dis* 1994;**21**:213–34.
267. Naamara W, Plummer F, Greenblatt R, *et al*. Treatment of chancroid with ciprofloxacin. A prospective, randomized clinical trial. *Am J Med* 1987;**82**:317–20.
268. Martin D, Sargent S, Wendel G, *et al*. Comparison of azithromycin and ceftriaxone for the treatment of chancroid. *Clin Infect Dis* 1995;**21**:409–14.
269. Fast M, Nsanze H, D'Costa L, *et al*. Treatment of chancroid by clavulanic acid with amoxycillin in patients with beta-lactamase-positive *Haemophilus ducreyi* infection. *Lancet* 1982;**2**:509–11.
270. Traisupa A, Ariyarit C, Metheeprapha C, *et al*. Treatment of chancroid with spectinomycin or co-trimoxazole. *Clin Ther* 1990;**12**:200–5.
271. Ballard R, da L'Exposto F, Dangor Y, *et al*. A comparative study of spectinomycin and erythromycin in the treatment of chancroid. *J Antimicrob Chemother* 1990;**26**:429–34.
272. Ernst AA, Marvez-Valls E, Martin DH. Incision and drainage versus aspiration of fluctuant buboes in the emergency department during an epidemic of chancroid. *Sex Transmit Dis* 1995;**21**:217–20.
273. Handsfield HH. Clinical presentation and natural course of anogenital warts. *Am J Med* 1997;**102**:16–20.
274. Oriel D. Genital human papillomavirus infection. In: Holmes K, Mardh PA, Sparling P, *et al*., eds. *Sexually Transmitted Diseases*. New York: McGraw-Hill, 1990.
275. Fife K, Ferenczy A, Douglas JM, Jr, *et al*. Treatment of external genital warts in men using 5% imiquimod cream applied three times a week, once daily, twice daily, or three times daily. *Sex Transmit Dis* 2001;**28**:226–31.
276. Stone K, Becker T, Hadgu A, Kraus S. Treatment of external genital warts: a randomized clinical trial comparing podophyllin, cryotherapy, and electrodessication. *Genitourin Med* 1990;**66**:16–19.
277. Connolly M, Bazmi K, O'Connell M, *et al*. Cryotherapy of viral warts: a sustained 10-s freeze is more effective than the traditional method. *Br J Dermatol* 2001;**145**:554–7.
278. Godley M, Bradbeer C, Gellan M, Thin R. Cryotherapy compared with trichloroacetic acid in treating genital warts. *Genitourin Med* 1987;**63**:390–2.
279. Abdullah A, Walzman M, Wade A. Treatment of external genital warts comparing cryotherapy (liquid nitrogen) and trichloroacetic acid. *Sex Transmit Dis* 1993;**20**:344–5.
280. Duus B, Philipsen T, Christensen J, *et al*. Refractory condylomata acuminata: a controlled clinical trial of carbon dioxide laser versus conventional surgical treatment. *Genitourin Med* 1985;**61**:59–61.
281. Simmons P, Langlet F, Thin R. Cryotherapy versus electrocautery in the treatment of genital warts. *Br J Vener Dis* 1981;**57**:273–4.
282. Jensen S. Comparison of podophyllin application with simple surgical excision in clearance and recurrence of perianal condyloma acuminata. *Lancet* 1985;**2**:1146–8.
283. Syed TA, Khayyami M, Kriz D, *et al*. Management of genital warts in women with human leukocyte interferon-alpha vs. podophyllotoxin in cream: a placebo-controlled, double-blind, comparative study. *J Mol Med* 1995;**73**:255–8.
284. Syed TA, Cheema KM, Khayyami M, *et al*. Human leukocyte interferon-alpha versus podophyllotoxin in cream for the treatment of genital warts in males. A placebo-controlled, double-blind, comparative study. *Dermatology* 1995;**191**:129–32.
285. Douglas JM, Jr, Eron LJ, Judson FN, *et al*. A randomized trial of combination therapy with intralesional interferon alpha 2b and podophyllin versus podophyllin alone for the therapy of anogenital warts. *J Infect Dis* 1990;**162**:52–9.

286. Olmos L, Vilata J, Rodriguez PA, *et al.* Double-blind, randomized clinical trial on the effect of interferon-beta in the treatment of condylomata acuminata. *Int J STD AIDS* 1994;**5**:182–5.

287. Gentile G, Formelli G, Busacchi P, Pelusi G. Systemic interferon therapy for female florid genital condylomata. Clin Exp *Obstet Gynecol* 1994;**21**:198–202.

288. Reichman RC, Oakes D, Bonnez W, *et al.* Treatment of condyloma acuminatum with three different interferon-alpha preparations administered parenterally: a double-blind, placebo-controlled trial. *J Infect Dis* 1990;**162**:1270–6.

289. Armstrong DK, Maw RD, Dinsmore WW, *et al.* Combined therapy trial with interferon alpha-2a and ablative therapy in the treatment of anogenital warts. *Genitourin Med* 1996;**72**:103–7.

290. Armstrong DK, Maw RD, Dinsmore WW, *et al.* A randomized, double-blind, parallel group study to compare subcutaneous interferon alpha-2a plus podophyllin with placebo plus podophyllin in the treatment of primary condylomata acuminata. *Genitourin Med* 1994;**70**:389–93.

291. Bonnez W, Oakes D, Bailey-Farchione A, *et al.* A randomized, double-blind, placebo-controlled trial of systemically administered interferon-alpha, -beta, or -gamma in combination with cryotherapy for the treatment of condyloma acuminatum. *J Infect Dis* 1995;**171**:1081–9.

292. Gilson RJ, Shupack JL, Friedman-Kien AE, *et al.* A randomized, controlled, safety study using imiquimod for the topical treatment of anogenital warts in HIV-infected patients. Imiquimod Study Group. *AIDS* 1999;**13**:2397–404.

293. Orlando G, Fasolo MM, Beretta R, *et al.* Combined surgery and cidofovir is an effective treatment for genital warts in HIV-infected patients. *AIDS* 2002;**16**:447–50.

294. Wilson JD, Brown CB, Walker PP. Factors involved in clearance of genital warts. *Int J STD AIDS* 2001;**12**:789–92.

295. Thin RN, Symonds MA, Booker R, *et al.* Double-blind comparison of a single dose and a five-day course of metronidazole in the treatment of trichomoniasis. *Br J Vener Dis* 1979;**55**:354–6.

296. Hager WD, Brown ST, Kraus SJ, *et al.* Metronidazole for vaginal trichomoniasis. Seven-day vs single-dose regimens. *JAMA* 1980;**244**:1219–20.

297. Austin TW, Smith EA, Darwish R, *et al.* Metronidazole in a single dose for the treatment of trichomoniasis. Failure of a 1-g single dose. *Br J Vener Dis* 1982;**58**:121–3.

298. Spence MR, Harwell TS, Davies MC, Smith JL. The minimum single oral metronidazole dose for treating trichomoniasis: a randomized, blinded study. *Obstet Gynecol* 1997;**89**:699–703.

299. Anjaeyulu R, Gupte SA, Desai DB. Single-dose treatment of trichomonal vaginitis: a comparison of tinidazole and metronidazole. *J Int Med Res* 1977;**5**:438–41.

300. Manorama HT, Shenoy DR. Single-dose oral treatment of vaginal trichomoniasis with tinidazole and metronidazole. *J Int Med Res* 1978;**6**:46–9.

301. Gabriel G, Robertson E, Thin RN. Single dose treatment of trichomoniasis. *J Int Med Res* 1982;**10**:129–30.

302. Sobel JD, Nyirjesy P, Brown W. Tinidazole therapy for metronidazole-resistant vaginal trichomoniasis. *Clin Infect Dis* 2001;**33**:1341–6.

303. duBouchet L, Spence MR, Rein MF, *et al.* Multicenter comparison of clotrimazole vaginal tablets, oral metronidazole, and vaginal suppositories containing sulfanilamide, aminacrine hydrochloride, and allantoin in the treatment of symptomatic trichomoniasis. *Sex Transmit Dis* 1997;**24**:156–60.

304. duBouchet L, McGregor JA, Ismail M, McCormack WM. A pilot study of metronidazole vaginal gel versus oral metronidazole for the treatment of *Trichomonas vaginalis* vaginitis. *Sex Transmit Dis* 1998;**25**:176–9.

305. Antonelli NM, Diehl SJ, Wright JW. A randomized trial of intravaginal nonoxynol 9 versus oral metronidazole in the treatment of vaginal trichomoniasis. *Am J Obstet Gynecol* 2000;**182**:1008–10.

306. Lyng J, Christensen J. A double-blind study of the value of treatment with a single dose tinidazole of partners to females with trichomoniasis. *Acta Obstet Gynecol Scand* 1981;**60**:199–201.

307. Shain RN, Perdue ST, Piper JM, *et al.* Behaviors changed by intervention are associated with reduced STD recurrence: the importance of context in measurement. *Sex Transm Dis* 2002;**29**:520–9.

308. Kissinger P, Brown R, Reed K, *et al.* Effectiveness of patient delivered partner medication for preventing recurrent *Chlamydia trachomatis*. *Sex Transm Infect* 1998;**74**:331–3.

309. Ramstedt K, Forssman L, Johannisson G. Contact tracing in the control of genital *Chlamydia trachomatis* infection. *Int J STD AIDS* 1991;**2**:116–18.
310. Schillinger JA, Kissinger P, Calvet H, *et al.* Patient-delivered partner treatment with azithromycin to prevent repeated *Chlamydia trachomatis* infection among women: a randomized, controlled trial. *Sex Transmit Dis* 2003;**30**:49–56.
311. Coutinho R, Lelie N, Albrecht-Van Lent P, *et al.* Efficacy of a heat inactivated hepatitis B vaccine in male homosexuals: outcome of a placebo controlled double blind trial. *BMJ* 1983;**286**:1305–8.
312. Szmuness W, Stevens C, Harley E, *et al.* Hepatitis B vaccine: demonstration of efficacy in a controlled clinical trial in a high-risk population in the United States. *N Engl J Med* 1980;**303**:833–41.
313. Halliday M, Rankin J, Bristow N, *et al.* A randomized double-blind clinical trial of a mammalian cell-derived recombinant DNA hepatitis B vaccine compared with a plasma-derived vaccine. *Arch Intern Med* 1990;**150**: 1195–2000.
314. Sagliocco L, Amoroso P, Stroffolini T, *et al.* Efficacy of hepatitis A vaccine in prevention of secondary hepatitis A infection: a randomized trial. 1999;**353**:1139.
315. Innis BL, Snitbhan R, Kunasol P, *et al.* Protection against hepatitis A by an inactivated vaccine. *JAMA* 1994;**271**: 1328–34.
316. Roumeliotou-Karayannis A, Papaevangelou G, Tassopoulos N, *et al.* Post-exposure active immunoprophylaxis of spouses of acute viral hepatitis B patients. *Vaccine* 1985;**3**:31–4.
317. Stanberry L, Spruance S, Cunningham A, *et al.* Glycoprotein-d-adjuvant vaccine to prevent genital herpes. *N Engl J Med* 2002;**347**:1652–61.
318. Koutsky LA, Ault KA, Wheeler CM, *et al.* A controlled trial of a human papillomavirus type 16 vaccine. *N Engl J Med* 2002;**347**:1645–51.
319. Turner CF, Rogers SM, Miller HG, *et al.* Untreated gonococcal and chlamydial infection in a probability sample of adults. *JAMA* 2002;**287**:726–33.
320. Ku L, St Louis M, Farshy C, *et al.* Risk behaviors, medical care, and chlamydial infection among young men in the United States. *Am J Publ Health* 2002;**92**:1140–3.
321. Scholes D, Stergachis A, Heidrich FE, *et al.* Prevention of pelvic inflammatory disease by screening for cervical chlamydial infection. *N Engl J Med* 1996;**334**:1362–6.
322. Howell MR, Quinn TC, Gaydos CA. Screening for *Chlamydia trachomatis* in asymptomatic women attending family planning clinics. A cost-effectiveness analysis of three strategies. *Ann Intern Med* 1998;**128**:277–84.
323. Wawer MJ, Sewankambo NK, Serwadda D, *et al.* Control of sexually transmitted diseases for AIDS prevention in Uganda: a randomized community trial. Rakai Project Study Group. *Lancet* 1999;**353**:525–35.
324. Gray RH, Wabwire-Mangen F, Kigozi G, *et al.* Randomized trial of presumptive sexually transmitted disease therapy during pregnancy in Rakai, Uganda. *Am J Obstet Gynecol* 2001;**185**:1209–17.
325. Gichangi PB, Ndinya-Achola JO, Ombete J, *et al.* Antimicrobial prophylaxis in pregnancy: a randomized, placebo-controlled trial with cefetamet-pivoxil in pregnant women with a poor obstetric history. *Am J Obstet Gynecol* 1997;**177**:680–4.
326. Temmerman M, Njagi E, Nagelkerke N, *et al.* Mass antimicrobial treatment in pregnancy. A randomized, placebo-controlled trial in a population with high rates of sexually transmitted diseases. *J Reprod Med* 1995; **40**:176–80.
327. Holmes KK, Johnson DW, Kvale PA, *et al.* Impact of a gonorrhea control program, including selective mass treatment, in female sex workers. *J Infect Dis* 1996;**174**(Suppl.2):S230–S239.
328. Jaffe HW, Rice DT, Voigt R, *et al.* Selective mass treatment in a venereal disease control program. *Am J Publ Health* 1979;**69**:1181–2.
329. Rekart M, Patrick D, Chakraborty B, *et al.* Targeted mass treatment for syphilis with oral azithromycin. *Lancet* 2003;**361**:313–14.
330. Kamb ML, Fishbein M, Douglas JM, Jr, *et al.* Efficacy of risk-reduction counseling to prevent human immunodeficiency virus and sexually transmitted diseases: a randomized controlled trial. Project RESPECT Study Group. *JAMA* 1998;**280**:1161–7.
331. Oakeshott P, Kerry S, Hay S, Hay P. Condom promotion in women attending inner city general practices for cervical smears: a randomized controlled trial. *Fam Pract* 2000;**17**:56–9.

332. James NJ, Gillies PA, Bignell CJ. Evaluation of a randomized controlled trial of HIV and sexually transmitted disease prevention in a genitourinary medicine clinic setting. *AIDS* 1998;**12**:1235–42.

333. Pourbohloul B, Rekart ML, Brunham RC. Impact of mass treatment on syphilis transmission: a mathematical modeling approach. *Sex Transmit Dis* 2003;**30**:297–305.

334. Mayaud P, Changalucha J, Grosskurth H, *et al*. The value of urine specimens in screening for male urethritis and its microbial aetiologies in Tanzania. *Genitourin Med* 1992;**68**:361–5.

335. McNagny SE, Parker RM, Zenilman JM, Lewis JS. Urinary leukocyte esterase test: a screening method for the detection of asymptomatic chlamydial and gonococcal infections in men. *J Infect Dis* 1992;**165**: 573–6.

336. Cacciatore B, Leminen A, Ingman-Friberg S, *et al*. Transvaginal sonographic findings in ambulatory patients with suspected pelvic inflammatory disease. *Obstet Gynecol* 1992;**80**:912–16.

337. Tukeva TA, Aronen HJ, Karjalainen PT, *et al*. MR imaging in pelvic inflammatory disease: comparison with laparoscopy and US. *Radiology*. 1999;**210**: 209–16.

338. Boardman LA, Peipert JF, Brody JM, *et al*. Endovaginal sonography for the diagnosis of upper genital tract infection. *Obstet Gynecol* 1997;**90**:54–7.

339. Jue R, Puffer J, Wood RM, *et al*. Comparison of fluorescent and conventional darkfield methods for the detection of *Treponema pallidum* in syphilitic lesions. *Tech Bull Regist Med Technol* 1967;**37**:123–5.

340. Jethwa HS, Schmitz JL, Dallabetta G, *et al*. Comparison of molecular and microscopic techniques for detection of *Treponema pallidum* in genital ulcers. *J Clin Microbiol* 1995;**33**:180–3.

341. Larsen S, Hambie E, Pettit D, *et al*. Specificity, sensitivity, and reproducibility among the fluorescent treponemal antibody-absorbtion test, the microhemagglutionation assay for *Treponema pallidum* antibodies, and the hemagglutination treponemal test for syphilis. *J Clin Microbiol* 1981;**14**:441–5.

342. Huber T, Storms S, Young P, *et al*. Reactivity of microhemaagglutination, fluorescent treponemal antibody absorbtion, Venereal Disease Research Laboratory, and rapid plasma reagin tests in primary syphilis. *J Clin Microbiol* 1983;**17**:405–9.

343. Augenbraun M, Rolfs R, Johnson R, *et al*. Treponemal specific tests for the serodiagnosis of syphilis. *Sex Transmit Dis* 1998;**25**:549–52.

344. Rodriguez I, Alvarez E, Fernandez C, Miranda A. Comparison of a recombinant-antigen enzyme immunoassay with *Treponema pallidum* hemagglutination test for serological confirmation for serological confirmation of syphilis. *Mem Inst Oswaldo Cruz* 2002;**97**:347–9.

345. Sambri V, Marangoni A, Simone M, *et al*. Evaluation of recomWell Treponema, a novel recombinant antigen-based enzyme-linked immunosorbent assay for the diagnosis of syphilis. *Clin Microbiol Infect* 2001;**7**:200–5.

346. Young H, Moyes A, Seagar L, McMillan A. Novel recombinant-antigen enzyme immunoassay for serological diagsnosis of syphilis. *J Clin Microbiol* 1998;**36**:913–17.

347. Castro R, Prieto E, Santo I, *et al*. Evaluation of an enzyme immunoassay technique for detection of antibodies against *Treponema pallidum*. *J Clin Microbiol* 2003;**41**:250–3.

348. Farshy CE, Hunter EF, Helsel LO, Larsen SA. Four-step enzyme-linked immunosorbent assay for detection of *Treponema pallidum* antibody. *J Clin Microbiol* 1985;**21**:387–9.

349. Lefevre JC, Bertrand MA, Bauriaud R. Evaluation of the Captia enzyme immunoassays for detection of immunoglobulins G and M to *Treponema pallidum* in syphilis. *J Clin Microbiol* 1990;**28**:1704–7.

350. Backhouse J, Nesteroff S. *Treponema pallidum* western blot: comparison with the FTA-ABS test as a confirmatory test for syphilis. *Diagn Microbiol Infect Dis* 2001;**39**:9–14.

351. Byrne RE, Laska S, Bell M, *et al*. Evaluation of a *Treponema pallidum* western immunoblot assay as a confirmatory test for syphilis. *J Clin Microbiol* 1992;**30**:115–22.

352. Sambri V, Marangoni A, Eyer C, *et al*. Western immunoblotting with five *Treponema pallidum* recombinant antigens for serologic diagnosis of syphilis. *Clin Diagn Lab Immunol* 2001;**8**:534–9.

353. Plummer F, Maggwa N, D'Costa L, *et al.* Cefotaxime treatment of *Haemophilus ducreyi* infection in Kenya. *Sex Transmit Dis* 1984;**11**:304–7.

354. von Krogh G, Szpak E, Andersson M, Bergelin I. Self-treatment using 0.25%-0.50% podophyllotoxin-ethanol solutions against penile condylomata acuminata: a placebo-controlled comparative study. *Genitourin Med* 1994;**70**:105–9.

355. Beutner K, Conant M, Friedman-Kien A, *et al.* Patient applied podfilox for treatment of genital warts. *Lancet* 1989;**1**:831–4.

356. Greenberg MD, Rutledge LH, Reid R, *et al.* A double-blind, randomized trial of 0.5% podofilox and placebo for the treatment of genital warts in women. *Obstet Gynecol* 1991;**77**:735–9.

357. Kirby P, Dunne A, King DH, Corey L. Double-blind randomized clinical trial of self-administered podofilox solution versus vehicle in the treatment of genital warts. *Am J Med* 1990;**88**:465–9.

358. Edwards L, Ferenczy A, Eron L, *et al.* Self-administered topical 5% imiquimod cream for external anogenital warts. HPV Study Group. Human PapillomaVirus. *Arch Dermatol* 1998;**134**:25–30.

359. Beutner K, Tyring S, Trofatter K, *et al.* Imiquimod, a patient-applied immune-response modifier for treatment of external genital warts. *Antimicrob Agents Chemother* 1998;**42**:789–94.

360. Syed TA, Ahmadpour OA, Ahmad SA, Ahmad SH. Management of female genital warts with an analog of imiquimod 2% in cream: a randomized, double-blind, placebo-controlled study. *J Dermatol* 1998;**25**:429–33.

361. Syed TA, Hadi SM, Qureshi ZA, *et al.* Treatment of external genital warts in men with imiquimod 2% in cream. A placebo-controlled, double-blind study. *J Infect* 2000;**41**:148–51.

362. Eron LJ, Judson F, Tucker S, *et al.* Interferon therapy for condylomata acuminata. *N Engl J Med* 1986;**315**: 1059–64.

363. Friedman-Kien AE, Eron LJ, Conant M, *et al.* Natural interferon alfa for treatment of condylomata acuminata. *JAMA* 1988;**259**:533–8.

364. Vance JC, Bart BJ, Hansen RC, *et al.* Intralesional recombinant alpha-2 interferon for the treatment of patients with condyloma acuminatum or verruca plantaris. *Arch Dermatol* 1986;**122**:272–7.

365. Welander CE, Homesley HD, Smiles KA, Peets EA. Intralesional interferon alfa-2b for the treatment of genital warts. *Am J Obstet Gynecol* 1990;**162**:348–54.

11
Human immunodeficiency virus (HIV)

Brian J Angus, Timothy EA Peto

Primary HIV infection

Case presentation 1

A 52-year-old homosexual man is feeling unwell with fever, malaise, a diffuse maculopapular rash and lymphadenopathy. He holidays regularly in Thailand and has had unprotected sexual intercourse with a regular Thai partner as well as with five commercial sex workers in Bangkok. You suspect he has primary HIV infection, ask how best to make the diagnosis and whether he should be treated with antiretroviral drugs immediately.

Diagnostic confirmation

A recent study compared the sensitivity and specificity of clinical symptoms, three HIV-1 RNA viral load assays, a p24 antigen enzyme immunoassay (EIA), and a third-generation enzyme immunoassay antibody test for diagnosis of primary HIV infection.[1] Of 258 eligible persons screened 40 had primary/early infection (22 pre-seroconversion, 18 within 6 months of seroconversion) and 218 did not. Primary HIV infection (PHI) was defined as a negative or indeterminate antibody test with subsequent seroconversion. The symptoms most strongly associated with PHI in multivariate analysis were fever (OR 5·2; 95% CI 2·3–11·7) and rash (OR 4·8; 95% CI 2·4–9·8). The sensitivity and specificity, respectively, for detecting pre-seroconversion HIV infection were: p24 antigen, 79% and 99%; third-generation EIA, 79% and 97%; HIV-1 RNA by branched chain DNA 100% and 95%; HIV-1 RNA by polymerase chain reaction 100% and 97%; HIV-1 RNA by transcription-mediated amplification testing, 100% and 98%. False-positive HIV-1 RNA tests were not reproducible and had values < 3000 copies/mL, while only one person with confirmed PHI was in this range.

Early treatment

In primary PHI there are no data on long-term clinical outcomes. Any perceived benefit comes from *in vitro* studies showing better immunological responses.[2,3] There is one study of zidovudine monotherapy in PHI from 1993 in which 77 patients were randomly assigned to receive either zidovudine (250 mg twice daily; N = 39) or placebo (N = 38) for 6 months.[4] Among the 43 patients who were still symptomatic at the time of enrolment, there was no difference in the mean duration of the retroviral syndrome of 15 days. During a mean follow up period of 15 months, minor opportunistic infections developed in eight patients: oral candidiasis in four, herpes zoster in two, and oral hairy leukoplakia in two. Disease progression was significantly less frequent in the zidovudine group (one opportunistic infection) than in the placebo group (seven opportunistic infections; $P = 0{\cdot}009$ by the log-rank test). After adjustment for the base-line CD4 cell count, the patients treated with zidovudine had an average gain of 8·9 CD4 cells/mm^3 per month (95% CI 1·4–19·1) during the first 6 months of the study, whereas those receiving placebo had an average loss of 12·0 CD4 cells/mm^3 per month (95% CI 5·2 to 18·7), for a between-group difference of 20·9 CD4 cells/mm^3 per month (95% CI 8·5–33·2; $P = 0{\cdot}001$). No long-term clinical benefits have been found.

Asymptomatic HIV infection

There is no good clinical evidence for when to start antiretroviral drug therapy in asymptomatic HIV-positive individuals. There is one Cochrane review (search date not stated, five randomized controlled trials (RCTs), 7722 people with asymptomatic HIV mainly with CD4 counts > 200 mm^3) comparing zidovudine given immediately versus zidovudine deferred until the early signs of AIDS.[5] It found that immediate versus deferred treatment significantly increased AIDS-free survival at 1 year (78/4431 [1·76%] with immediate zidovudine *v* 131/3291 [3·98%] with deferred zidovudine; OR 0·52; 95% CI 0·39–0·68), but the difference was not significant at the end of the RCTs (median follow up of 50 months; 1026/4431 [23·2%] with immediate zidovudine *v* 882/3291 [26·8%] with deferred zidovudine; OR 0·96; 95% CI 0·87–1·05). Overall survival was similar in the two groups at 1 year (24/4431 [5·4%] with immediate zidovudine *v* 18/3291 [5·5%] with deferred zidovudine; OR 1·22; 95% CI 0·67–2·25) and at the end of the RCTs (734/4431 [16·6%] with immediate zidovudine *v* 617/3291 [18·7%] with deferred zidovudine; OR 1·04; 95% CI 0·93–1·16). The conclusion was that, although an initial effect was seen, this was not sustained. There is as yet no similar evidence for so-called triple or highly active antiretroviral therapy (HAART).

As far as harm from early zidovudine is concerned there is a meta-analysis of pooled toxicity data in terms of events per 100 patient-years. Longest follow up was 3 years.[6] In asymptomatic people, early treatment conferred a small but significant increase in the risk of anemia (RR of hemoglobin < 8·0 g/dL, early *v* deferred treatment 2·1; 95% CI 1·1–4·1; AR 0·4 events per 100 person-years). There was also a small increase in risk of neutropenia with early treatment (AR 1·1 events per 100 person-years; $P = 0·07$).

Prognostic features for progression of disease

There is conflicting evidence about the value of viral load at baseline. Early studies suggested that high viral load was associated with an increased risk of death[7] and it is certainly associated with a more rapid fall in CD4 count. However, a meta-analysis of outcomes for people starting HAART was published recently[8] and showed only a small effect of viral load influencing outcome. The analysis included 12 574 people, 79% of whom were men: 21% had HIV disease classified as CDC stage 3 (AIDS); 80% began therapy with a protease inhibitor and two nucleoside analogues. At baseline, the median CD4 count was 250 cells, and the median viral load was 4·9 log. After 6 months of treatment, the median CD4 count had increased to 343 cells, and 73% of the cohort had a viral load below 400 copies.

During 24 310 person-years of follow up, there were 870 AIDS events and 344 deaths (a total of 1094 events of either AIDS or death). The researchers calculated the risk of disease progression at 1, 2 or 3 years after beginning treatment according to five key baseline variables: CD4 count, viral load, age, transmission category, and CDC stage.

Overall, a CD4 count < 200, viral load > 5 log (100 000 copies), age > 50, being an injecting drug user, and being in CDC stage 3 predicted a poorer outcome. There is a useful online risk calculator at http://www.art-cohort-collaboration.org

Summary

Nucleic acid-based tests are sensitive and specific for the diagnosis of primary HIV infection. There are no RCTs evaluating delayed versus early treatment with three drug regimens, although most guidelines suggest treatment for symptomatic early disease.[9,10] These studies, although necessary, are unlikely to be conducted in the near future. RCTs conducted when zidovudine was the only drug available found no significant difference between immediate versus delayed treatment in survival at 1 year despite early changes in surrogate markers.

Case presentation 1 (continued)

The patient tests positive for HIV antibody. His CD4 count is 560 cells/mL with a HIV viral load of 100 000 copies/mL by PCR. He is offered treatment because he is symptomatic but declines it. He has a calculated risk of AIDS after starting HAART of 6·0% (95% CI 4·8–7·6) and of death of 2·0% (95% CI 1·5–3·4) at the end of year 3 of treatment.

Tuberculosis

Case presentation 2

A 38-year-old female asylum seeker from Ethiopia is admitted directly from an airport health-screening clinic. She is said to have an abnormal chest *x* ray film with a cough, hemoptysis, and weight loss. On examination she has a fever with a temperature of 38·2°C, a pulse of 80 per minute, BP 142/80 mmHg, and respiratory rate of 24 per minute. She looks pale and has widespread lymphadenopathy and hepatosplenomegaly. Her full blood count shows a hemoglobin of 8·4, white cell count of 4·3, platelets of 166. Blood film is normochromic and normocytic and there are no malarial parasites seen on three occasions. Biochemistry is normal. Her chest *x* ray film shows left apical infiltration. She tests seropositive for HIV-1 infection, hepatitis B surface and core antibody positive, but she is antigen negative. She is hepatitis C seronegative and VDRL negative. CD4 count is 310, viral load 70 000 copies/mL. You suspect she has *Mycobacterium tuberculosis* infection complicating HIV infection. She has evidence of previous hepatitis B infection. You question how best to confirm the diagnosis of tuberculosis (TB) and what your treatment options are.

The prevalence of *Mycobacterium tuberculosis* (MTB)/HIV coinfection worldwide is 0·18% and 640 000 incident TB cases (8%) have HIV infection.[11] There are currently estimated to be 40 million people living with HIV infection, 28·5 million of them in Africa.[12] An estimated 1·87 million (1·4–2·8 million) people have died of TB and the global case fatality rate is 23% but exceeds 50% in some African countries with high HIV rates, for example Ethiopia; 80% of all incident TB cases have been found in 22 developing countries. Nine of 10 countries with the highest incidence rates per capita were in Africa.

Diagnosis

Significant clinical differences have been found between patients who are sputum smear-positive with acid alcohol fast bacilli (AFB) and those who are smear-negative with respect to cough, sputum production, and typical chest *x* ray film appearance (79%, 76%, and 79% sensitivity, respectively). There was no difference between HIV seropositive and seronegative patients.[13]

Sputum samples are just as likely to be AFB-positive in HIV-positive as -negative patients[14] and induced sputum may increase the yield.[15] Concentration methods of liquefied sputum in a large cohort of consecutive patients with suspected pulmonary TB showed that the overall sensitivity increased from 54·2% using conventional direct microscopy to 63·1% after concentration ($P < 0·0015$). In HIV-positive patients, sensitivity increased from 38·5% to 50·0% ($P < 0·0034$).[16]

Treatment

The efficacy of a 6-month short-course quadruple drug regimen of chemotherapy for pulmonary TB in the presence of HIV infection was confirmed in a study performed in Kinshasa, Zaire. After 6 months, 260 of 335 HIV-seropositive and 186 of 188 HIV-seronegative participants could be evaluated, and their rates of treatment failure were similar at 3·8 and 2·7%, respectively. At 24 months, the HIV-seropositive patients who received 6 months' extended treatment of rifampicin and isoniazid twice weekly had a relapse rate of 1·9%, as compared with 9% among the HIV-seropositive patients who received placebo for the second 6 months ($P < 0{\cdot}01$). Extended treatment, however did not improve survival.[17]

Antituberculosis prophylaxis

Without prophylaxis, people who are HIV- and tuberculin skin test-positive have a 50% or more lifetime risk of developing active TB compared with a 10% lifetime risk in people who are HIV-positive but tuberculin skin test-negative.[18] Two systematic reviews have found that anti-TB prophylaxis reduces the rate of developing active TB and death in the short term in people who are HIV- and tuberculin skin test-positive. A Cochrane review identified six well-conducted RCTs in 4652 HIV-positive adults from Haiti, Kenya, USA, Zambia, and Uganda.[19] All compared isoniazid (6–12 months) or combination therapy (3 months) with placebo. Mean follow up was 2–3 years, and the main outcomes, stratified by tuberculin skin test positivity, were TB (either microbiological or clinical) and death. Among tuberculin skin test-positive adults, anti-TB prophylaxis significantly reduced the incidence of TB (RR compared with placebo 0·24; 95% CI 0·14–0·40) and was associated with a trend towards reducing the risk of death (RR compared with placebo 0·77; 95% CI 0·58–1·03). Among tuberculin skin test-negative adults, there was no significant difference in risk of TB (RR compared with placebo 0·87; 95% CI 0·56–1·36) or death (RR compared with placebo 1·07; 95% CI 0·88–1·30). There was a significant increase in adverse drug reactions requiring cessation of treatment on isoniazid compared with placebo (RR 1·75; 95% CI 1·23–2·47).

The second review of seven trials with 4529 people compared isoniazid with placebo or no treatment.[20] Among tuberculin skin test-positive participants the incidence of TB was significantly reduced (RR compared with placebo 0·40; 95% CI 0·24–0·65), but this was not so among tuberculin skin test-negative participants (RR compared with placebo 0·84; 95% CI 0·54–1·30). This review found no evidence of any impact on mortality. In this analysis, the estimated RR of stopping treatment because of adverse reactions was 1·36 (95% CI 1·00–1·86).[20]

There is insufficient evidence about the long-term effects of prophylaxis on rates of TB and death and the reviews found no evidence of benefit in people who are HIV-positive but tuberculin skin test-negative. There is evidence from RCTs that regimens using combinations of TB drugs for 2–3 months for prophylaxis have similar effectiveness as those using isoniazid alone for 6–12 months. One RCT has found that adverse reactions causing cessation of treatment are more common with multidrug regimens.[20]

Summary

TB remains one of the commonest causes of illness in the world both in HIV-infected and uninfected individuals. The diagnostic and therapeutic approach should be the same. Anti-TB chemoprophylaxis may be useful in HIV-positive people who are also tuberculin skin test-positive. However, in areas with constantly high rates of TB exposure, the impact of this is not clear.

Case presentation 2 (continued)

Her sputum is positive for AFB and she is commenced on rifampicin, isoniazid, pyrazinamide, and ethambutol orally for 6 months. Sputum culture is positive for *Mycobacterium tuberculosis* which is fully sensitive to rifampicin, isoniazid, streptomycin, pyrazinamide, and ethambutol.

The main concern in this patient is to treat her TB infection effectively. She is at some risk of hepatotoxicity (see later). Since this patient's CD4 count is adequate it would be prudent not to commence any other potentially hepatotoxic drugs or drugs that potentially may interact with her anti-TB therapy; starting HAART can probably be safely deferred.

Pneumocystis carinii pneumonia

Case presentation 3

A 42-year-old Zimbabwean male nurse presents to the Accident and Emergency Department. He is short of breath on exertion and has a fever of 39°C, pulse 110 per minute, and a blood pressure of 110/76 mmHg. Pulse oximetry shows an oxygen saturation of 83% on room air. You suspect *Pneumocystis carinii* pneumonia (PCP) and wonder how best to investigate and manage him?

PCP remains the most common AIDS-related opportunistic infection (OI), usually occurring among those not receiving primary care.[21]

Diagnosis

Kovacs[22] described the differences between the clinical characteristics of PCP in 49 HIV-infected and those in 39 HIV-negative persons. At presentation, patients with AIDS had a longer median duration of symptoms (28 *v* 5 days) and higher median room air arterial oxygen tension (69 *v* 52 mmHg [9·2–6·9 kPa]). The sensitivities for detection of *P. carinii* in induced sputum were 92% with silver stain, 97% with direct immunofluorescent antibody (DFA), 97% with indirect immunofluorescent antibody (IFA), and 92% with Diff-Quik (DQ) (a modified Giemsa stain). The sensitivities for detection in bronchoalveolar lavage (BAL) were 86% with silver stain, 90% with DFA, 86% with IFA, and 81% with DQ.[23] PCR seems to be more sensitive than any of these methods.[24] The sensitivity of induced sputum for the diagnosis of *P. carinii* was 13% and of BAL 77%. In the subgroup of patients with an adequate induced sputum sample, the sensitivity of induced sputum was 28%.[25]

Treatment

In the pre-AIDS era, an early study showed that co-trimoxazole (trimethoprim-sulfamethoxazole, TMP-SMX) was as effective as pentamidine in children with PCP and with fewer side effects. Of the 26 patients initially treated with co-trimoxazole, 20 recovered, 17 after co-trimoxazole alone and three of nine who were crossed over to pentamidine. Of the 24 patients initially treated with pentamidine, 18 recovered: 14 of 15 who received only pentamidine and four of nine who were crossed over to co-trimoxazole.[26] This was confirmed in the treatment of AIDS when 36 recipients of TMP-SMX and 33 recipients of pentamidine completed therapy without crossover. Co-trimoxazole caused a rash (44%) and anemia (39%) more frequently ($P < 0{\cdot}03$), whereas pentamidine caused nephrotoxicity (64%), hypotension (27%), or hypoglycemia (21%) more frequently ($P < 0{\cdot}01$). The arterial alveolar oxygen gradient ([A–a] DO_2) improved by greater than 1·3 kPa (10 mmHg) 8 days earlier for co-trimoxazole recipients (95% CI for the difference in response, −1,17; $P = 0{\cdot}04$). Thirty-one (86%) patients treated with co-trimoxazole and 20 (61%) with pentamidine survived and were without respiratory support at completion of treatment (95% CI for the difference in response, 5,45%; $P = 0{\cdot}03$).[27]

There is evidence from RCTs that corticosteroids are a useful adjunct to therapy in severe PCP: 10 patients with AIDS and deteriorating PCP had 7 days of intravenous methylprednisolone added to their antibiotic regimen; eight similar patients were treated with co-trimoxazole alone; nine of the 10 methylprednisolone-treated patients survived their episode of PCP, compared with two of the eight conventionally treated patients. Clinical improvement was evident within 2 days of the start of steroid therapy, and in none of the 10 patients did clinical deterioration or recurrence of PCP occur on cessation of steroid therapy. In one steroid-treated patient disseminated herpes zoster developed 2 days after discontinuation of methylprednisolone.[28]

In a double-blind, placebo-controlled trial patients with marked abnormalities in gas exchange, who had been treated with antibiotics for < 72 hours, were randomly assigned to receive either methylprednisolone (40 mg) or placebo every 6 hours for 7 days, in addition to treatment for 21 days with TMP-SMX: nine out of 12 patients treated with steroids (75%) survived until hospital discharge, as compared with only two of 11 placebo recipients (18%) ($P < 0{\cdot}008$). Respiratory failure developed in nine placebo recipients, as compared with only three patients treated with corticosteroids ($P < 0{\cdot}008$). No patient required the interruption or discontinuation of corticosteroid or antibiotic treatment because of toxicity or a complicating event. Because of the marked difference in survival, it was deemed unethical to continue the trial, and the study was terminated.[29]

A total of 333 patients with AIDS and PCP received standard treatment and were randomly assigned to receive either 40 mg of prednisolone twice daily or no additional therapy. The primary endpoints in this unblinded trial were the occurrence of respiratory failure (hypoxemia ratio [partial pressure of arterial oxygen divided by fraction of inspired oxygen] < 75, intubation, or death), death, and dose-limiting toxicity of the initial standard therapy. Of the patients with confirmed or presumed PCP (N = 225 and N = 26, respectively), those assigned to treatment with corticosteroids had a lower cumulative risk at 31 days of respiratory failure (0·14 *v* 0·30, $P = 0{\cdot}004$) and of death (0·11 *v* 0·23, $P = 0{\cdot}009$), as well as a lower risk of death within 84 days (0·16 *v* 0·26, $P = 0{\cdot}026$). The frequency of dose-limiting toxicity of the standard therapy was similar in the two treatment groups. Intention-to-treat analyses of the entire cohort confirmed these findings. Clinical benefit could not be demonstrated, however, for patients with mild disease (hypoxemia ratio, > 350), equivalent to a partial pressure of oxygen > 9·9 kPa (75 mmHg) on room air. The patients assigned to corticosteroid treatment had an excess of localized herpetic lesions (26% *v* 15%, $P = 0{\cdot}04$) but not of other infections or of neoplasms.[30]

Fifty-nine HIV-1 infected patients with a microscopically proven first episode of moderate to severe PCP were enrolled into a randomized European multicenter study. The effect of adjunctive corticosteroid (CS) therapy was assessed on: survival to discharge, need for mechanical ventilation (MV) and survival at day 90.

Intravenous methylprednisolone 2 mg/kg was given within 24 hours of standard therapy daily for 10 days. All patients received co-trimoxazole as standard treatment. Inclusion criteria were a $Pa\text{O}_2$ < 9·0 kPa (67·5 mmHg) and/or a $Pa\text{CO}_2$ < 4·0 kPa (30·0 mmHg). During the acute episode of PCP, nine (31%) of the 29 control patients died versus three (10%) of the 30 CS-treated patients ($P = 0{\cdot}01$). Mechanical ventilation was necessary in 15 patients; 12 (41%) in the control group and three (10%) in the steroid group ($P = 0{\cdot}01$). The 90-day survival was 69% in patients receiving co-trimoxazole alone versus 87% in patients receiving adjunctive therapy ($P = 0{\cdot}07$).[31]

Although the addition of early short-term high-dose methylprednisolone did not significantly affect the outcome of PCP in 78 patients with HIV and a $P\text{O}_2$ < 9·3 kPa (70 mmHg) on room air at presentation, it did lower the incidence of hypersensitivity reactions to co-trimoxazole. Patients were randomized to receive methylprednisolone (40 mg) or placebo parenterally twice daily for 10 days within 24 hours of the first dose of antimicrobial therapy for PCP. The primary endpoint included death, need for mechanical ventilation for >6 days, or a partial Pao_2 < 70 mmHg while breathing room air 10 days after initiation of treatment. There was no statistically significant difference in the primary endpoint between patients randomized to CS or placebo ($P = 0{\cdot}522$; 95% CI = −0·30, 0·16). The incidence of superinfections during therapy or of other HIV-associated infections or malignancies in the 6 months following treatment for PCP was not significantly different between the two groups. More patients randomized to placebo had to discontinue treatment with co-trimoxazole because of hypersensitivity than those randomized to corticosteroids ($P = 0{\cdot}039$).[32]

In mild disease (O_2 saturations >90% by pulse oximetry), early deterioration developed in 7/12 patients on placebo and 1/11 patients taking 60 mg per day oral prednisolone respectively ($P = 0{\cdot}027$). Even though patients suffering early deterioration in the placebo group were switched to corticosteroids, significant differences between the groups remained at day 30 with regard to exercise tolerance. More than half of patients assigned to the corticosteroid group exercised for a median of 6·5 minutes on day 30 ($P = 0{\cdot}017$).[33]

Alternative treatments

The combination of clindamycin plus primaquine appears to be the most effective alternative treatment for patients with PCP who are unresponsive to first-line therapy.[34] In a meta-analysis of 27 published clinical drug trials, case series, and case reports 497 patients with microbiologically confirmed PCP (456 with HIV), whose initial antipneumocystis treatment had failed and who required alternative drug therapy, were reviewed. Failed regimens included co-trimoxazole (160 patients), intravenous pentamidine (63 patients), co-trimoxazole and/or pentamidine (258 patients), aerosolized pentamidine (six patients), atovaquone (three patients), dapsone (three patients), a combination product of trimethoprim and dapsone (two patients), and co-trimoxazole followed by a combination of clindamycin and primaquine phosphate (two patients). Efficacies of salvage regimens were as follows: clindamycin-primaquine [42–44 [88–92%] of 48 patients; $P < 10^{-8}$], atovaquone [4/5 [80%]], eflornithine hydrochloride [40/70 [57%]; $P < 0{\cdot}01$], co-trimoxazole [27/51 [53%]; $P < 0{\cdot}08$], pentamidine [64/164[39%]], and trimetrexate [47/159 [30%]].

Summary

PCP remains the most common AIDS-related OI and there is evidence supporting the use of co-trimoxazole and steroids for its treatment.

Case presentation 3 (continued)

PCP is suspected on CXR and confirmed on silver staining of BAL fluid and he recovers well with intravenous co-trimoxazole therapy and steroids. He is continued on oral co-trimoxazole as secondary prophylaxis.

Adherence to regimen

Case presentation 4

A 28-year-old homeless, intravenous drug user is admitted with widespread psoriasis to the dermatology ward. He is found to have diffuse generalized lymphadenopathy and oral candidiasis. He is tested for HIV and found to be positive. His CD4 count is now measured at 120 cells/mL and the viral load is 1 000 000 copies/mL. He is hepatitis C antibody-positive, HCV RNA-positive and hepatitis B surface antigen-negative. He wants to know what treatment you would recommend and you wonder what might be useful in helping him to adhere to the treatment plan.

The question of which drugs to start in the treatment of naive patients is still unanswered and unlikely to be addressed in a large enough trial; however, a recent large Cochrane meta-analysis has provided evidence that three drugs are better than two, and two better than monotherapy.[35] There were 20 404 patients included in the 54 randomized controlled trials with 66 comparison groups included in the analysis. For both the clinical outcomes and surrogate markers, combinations with up to, and including, three drugs (HAART) were progressively and significantly more effective. The odds ratio for disease progression or death for triple therapy compared with double therapy was 0·6 (95% CI 0·5–0·8). There was heterogeneity in effect sizes probably related to the different drugs used and differences in trial design. The question of which three drugs should be used initially or even from which class they should come remains unanswered.

There are no data concerning which drugs have superior clinical outcomes. Recent studies looking at surrogate markers, in particular a drop in viral load to below a detectable level at 48 weeks seem to favor a combination of zidovudine/lamivudine and efavirenz. ACTG 384 enrolled 980 naive patients with a CD4 count of around 278 and viral load of 87 000 copies and compared six arms involving zidovudine/ lamivudine versus stavudine/didanosine with either efavirenz and/or nelfinavir.[36] It showed a trend favoring zidovudine/lamivudine/efavirenz at 28 months. Preliminary results from the CLASS study in 297 naive patients with relatively high viral loads of 4·9 log and CD4 counts around 300, randomized to ritonavir-amprenavir, efavirenz or stavudine plus abacavir/lamivudine at 48 weeks, again showed the efavirenz group more likely to achieve viral suppression (76% *v* 53% *v* 62% respectively).[37] It needs to be emphasized that these results relate to surrogate markers and not to clinical outcome. It has not been established that early virological suppression is associated with a better clinical outcome.

There are obviously other considerations about which drug is suitable for individual patients, for example the teratogenicity of efavirenz makes it less attractive for women of childbearing age. Zidovudine is usually avoided in patients with anemia or when anemia can be predicted to occur with treatment such as ribavirin for HCV or chemotherapy for lymphoma. Nevirapine is more likely to cause severe rashes in women rather than men.[38]

Compliance has been shown to be an important factor in the long-term outcome of treatment. It may be that the easiest drug combination to comply with will be the most effective irrespective of drug potency or resistance profile. Adherence to any long-term drug regimen is difficult; however, it is of particular importance in the treatment of HIV because of the propensity of the virus to mutate and escape drug control. Good adherence can predict for viral suppression[39] and the development of viral resistance is associated with low blood drug levels usually owing to poor adherence.[40,41] There have been observations that even a 10% increase in adherence can lead to a 20% reduction in disease progression[42] and there are suggestions that with 100% adherence results are even better.[43]

To assess the effect of HAART adherence on survival in HIV-infected patients, a cohort study was performed on patients who began ART during the period 1990–1999. Patients were considered non-adherent if the total dose of antiretroviral drug was less than 90% of that prescribed. Adherence was assessed through self-reporting and hospital pharmacy appointments. A total of 1219 patients were included. The first drug regimen was with monotherapy in 23·7% of cases, with two drugs in 30·5%, and with triple therapy (HAART) in

45·8%. In multivariate analysis, the variables that presented significant differences with respect to mortality were clinical stage at the beginning of treatment (AIDS: relative hazard [RH] = 2·97; 95% CI 2·14–4·13), CD4 cell count (< 200 cells/microliter^{-1}: RH = 5·89; 95% CI 3·44–10·10), type of treatment (monotherapy: RH = 9·76; 95% CI 4·56–20·9); bi-therapy (RH = 9·12; 95% CI 4·23–19·64), and adherence (non-adherence: RH = 3·87; 95% CI 1·77–8·46).[44] A systematic review of 76 studies showed that once or twice a day was better than more frequent dosing (compliance with one dose = 79% ± 14%; two doses = 69% ± 15%; three doses = 65% ± 16%; four doses = 51% ± 20% (P < 0·001 among dose schedules, no significant difference between one and two doses).[45]

The principal factors associated with non-adherence for HAART appear to be mainly patient-related, reflecting the types of individuals affected by HIV including homelessness and substance and alcohol abuse. Increased community and social input can help.[46] However, other factors may also contribute, such as inconvenient dosing frequency, dietary restrictions, pill burden, side effects,[47] patient healthcare provider relationships, and the system of care.[48]

As far as HAART adherence specifically is concerned, there have been eight RCTs focusing on education, the use of electronic monitoring devices, and social programs. The first, a prospective, randomized, two-arm controlled study, included patients starting their first-or second-line HAART and who were randomized to receive psychoeducative intervention to implement adherence (experimental group, EG) or a usual medical follow up (control group, CG). Self-reported adherence was registered at each visit and its "veracity" was tested by randomized blood analyzes performed without previous warning in 40% of patients. Appropriate adherence was defined as the consumption of > 95% of medication prescribed. A total of 116 patients were included and at week 48, 94% of patients in the EG versus 69% in the CG achieved 95% adherence (P = 0·008); 89% of patients in the EG versus 66% in the CG had HIV-1 RNA levels < 400 copies/mL (P = 0·026). Overall, 85% of patients with good adherence but only 45% of those with poor adherence had undetectable viral load (P = 0·008). In a multivariate analysis, variables significantly related to adherence were: having received a psychoeducative intervention (OR 6·58; P = 0·04), poor effort to take medication (OR 5·38; P = 0·03), and high self-perceived capacity to follow the regimen (OR 13·76; P = 0·04). Self-reported adherence and drug plasma levels coincided in 93% of cases. However, differences in adherence did not reach statistical significance in the ITT analysis although a clear tendency toward benefit was observed in the EG.[49]

Knobel randomized 170 people (2:1) taking zidovudine/lamivudine/indinavir to receive standard care or to receive detailed information on their therapy and for it to be adapted to their lifestyle. Adherence was measured by structured interview and pill counts. Patients who took more than 90% of their doses were defined as adherent. After 24 weeks, there was a significant difference in adherence between groups (76·7% intervention *v* 52·7% control), but no difference in proportions with viral load < 50 copies.[50] Gifford randomized 168 people taking HAART to either a group-based patient education program (SME), a social support (SS) control, or a printed materials (PM) control group. A trained nurse and peer educator taught adherence and self-care skills-led SME over six 2-hour sessions. Adherence was measured by self-report and summarized as excellent (100%); fair (80–99%); or poor (< 80%). Self-report was associated with serum drug levels. Immediately after the intervention, adherence levels were better in SME compared with PM, but no different to SS, regardless of baseline level. After 6 months' follow up, there was no difference in adherence level between the three groups at any baseline adherence level. The authors conclude that benefits gained from adherence interventions may not persist over the longer term without reinforcement.[51]

A study was made of 365 HAART recipients who were randomized to take part in a Treatment Education Program (TEP) or to a control arm that received standard follow up. The TEP included four face-to-face educational sessions of 1 hour each, conducted by doctor or a nurse, using a toolkit called "Ciel Bleu", designed to teach patients about HIV pathogenesis, disease progression, the rationale for anti-HIV therapy, and the importance of adherence. TEP patients also received a beeper pillbox, and a number of devices to aid treatment scheduling. Every 6 months, participants self-reported adherence over the previous week via a questionnaire. At entry, mean viral load was 2·42 log, mean duration of prior treatment was 4 years, 57% had viral load below 200 copies, and adherence levels were comparable across the two arms, with 46% belonging to the upper level adherence stratum. Over 6 months' follow up, adherence levels improved in the TEP group, and fell in the control arm but this was not translated into appreciable changes in viral load and CD4 count in either group.[52]

After a 2-week period where adherence to HAART was monitored using an electronic pill cap, 71 people who recorded < 90% adherence were randomized to continued monitoring or to receive a pager (MediMom, an internet-based paging system). Adherence level at randomization was 56%. The pager was associated with improved adherence at week 2 (70% *v* 56% in the non-pager group), and at week 12 (64% *v* 52% respectively). It was noted that adherence in this population remained inadequate even following the intervention.[53]

In a comparative HAART trial (ACTG 388), 282 individuals were enrolled to standard adherence care versus standard care plus scripted telephone calls (16 calls over 96 weeks). Adherence was measured at clinic visits by self-report over the previous 4 days; 73% of phone calls were completed successfully. Over 64% of subjects in each arm reported > 95% adherence, and > 61% reported 100% adherence; 34% of subjects met criteria for virological failure. There was no difference in time to virological failure between arms. The authors concluded that within a clinical trial setting, telephone calls did not improve high levels of reported adherence, or virological outcome.[54]

HIV-infected predominantly African American males (N = 55) who had histories of heroin or cocaine use (80%) on stable HAART regimens had 4-weekly sessions of either non-directive inquiries about adherence (control group, C), cue-dose training, which consisted of the use of personalized cues for remembering particular dose times, and feedback about medication taking using Medication Event Monitoring System (MEMS) pill bottle caps, which record time of bottle opening (CD group), or cue-dose training combined with cash reinforcement for correctly timed bottle opening (CD + CR). Opening of the pill bottle within 2 hours before or after a predetermined time was measured by MEMS. Adherence to the medication as documented by MEMS was significantly enhanced during the 4-week training period in the CD + CR group, but not in the CD group, compared with the control group. Improvement was also seen in adherence to antiretroviral drugs that were not the object of training and reinforcement. Following discontinuation of training and reinforcement at 8 weeks, adherence in the cash-reinforced group returned to near-baseline levels.[55]

Wall randomized 27 individuals undergoing methadone maintenance treatment with low adherence to AZT monotherapy to receive either 8 weeks of weekday supervised dispensing of therapy or standard care. Adherence was measured by self-report, erythrocyte mean corpuscular volume (MCV), MEMS, and pills counting. MCV levels were significantly higher in the intervention group during the intervention period, and MEMS demonstrated higher adherence in the intervention group on weekdays during this period, although not at weekends. There were no significant differences regarding the other measures, and no differences in any measure after 1 month of follow up.[56]

Finally Samet randomized 151 people with a history of alcohol problems who were receiving HAART to usual follow up or an intervention (four meetings with a nurse trained in motivational interviewing who addressed alcohol problems, provided a programmable watch, and enhanced perception of treatment efficacy). Adherence was measured by self-reported 30-day recall. After 13 months' follow up, there were no differences in adherence between the two groups, or in other outcome measures (CD4 count, viral load, and alcohol consumption).[57]

As mentioned previously toxicity is also a determinant of a successful regimen both in terms of tolerability and adherence. Liver enzyme elevation (LEE) defined as transaminases greater than five times baseline or > 100 IU/mL is commonly observed after combination HAART is begun. Potential risk factors after treatment with ritonavir and saquinavir with or without stavudine were investigated in 208 HIV-infected patients, by use of the Cox proportional hazard model: 18 patients (9%) developed LEE during the 48-week follow up. Multivariate analysis, adjusted for baseline levels of alanine aminotransferase (ALT) and aspartate aminotransferase (AST), showed that hepatitis B surface antigen (HBsAg) positivity (RR 8·8; 95% CI 3·3–23·1) and the use of stavudine (RR, 4·9; 95% CI 1·5–16·0) were the only significant risk factors for developing LEE. After LEE occurred, ALT and AST concentrations decreased by > 50% in 13 of 14 patients who continued ARVT during LEE. Therefore in this study, it appeared safe to continue ARVT during LEE; however, more data from larger studies are required to confirm this finding.[58]

In a retrospective study 65 patients taking HAART were evaluated and 24 were identified to have antiretroviral hepatotoxicity. An age over 40 years ($P = 0{\cdot}019$), an absolute CD4 count of < 310 cells/mL ($P = 0{\cdot}002$) and coexisting hepatitis C infection ($P = 0{\cdot}035$) were significantly associated with hepatotoxicity. Patients older than 40 years had a 7-fold increased risk (RR 6·9; 95% CI 1·7–27·3) and those with an absolute CD4 count of < 310 cells/mL had a 10-fold increased risk (RR 10·2; 95% CI 2·5–41·9) for antiretroviral hepatotoxicity, in comparison with those who were younger or who had a greater absolute CD4 count. Of the eight patients documented to have coexisting hepatitis C infection, six (75%) were in the antiretroviral hepatotoxicity group.[59]

In another retrospective study of 394 patients 7% were HBsAg-positive and 14% were anti-HCV-positive. Patients with chronic hepatitis had a higher risk for LEE compared with patients without coinfection: 37% versus 12% respectively. After adjustment for higher baseline transaminases, the presence of HBsAg or anti-HCV remained associated with an increased risk of LEE (RR 2·78; 95% CI 1·50–5·16 and RR 2·46; 95% CI 1·43–4·24, respectively). In patients with LEE, transaminases declined whether HAART was continued or modified. Of patients with chronic HBV infection 38% lost HBeAg or developed anti-HBe after initiation of HAART, and one seroconverted from HBsAg-positive to anti-HBs-positive. However, there was no clear relationship with LEE.[60]

Finally in the Swiss cohort, a prospective analysis revealed 1157 patients (37·2%) were coinfected with HCV, 1015 of whom (87·7%) had a history of intravenous drug use. In multivariate Cox's regression, the probability of progression to a new AIDS-defining clinical event or to death was independently associated with HCV seropositivity (HR 1·7; 95% CI 1·26–2·30), and with active intravenous drug use (HR 1·38; 95% CI 1·02–1·88). Virological response to HAART and the probability of treatment change were not associated with HCV serostatus. In contrast, HCV seropositivity was associated with a smaller CD4 cell recovery (HR for a CD4 cell count increase of at least 50 cells/mm^3 = 0·79; 95% CI 0·72–0·87).[61]

There is a significantly elevated risk of severe liver disease in persons who are coinfected with HIV and HCV. A meta-analysis to quantify the effect of HIV coinfection on progressive liver disease in persons with HCV revealed eight studies that included outcomes of histological cirrhosis or decompensated liver disease. These studies yielded a combined adjusted RR of 2·92 (95% CI 1·70–5·01). Studies that examined decompensated liver disease had a combined RR of 6·14 (95% CI 2·86–13·20), whereas studies that examined histological cirrhosis had a pooled RR of 2·07 (95% CI 1·40–3·07).[62] There are data that suggest that the responses to therapy with interferon and ribivarin are similar to those in non-HIV infected patients and dependent on HCV genotype.[63,64]

Summary

There is no evidence as to which drug regimen is most efficacious clinically. Adherence to HAART is important and, to facilitate this, drug regimens are becoming simpler, many with once a day drugs and no food or fluid restrictions. There is still no consensus on how best to measure adherence. Once a day medications can be given as directly observed therapy combined for example with methadone[65] (although there are important interactions with methadone and HAART[66]). The studies to try to improve adherence through social and education means have been disappointing and short lived but there is no doubt that they are important. Hepatotoxicity remains a challenge especially in the many patients who have coexisting liver disease and may be taking other hepatotoxic drugs. The daily problems that patients face with their medication needs to be kept in mind constantly by the physician.

Opportunistic infection prophylaxis

Although the risk of opportunistic infection has fallen in recent years it increases dramatically once a patient's CD4 count is less than 200.[21] In the United Kingdom around 50% of patients present with a CD4 < 350 and 30% with a CD4 < 200 cells/mm^3.[67]

Prophylaxis for PCP

There are two systematic reviews: Ioannidis *et al.* searching in 1995 and covering 35 RCTs[68] and Bucher *et al.* from 1997[69] covering 22 trials. Both of these were before the widespread introduction of HAART. Since then the incidence of OIs in HIV patients has fallen so much that further studies are unlikely. The main focus recently has been on stopping prophylaxis after immune restoration.

Co-trimoxazole versus placebo

The first systematic review found that prophylaxis with co-trimoxazole (or aerosolized pentamidine) reduced the incidence of PCP more than placebo (RR 0·32; 95% CI 0·23–0·46). There were no placebo controlled data on the incidence of toxoplasmosis. They found that severe adverse effects (predominantly rash, fever, and hematological effects leading to discontinuation within 1 year) occurred in more people taking higher doses of co-trimoxazole than lower doses (25% *v* 15%).[68]

One subsequent RCT of 545 people in sub-Saharan Africa with symptomatic disease, second or third clinical stage disease in the WHO staging system regardless of CD4 cell count, comparing co-trimoxazole with placebo, found no significant difference in incidence of PCP or toxoplasmosis. Patients taking co-trimoxazole were less likely to suffer a serious event (death or hospital admission, irrespective of the cause) than those on placebo regardless of their initial CD4 cell count (84 *v* 124; HR 0·57; 95% CI 0·43–0·75; P < 0·001). This implies that in Africa the effect of co-trimoxazole is on preventing bacterial infections, not PCP. Moderate neutropenia occurred more frequently with co-trimoxazole (neutropenia AR 62/271 [23%] with co-trimoxazole *v* 26/244 [10%] with placebo; RR 2·1; 95% 1·4–3·3; NNH 8; 95% CI 5–14).[70]

Co-trimoxazole versus aerosolized pentamidine

The first review also found that co-trimoxazole was more effective at preventing PCP than aerosolized pentamidine (RR 0·58; 95% CI 0·45–0·75). Bronchospasm occurred in 3% of people taking aerosolized pentamidine 300 mg monthly.[68] A second systematic review found that co-trimoxazole was more effective at preventing toxoplasmosis than aerosolized pentamidine (RR 0·78; 95% CI 0·55–1·11).[69]

Co-trimoxazole versus dapsone (with or without pyrimethamine)

The first review found that co-trimoxazole compared with dapsone (with or without pyrimethamine) reduced the incidence of PCP, but the result did not reach significance (RR 0·61; 95% CI 0·34–1·10).[68] The second review found that co-trimoxazole was significantly more effective in preventing PCP than dapsone/pyrimethamine (RR 0·49; 95% CI 0·26–0·92). It found no significant difference between co-trimoxazole and dapsone/pyrimethamine in preventing toxoplasmosis (RR 1·17; 95% CI 0·68–2·04).[69]

High- versus low-dose co-trimoxazole

The first systematic review found no significant difference in the rate of PCP infection between lower dose (160/800 mg three times weekly or 80/400 mg daily) and higher dose (160/800 mg daily) of co-trimoxazole (failure rate per 100 person-years was 1·6; 95% CI 0·9–2·5 with lower dose *v* 0·5; 95% CI 0–2·9 with higher dose).[68] One subsequent RCT (2625 people) also found no significant difference in the rate of PCP infection in people receiving co-trimoxazole 160/800 mg daily compared with three times weekly (3·5 *v* 4) or the reduction in incidence of PCP or toxoplasmosis on pentamidine or placebo. One systematic review has found no significant difference between high and low-dose co-trimoxazole for PCP, although adverse effects are more common with the higher dose group.[68] Discontinuation because of adverse effects was significantly more common in people taking higher doses of co-trimoxazole (RR 2·14; $P < 0·001$).[71]

Summary

Systematic reviews have found that co-trimoxazole is the most effective prophylactic agent for PCP.

Adverse reactions

Case presentation 4 (continued)

He is started on co-trimoxazole initially. He develops a widespread maculopapular rash with nausea and vomiting. A diagnosis of co-trimoxazole hypersensitivity is made. What are the options for patients who cannot tolerate TMX/SMX?

Adverse reactions to co-trimoxazole

One RCT of 372 people found that gradual initiation of co-trimoxazole may improve tolerance of the regimen (17% *v* 33% at 12 weeks).[72] Two RCTs (238 people; 50 people) found no significant benefit from acetylcysteine in preventing co-trimoxazole hypersensitivity reactions in HIV infected people.[73,74]

Atovaquone versus dapsone

There is one RCT of atovaquone in 1057 people intolerant of co-trimoxazole, of whom 298 had a history of PCP.[75] When compared with dapsone they found no significant difference between atovaquone 1500 mg daily compared with dapsone 100 mg daily (15·7 *v* 18·4 cases of PCP per 100 person-years; $P = 0{\cdot}20$). The overall risk of stopping treatment because of adverse effects was similar in the two arms (RR 0·94; 95% CI 0·74–1·19). Atovaquone was stopped more frequently than dapsone in people who were receiving dapsone at baseline (RR 3·78; 95% CI 2·37–6·01; $P < 0{\cdot}001$), and less frequently in people not receiving dapsone at baseline (RR 0·42; 95% CI 0·30–0·58; $P < 0{\cdot}001$).

Atovaquone versus pentamidine

One RCT with 549 people intolerant of co-trimoxazole compared high dose with low-dose atovaquone (1500 mg daily *v* 750 mg daily) with monthly aerosolized pentamidine (300 mg). It found no significant difference between the groups in the incidence of PCP (26% *v* 22% *v* 17%) or mortality (20% *v* 13% *v* 18%) after a median follow up of 11·3 months.[76]

Azithromycin

One RCT with 693 people compared azithromycin, rifabutin, and both drugs in combination, in people who were already receiving standard PCP prophylaxis. It found that azithromycin, either alone or in combination with rifabutin, reduced the risk of developing PCP by 45% when compared with rifabutin alone ($P = 0{\cdot}008$).[77] Gastrointestinal side effects are common with azithromycin, but they are usually mild and do not lead to stopping treatment when used for mycobacterial infection. The addition of rifabutin significantly increased the risk of stopping treatment (RR 1.67; $P = 0{\cdot}03$).[78]

Dapsone

A meta-analysis of 16 trials with 4267 patients evaluating dapsone toxicity found no significant difference in mortality for dapsone (OR for mortality for dapsone *v* other primary prophylaxis 1·11; 95% CI 0·96–1·29).[79] Detels *et al.* found that adverse effects were dose-related for dapsone (low *v* high dose: 29% *v* 12%).[80]

Concomitant coverage for toxoplasmosis

Standard co-trimoxazole prophylaxis or dapsone should offer adequate coverage for toxoplasmosis. Pentamidine has no intrinsic activity against *Toxoplasma gondii.* Toxoplasmosis risk is probably clinically meaningful only with CD4 < 100/mm^3 and positive toxoplasma serology.[81]

Case presentation 4 (continued)

He is commenced on dapsone and then 2 weeks later zidovudine, lamivudine, and efavirenz. His viral load falls to undetectable and CD4 count climbs to 320 cells within 6 months. He has some problems with recurrent cold sores. You wonder how to manage his herpes infection and when his PCP prophylaxis can be safely stopped.

Treatment of herpes simplex

The only studies are with famciclovir for the suppression of herpes simplex virus reactivation; however, acyclovir or valaciclovir are also used.[82]

Stopping Pneumocystis prophylaxis

In the meta-analysis of 14 randomized and non-randomized studies with 3584 subjects who had discontinued prophylaxis when their CD4 count was sustained > 200 for 3 months, eight cases of PCP occurred during 3449 person-years (0·23 cases per 100 person-years; 95% CI 0·10–0·46).[83] In the decision analysis, mortality and time spent alive without immunodeficiency in the modelled discontinuation strategy were similar to those in the continuation strategy. For patients who received primary prophylaxis, the discontinuation strategy led to slightly fewer episodes of PCP and fewer toxicity-related prophylaxis withdrawals (8·6 *v* 34·5 cases per 100 patients during a 10-year period). Comparative results were similar for patients on secondary prophylaxis. The review found a low incidence of PCP in people discontinuing both primary and secondary prophylaxis after a mean of 1·5 years (7/3035 [0·23%] with discontinuing primary prophylaxis and 1/549 [0·18%] discontinuing secondary prophylaxis; mean annual incidence over 1·5 years 0·23%; 95% CI 0·10–0·46%; no statistical heterogeneity among studies). Neither of the two RCTs identified in the review found any cases of PCP after discontinuation. (First RCT: 587 people with satisfactory response to HAART, CD4 > 200 mm^3, and viral load < 5000 copies/mL for > 3 months; absolute risk for PCP or toxoplasma encephalitis at median 20 months = 0%, whether or not prophylaxis continued.[84] Second RCT: 708 people taking HAART, CD4 > 200 mm^3 for 3 months; absolute risk for PCP at 6 months = 0%).[85]

Toxoplasmosis

There are two RCTs. The first, which was included in the systematic review, found no cases of toxoplasma encephalitis at 6 months in people discontinuing prophylaxis (see PCP above).[85] The second RCT (302 people with a satisfactory response to HAART) compared discontinuation with continuation of toxoplasma prophylaxis.[86] After a median of 10 months it found no episodes of toxoplasma encephalitis in either group.

Case presentation 4 (continued)

He returns after 6 months with CD4 now 400 cells/mm^3 and viral load undetectable. However after the death of a close friend it soon becomes apparent that he has developed a chaotic lifestyle, abusing substances, and has problems with taking regular medication. He decides not to attend the clinic for a while and is lost to follow up. After 3 years he returns with a CD4 count of 50 cells and an increasing viral load. He has been intermittently attending another clinic and his current medication is stavudine, didanosine, abacavir, ritonavir, and amprenavir. Viral resistance testing, viral phenotyping, and therapeutic drug monitoring may be used to guide therapy in this situation but the situation is far from clear.

Genotypic resistance testing

There are three RCTs showing a benefit of genotypic resistance testing plus expert advice for patients failing HAART. A total of 326 HIV-1 infected patients on stable HAART with virological failure were studied. The baseline CD4 cell count and plasma HIV-1 RNA were 387(± 224) × 10^6 cells/liter and 4(± 1) log respectively. The proportion of patients with plasma HIV-1 RNA < 400 copies/mL at 24 weeks differed between genotyping and no genotyping arms (48·5 and 36·2%; $P < 0·05$). Factors associated with a higher probability of plasma HIV-1 RNA < 400 copies/mL were HIV-1 genotyping (OR 1·7; 95% CI 1·1–2·8; $P = 0·016$) and the expert advice in patients failing a second-line HAART (OR, 3·2; 95% CI 1·2–8·3; $P = 0·016$).[87]

To compare standard care (control, N = 43) or treatment according to the resistance mutations in protease and reverse-transcriptase genes (genotypic group, N = 65), 108 patients were enrolled in the VIRADAPT study. All patients were similar for risk factors, age, sex, previous treatment, CD4 cell count (214/microliter [SD 14]) and log HIV-1 RNA viral load at baseline (4.7 log copies/mL [0.1]). At month 3, the mean change in HIV-1 RNA was – 1·04 log in the study group compared with – 0·46 log in the control group (mean difference 0·58 log; 95% CI 0·14–1·02; $P = 0{\cdot}01$). At month 6, changes were – 1·15 (0·15) log copies/mL, and – 0·67 (0·19) log copies/mL in the genotypic group and the control group, respectively (mean difference 0·48 log; $P = 0{\cdot}05$). Difference in the drop in viral load combined at 3 months and 6 months was significant ($P = 0{\cdot}015$). At month 3, HIV-1 RNA was lower than detection level (200 copies/mL) in 29% (19/65) of patients in the genotypic group versus 14% (6/43) in the control group ($P = 0{\cdot}017$). At month 6, the values were 32% (21/65) and 14% (6/43) ($P = 0{\cdot}067$) for the genotypic group and the control group, respectively. Therapy was generally well tolerated, with 10 patients (six in the genotypic group, four in the control group) requiring toxic effect-related drug modification.[88]

In the genotypic antiretroviral resistance testing (GART) study, 153 HIV-infected adults, with a 3-fold or greater rise in plasma HIV-1 RNA on at least 16 weeks of combination HAART, were randomized either to a GART group, where genotype interpretation and suggested regimens were provided to clinicians, or to a no-GART group, where treatment choices were made without such input. Plasma HIV-1 RNA levels and CD4 cell counts were measured at 4, 8, and 12 weeks following randomization. The primary endpoint was change in HIV-1 RNA levels from baseline to the average of the 4- and 8-week levels. The average baseline CD4 cell count was 230×10^6 cells/liter and the median HIV-1 RNA was 28 085 copies/mL. At entry, 82 patients were failing on regimens containing indinavir, 51 on nelfinavir, 11 on ritonavir, and nine on saquinavir. HIV-1 RNA, averaged at 4 and 8 weeks, decreased by 1·19 log for the 78 GART patients and – 0·61 log for the 75 no-GART patients (treatment difference: – 0·53 log; 95% CI – 0·77, – 0·29; $P = 0{\cdot}00001$). Overall, the best virological responses occurred in patients who received three or more drugs to which their HIV-1 appeared to be susceptible.[89] A note of caution is given here since a recent paper showed discrepant results in "expert" interpretation of genotype resistance data.[90]

Viral phenotyping

A total of 272 subjects who failed to achieve or maintain virological suppression (HIV-1-RNA plasma level > 2000 copies/mL) with previous exposure to two or more nucleoside reverse transcriptase inhibitors and one protease inhibitor were randomized to HAART guided by phenotyping or standard of care. The percentage of subjects with HIV-1-RNA plasma levels < 400 copies/mL at week 16 (primary), change from baseline in HIV-1-RNA plasma levels and number of "active" (less than 4-fold resistance) antiretroviral agents used (secondary) were measured. At week 16, using intent-to-treat (ITT) analysis, a greater proportion of subjects had HIV-1-RNA levels < 400 copies/mL in the phenotyping than in the standard of care arm ($P = 0{\cdot}036$, ITT observed; $P = 0{\cdot}079$, ITT missing equals failure). An ITT-observed analysis showed that subjects in the phenotyping arm had a significantly greater median reduction in HIV-1-RNA levels from baseline than the standard of care arm ($P = 0{\cdot}005$ for 400 copies/mL; $P = 0{\cdot}049$ for 50 copies/mL assay detection limit). Significantly more subjects in the phenotyping arm were treated with two or more "active" antiretroviral agents than in the standard of care arm ($P = 0{\cdot}003$).[91]

Therapeutic drug monitoring

There are no randomized controlled data to support therapeutic drug monitoring but, in a pharmacological substudy of VIRADAPT, the impact of plasma protease inhibitor (PI) trough levels on changes in HIV RNA were assessed in 81 patients treated with genotypic-guided therapy. Linear regression analysis showed a significant relationship between PI concentration and HIV RNA in the plasma. "Suboptimal" concentration (SOC) was defined as at least two PI plasma levels $< 2 \times$ IC95 and patients were categorized into four groups: G1 (SOC/control), G2 (OC/control), G3 (SOC/genotype), andG4 (OC/genotype). OC and SOC were found in 67·9% (55/81) and 32·1% (26/81) of patients, respectively. Mean changes in HIV RNA from baseline at month 6 were:

$-0{\cdot}23 \pm 0{\cdot}29$ log copies/mL (G1);
$-0{\cdot}97 \pm 0{\cdot}28$ (G2);
$-0{\cdot}68 \pm 0{\cdot}37$ (G3);
$-1{\cdot}38 \pm 0{\cdot}20$ (G4).

Multivariate analysis showed PI plasma concentrations to be an independent predictor of HIV-RNA evolution ($P = 0{\cdot}017$).[92]

Structured treatment interruption

There has been some interest in structured treatment interruption (STI) since small cohorts of patients with viral resistance in Berlin and Harvard who stopped antiretroviral drugs showed a rise in CD4 count. Small studies have shown conflicting results on surrogate markers, which may be explained by the length of the treatment interruption (on average 8–16 weeks) or on the number of drugs commenced after it (so called mega or giga HAART).[93,94] There is a multinational clinical trial looking at the options in management with antiretrovirals (OPTIMA) in these so-called salvage therapy patients. This strategy is not recommended outside of the setting of a clinical trial. There is evidence from the large EUROSIDA cohort that even at low CD4 counts there is a benefit from not stopping therapy.[95]

Treatment and prophylaxis of opportunistic infections

Case presentation 4 (continued)

The patient decides not to continue with therapy and is adamant that he no longer wants any in the future. He is admitted with increasing confusion, fever, and neck stiffness. Fundoscopy reveals CMV retinitis but no papilledema. His CD4 count is 10 cells. You consider the possible conditions he is at risk of and how best to manage him.

Table 11.1 lists the usual pathogens related to CD4 count.

Cryptococcal meningitis needs to be excluded by lumbar puncture and staining of cerebrospinal fluid (CSF) with Indian ink.

Case presentation 4 (continued)

The opening pressure is 30 mm of CSF, and CSF is positive for *Cryptococcus* with a white cell count of 115, mainly lymphocytes; a CSF protein of 2·4 g/dL (range –1.6 g dL), and a glucose of 0·6 mmol/liter. A diagnosis of cryptococcal meningitis is made.

Treatment of cryptococcal meningitis

Amphotericin

In a double-blind multicenter study, patients with a first episode of AIDS-associated cryptococcal meningitis were randomly assigned to treatment with higher dose amphotericin B (0·7 mg/kg per day) with or without flucytosine (100 mg/kg per day) for 2 weeks (step 1), followed by 8 weeks of treatment with itraconazole (400 mg

Table 11.1 Pathogens related to CD4 counts

CD4 count	Infection	Non-infectious complications
> 500	Acute HIV syndrome	Progressive generalized lymphadenopathy
	Candida vaginitis	Polymyositis
		Aseptic meningitis
		Guillain–Barré syndrome
200–500	Pneumococcal and other bacterial pneumonia	Carcinoma in situ
	Pulmonary tuberculosis	Cervical cancer
	Kaposi sarcoma	Lymphocytic interstitial pneumonitis
	Herpes zoster	Mononeuritis multiplex
	Thrush	Anemia
	Cryptosporidiosis, self-limiting	Idiopathic thrombocytopenia purpura
	Oral hairy leukoplakia	
< 200	*Pnemocystis carinii* pneumonia	Wasting
	Candida esophagitis	B-cell lymphoma
	Disseminated/chronic herpes simplex	Cardiomyopathy
	Toxoplasmosis	Peripheral neuropathy
	Cryptococcosis	HIV-associated dementia
	Disseminated histoplasmosis	CNS lymphoma
	Disseminated coccidiomycosis	HIV-associated nephropathy
	Chronic cryptosporidiosis	
	Progressive multifocal leukoencephalopathy (PMLE)	
	Microsporidiosis	
	Miliary/extrapulmonary tuberculosis	
< 50	CMV disease	
	Disseminated *Mycobacteruim avium* complex	

Table reproduced by permission of Bartlett, JG. *Johns Hopkins Hospital 2002 Guide to Medical Care of Patients with HIV infection*, Philadelphia: Lippincott Williams & Williams, 2002.

per day) or fluconazole (400 mg per day) (step 2). Treatment was considered successful if CSF cultures were negative at 2 and 10 weeks, or if the patient was clinically stable at 2 weeks and asymptomatic at 10 weeks. At 2 weeks, the CSF cultures were negative in 60% of the 202 patients receiving amphotericin B plus flucytosine and in 51% of the 179 receiving amphotericin B alone ($P = 0{\cdot}06$). Elevated intracranial pressure was associated with death in 13 of 14 patients during step 1. The clinical outcome did not differ significantly between the two groups: 72% of the 151 fluconazole recipients and 60% of the 155 itraconazole recipients had negative cultures at 10 weeks (95% CI for the difference in percentages, − 100, 21). The proportion of patients who had clinical responses was similar with fluconazole (68%) and itraconazole (70%). Overall mortality was 5·5% in the first 2 weeks and 3.9% in the next 8 weeks, with no significant difference between the groups. In a multivariate analysis, the addition of flucytosine during the initial 2 weeks and treatment with fluconazole for the next 8 weeks were independently associated with CSF sterilization. As a result standard guidelines for treatment of cryptococcal meningitis recommend 2 weeks of amphotericin B at a dose of 0·7 mg/kg per day (with flucytosine) followed by fluconazole at a dose of 400 mg per day for another 8 weeks.[96]

There is one direct comparison between amphotericin B deoxycholate (0·7mg/kg per day) and liposomal amphotericin (AmBisome) (4mg/kg per day) in 27 patients showing that AmBisome therapy resulted in a CSF culture negativity within 7 days in six out of 15 patients versus one out of 12 amphotericin B-treated patients ($P = 0{\cdot}09$); within 14 days in 10 out of 15 AmBisome patients versus one out of nine amphotericin B patients ($P = 0{\cdot}01$); and within 21 days in 11 out of 15 AmBisome patients versus three out of eight amphotericin B patients ($P = 0{\cdot}19$).[97] The liposomal amphotericin was less nephrotoxic and this has been confirmed in other studies in HIV-positive patients.[98]

Azoles

Fluconazole had been used for treatment with better outcome than historical controls (20% survival) as either 400 mg daily with flucytosine (75% survival at 10 weeks, N = 32),[99] higher doses such as 800 mg alone (38% survival at 4·5 months, N = 8)[100] or intravenously 800–1000 mg (82% survival at 10 weeks, N = 14).[101] In the largest comparative study of 194 eligible patients, 131 received fluconazole and 63 received amphotericin B.[102] Treatment was successful in 25 of the 63 amphotericin B recipients (40%; 95% CI 26–53) and in 44 of the 131 fluconazole recipients (34%; 95% CI 25–42%; $P = 0{\cdot}40$). There was no significant difference between the groups in overall mortality owing to cryptococcosis (amphotericin *v* fluconazole, 9 of 63 [4%] *v* 24 of 131 [8%]; $P = 0{\cdot}48$); however, mortality during the first 2 weeks of therapy was higher in the fluconazole group (15% *v* 8%; $P = 0{\cdot}25$). The median length of time to the first negative CSF culture was 42 days (95% CI 28–71) in the amphotericin B group and 64 days (95% CI 53–67) in the fluconazole group ($P = 0{\cdot}25$). Multivariate analyses identified abnormal mental status (lethargy, somnolence, or obtundation) as the most important predictive factor of death during therapy ($P < 0{\cdot}0001$).[102]

In Africa 30 patients were randomized to receive combination therapy with fluconazole, 200 mg once a day for 2 months, and flucytosine, 150 mg/kg per day) for the first 2 weeks, and 28 to receive fluconazole alone. Patients in both groups who survived for 2 months continued fluconazole as maintenance therapy at a dose of 200 mg three times per week for 4 months. The combination therapy prevented death within 2 weeks and significantly increased the survival rate among patients (32%) at 6 months over that among patients receiving monotherapy (12%) ($P = 0{\cdot}022$).[103]

Oral itraconazole (200 mg twice a day) for 6 weeks was less effective than amphotericin B (0·3 mg/kg per day) plus flucytosine (150 mg/kg daily) in 28 patients.[104]

The importance of controlling the raised intracranial pressure associated with cryptococcal meningitis by repeated lumbar puncture or CSF drainage was established in a retrospective analysis of 221 patients in the van der Horst study.[96] After receiving antifungal therapy, those patients whose CSF pressure was reduced by > 10 mm or did not change had more frequent clinical response at 2 weeks than did those whose pressure increased > 10 mm ($P < 0{\cdot}001$). Patients with pretreatment opening pressure of < 250 mm H_2O had increased short-term survival compared with those with higher pressure.[105] This was confirmed in a small prospective study of 10 patients with raised ICP treated with CSF drainage.[106]

Prophylaxis against fungal infection

Fluconazole versus placebo

One RCT (323 women with CD4 ≤ 300/mm^3) found that fluconazole versus placebo significantly reduced the incidence of candidiasis (44% *v* 58% in those who suffered at least one episode of candidiasis; RR 0·56; 95% CI 0·41–0·77).[107]

Itraconazole versus placebo

One RCT (295 people with advanced HIV disease) found that itraconazole reduced the incidence of invasive fungal infections (6 *v* 19; *P* = 0·0007).[108] It found no significant effect on recurrent or refractory candidiasis.

High-dose versus low-dose fluconazole

One RCT (636 people) compared fluconazole 200 mg daily with 400 mg once weekly and found no difference in the rate of invasive fungal infections over a follow up of 74 weeks (8% *v* 6%; ARR 2·2%; 95% CI −1·7% to + 6.). However, the incidence of candidiasis was twice as common in people taking the weekly dose.[109]

Fluconazole versus clotrimazole

One RCT found that fluconazole reduced the incidence of invasive fungal disease and mucocutaneous candidal infections compared with clotrimazole (4% *v* 11%; RH 3·3; 95% CI 1·5–7·6).[110] None of the above RCTs found any difference in mortality.

Itraconazole versus placebo

One RCT (44 people with HIV infection and candidiasis, treated with itraconazole 200 mg for 4 weeks before randomization) compared prophylaxis with itraconazole versus placebo for 24 weeks. It found that itraconazole reduced the number of people who relapsed (5/24 [21%] with itraconazole *v* 14/20 [70%] with placebo; ARR 49%; 95% CI 19–64; NNT 2; 95% CI 2–5), and increased the time interval before relapse occurred (median time to relapse: itraconazole 8.0 weeks *v* placebo 10·4 weeks; *P* = 0·001).[111]

Itraconazole versus fluconazole

One RCT (108 people with HIV infection) found that itraconazole reduced relapses of successfully treated cryptococcal meningitis more than fluconazole (13/57 [23%] *v* 2/51 [4%]; ARR 19%; 95% CI 6·2–31·7; RR 0·17; 95% CI 0·04–0·71; NNT 5; 95% CI 3–16). The trial was stopped early because of the higher rate of relapse with fluconazole; two people discontinued itraconazole because of skin rashes, one because of severe anemia, and one because of gastrointestinal effects compared with none taking fluconazole.[112]

There is one open label uncontrolled study (44 people), which found that itraconazole may be effective in preventing the relapse of histoplasmosis.[113]

Mycobacterium avium complex

Treatment

HIV-positive patients (N = 246) with disseminated *Mycobacterium avium* complex (MAC) received either azithromycin 250 mg every day, azithromycin 600 mg every day, or clarithromycin 500 mg twice a day, each combined with ethambutol, for 24 weeks. The azithromycin 250 mg arm of the study was dropped after an interim analysis showed a lower rate of clearance of bacteremia. At 24 weeks of therapy, the likelihood of patients developing two consecutive negative cultures (46% *v* 56%; *P* = 0·24) or one negative culture (59% *v* 61%; *P* = 0·80) was similar for azithromycin 600 mg (N = 68) and clarithromycin (N = 57), respectively. The likelihood of relapse was 39% versus 27% (*P* = 0·21) on azithromycin compared with clarithromycin, respectively. Of the six patients who experienced relapse, none of those randomized to receive azithromycin developed isolates resistant to macrolides, compared with two of three patients randomized to receive clarithromycin (corrected). Mortality was similar in patients comprising each arm of the study (69% *v* 63%; HR [95% CI] 1·1 [0·7, 1·7]).[114]

AIDS patients with disseminated MAC disease (N = 85) were randomized to receive a three-drug regimen of clarithromycin, rifabutin or clofazimine, and ethambutol. Two dosages of clarithromycin, 500 or 1000 mg twice daily, were compared. The Data and Safety Monitoring Board recommended discontinuation of the clarithromycin dosage comparison and continuation of the rifabutin versus clofazimine comparison. After a mean follow up of 4·5 months, 10 (22%) of 45 patients receiving clarithromycin at 500 mg twice daily had died (70 deaths per 100 person-years) compared with 17 (43%) of 40 patients receiving clarithromycin at 1000 mg twice daily (158 deaths per 100 person-years) (RR 2·43; 95% CI 1·11–5·34; $P = 0·02$). After 10.4 months, 20 (49%) of 41 patients receiving rifabutin had died (81 deaths per 100 person-years) compared with 23 (52%) of 44 patients receiving clofazimine (94 deaths per 100 person-years) (RR 1·20; 95% CI 0·65–2·19; $P = 0·56$). Bacteriologic outcomes were similar among treatment groups. In treating MAC disease in AIDS patients, the maximum dose of clarithromycin should be 500 mg twice daily.[115]

The effect of two regimens for treatment of MAC bacteremia in an HIV-positive population on symptoms and health status outcomes were evaluated using a substudy of an open-label randomized controlled trial. The study was conducted in 24 hospital-based HIV clinics in 16 Canadian cities. Patients had HIV infection and MAC bacteremia and were given either rifampin 600 mg plus ethambutol 15 mg/kg daily plus clofazimine 100 mg daily plus ciprofloxacin 750 mg twice daily (four-drug arm), or rifabutin 600 mg daily (amended to 300 mg daily in mid-trial) plus ethambutol 15 mg/kg daily plus clarithromycin 1000 mg twice daily (three-drug arm). The primary health status outcome was the change on the 8-item symptom subscale of the Medical Outcome Study (MOS)-HIV Health Survey adapted for MAC. Patients on the three-drug arm had better outcomes on the MOS-HIV symptom subscale at 16 weeks ($P = 0·06$), with statistically significant differences restricted to night sweats and fever and chills ($P < 0·001$). Changes on other MOS-HIV subscales and on the Karnofsky score were also evaluated. The proportion of patients improving on the symptom subscale relative to baseline was 55% on the three-drug arm and 40% on the four-drug arm. Patients on the three-drug arm also had better Karnofsky score at 16 weeks ($P < 0·001$) and better outcomes on the social function, mental health, energy/fatigue, health distress, and cognitive function subscales of the MOS-HIV. The three-drug arm was superior to the four-drug arm in terms of impact on MAC-associated symptoms, functional status, and other aspects of health status.[116]

Prophylaxis

Prospective cohort studies have found that the risk of disseminated MAC disease increases substantially with a lower CD4 count but was clinically important only for CD4 $< 50/mm^3$.[81] Azithromycin and clarithromycin reduce the incidence of MAC more than placebo.

Azithromycin

One RCT (174 people with AIDS and CD4 $< 100/mm^3$) found that azithromycin once weekly reduced the incidence of MAC more than placebo (11% *v* 25%; $P = 0·004$). Gastrointestinal side effects were more likely with azithromycin than with placebo (71/90 [79%] *v* 25/91 [28%]; number needed to harm [NNH] 2), but they were rarely severe enough to cause discontinuation of treatment (8% *v* 2% in the two arms; $P = 0·14$).[117]

Clarithromycin

There is one systematic review (search date 1997) of prophylaxis and treatment of MAC.[118] It identified one RCT (682 people with advanced AIDS) that found that clarithromycin compared with placebo significantly reduced the incidence of MAC (6% *v* 16%; HR 0·31; 95% CI 0·18–0·53). It found no significant difference in the death rate (32% *v* 41%; HR 0·75; $P = 0·026$).[119] Adverse effects led to discontinuation of treatment in slightly more people taking clarithromycin than placebo (8% *v* 6%; *P* = 0·45). More people taking clarithromycin suffered altered taste (11% *v* 2%) or rectal disorders (8% *v* 3%).[117]

Clarithromycin plus rifabutin

We found no systematic review. One RCT (1178 people with AIDS) compared rifabutin versus clarithromycin versus clarithromycin plus rifabutin.[120] It found that the risk of MAC was significantly reduced in the clarithromycin alone group (relative risk reduction [RRR] 44% for clarithromycin *v* rifabutin; *P* = 0·005) and the combination group when compared with rifabutin alone (RRR 57% for combination *v* rifabutin; *P* = 0·0003). There was no significant difference in the risk of MAC between the combination and clarithromycin arms (*P* = 0·36).

Azithromycin plus rifabutin

One RCT (693 people) found that the combination of azithromycin plus rifabutin versus azithromycin alone significantly reduced the incidence of MAC at 1 year (15·3% with rifabutin *v* 7·6% for azithromycin *v* 2·8% with rifabutin plus azithromycin; *P* = 0·008 for rifabutin *v* azithromycin; *P* = 0·03 for combination *v* azithromycin). Dose limiting toxicity was more likely with azithromycin plus rifabutin than with azithromycin alone (HR 1·67; *P* = 0·03).[78]

In another RCT, adverse events occurred in 31% of people receiving the combination of clarithromycin and rifabutin compared with 16% on clarithromycin alone and 18% on rifabutin alone (*P* < 0·001).[118] Uveitis occurred in 42 people: 33 were on clarithromycin plus rifabutin, seven were on rifabutin alone, and two were on clarithromycin alone. This is confirmed by a review of 54 people with rifabutin associated uveitis which found that uveitis was dose dependent, occurred from 2 weeks to more than 7 months after initiation of rifabutin treatment, and was more likely in people taking rifabutin and clarithromycin. In most people, uveitis resolved 1–2 months after discontinuation of rifabutin.[121]

Other combinations

There are four RCTs. The first RCT (95 people) found that the combination of clarithromycin (1000 mg daily), clofazimine, and ethambutol was associated with significantly fewer relapses of MAC than the combination of clarithromycin plus clofazimine without ethambutol (68% relapsed in the three-drug regimen *v* 12% in the two-drug regimen at 36 weeks; *P* = 0·004).[122]

The second RCT (106 people) found that the addition of clofazimine to clarithromycin and ethambutol did not improve clinical response and was associated with higher mortality in the clofazimine arm (62% with clofazimine *v* 38% without clofazimine; *P* = 0·012).[123]

The third RCT (144 people) found that the combination of clarithromycin, rifabutin, and ethambutol reduced the relapse rate of MAC compared with clarithromycin plus clofazimine.[124]

The fourth RCT (198 people) found no significant difference in survival between people taking clarithromycin plus ethambutol and people taking clarithromycin plus ethambutol plus rifabutin.[125]

One RCT (85 people) comparing clarithromycin 500 mg twice daily versus 1000 mg twice daily found that after a median follow up of 4·5 months, more people died with the higher dose (17/40 [43%] with 1000 mg twice daily *v* 10/45 [22%] with 500 mg twice daily; ARI 20%; 95% CI 0·2–33; NNH 5; 95% CI 3–470).[115] A similar difference was seen in another RCT (154 people).[126] Combinations of drugs may lead to increased toxicity. Optic neuropathy may occur with ethambutol, but has not been reported in RCTs in people with HIV where the dose and symptoms were carefully monitored.

Stopping prophylaxis

In 643 HIV-1-infected patients, with a previous CD4 cell count < 50 cells/mm^3 and a sustained increase to > 10 cells/mm^3 during HAART, given azithromycin, 1200 mg once weekly (N = 321), or matching placebo (N = 322), a median follow up of 16 months showed two cases of MAC infection among the 321 patients assigned to placebo (incidence rate, 0·5 event per 100 person-years; 95% CI 0·06–1·83 events per 100 person-years) compared with no cases among the 322 patients assigned to azithromycin (95% CI 0–0·92 events per 100 person-years), resulting in a treatment difference of 0.5 events per 100 person-years (95% CI – 0·20 to 1·21 events per 100 person-years) for placebo versus azithromycin. Both cases were atypical in that MAC was localized to the vertebral spine. Patients receiving azithromycin were more likely than those receiving placebo to discontinue treatment with the study drug permanently because of adverse events (8% *v* 2%; HR 0·24; 95% CI 0·10–0·57).[127]

The second RCT (520 people without previous MAC disease, with CD4 > 100/mm^3 in response to HAART compared azithromycin with placebo. There were no episodes of confirmed MAC disease in either group over a median follow up of 12 months.[128] In both RCTs, adverse effects leading to discontinuation of treatment were more common with azithromycin than with placebo (7% *v* 1%; *P* = 0·002; 8% *v* 2%; P < 0·001).

Summary

RCTs have found that clarithromycin and ethambutol, with or without rifabutin, reduce the incidence of MAC. Clofazimine and high-dose clarithromycin are associated with increased mortality. Clarithromycin alone and clarithromycin plus rifabutin both reduce the incidence of MAC compared with rifabutin alone. Azithromycin plus rifabutin reduces the incidence of MAC compared with azithromycin alone but is associated with more side effects.

Treatment of cytomegalovirus

Ganciclovir and foscarnet have been the mainstays of treatment of cytomegalovirus (CMV) disease.[129] There has been a recent study comparing the effects of oral valganciclovir with those of intravenous ganciclovir as induction therapy for newly diagnosed CMV retinitis in 160 patients with AIDS. The primary endpoint was photographically determined progression of cytomegalovirus retinitis within 4 weeks after the initiation of treatment. Secondary endpoints included the achievement of a prospectively defined satisfactory response to induction therapy and the time to progression of cytomegalovirus retinitis. After 4 weeks, all patients received valganciclovir as maintenance therapy. Eighty patients were randomly assigned to each treatment group. Of the patients who could be evaluated, seven of 70 assigned to intravenous ganciclovir (10·0%) and seven of 71 assigned to oral valganciclovir (9·9%) had progression of cytomegalovirus retinitis during the first 4 weeks (difference in proportions, 0·1 percentage point; 95% CI – 9·7 to 10·0); 47 of 61 patients (77·0%) assigned to intravenous ganciclovir and 46 of 64 (71·9%) assigned to valganciclovir had a satisfactory response to induction therapy (difference in proportions, 5·2 percentage points; 95% CI – 20·4 to 10·1). The median times to progression of retinitis were 125 days in the group assigned to intravenous ganciclovir and 160 days in the group assigned to oral valganciclovir. The frequency and severity of adverse events were similar in the two treatment groups.[130]

Prophylaxis for CMV

Ganciclovir

One RCT (725 people with a median CD4 count of 22/mm^3) found that oral ganciclovir halved the incidence of CMV compared with placebo (event rate 16% *v* 30%; $P = 0{\cdot}001$). 25% of people who did not develop CMV developed severe neutropenia (and were then treated with granulocyte colony-stimulating factor).[131] A second RCT (994 HIV-1 infected people with CD4 < 100/mm^3 and CMV seropositivity) found no difference in the rate of CMV in people taking oral ganciclovir compared with placebo (event rates 13·1 *v* 14·6 per 100 person-years; HR 0·92; 95% CI 0·65–1·27).[132] Neither RCTs found a significant difference in overall mortality.

Acyclovir

There is one systematic review of individual patient data (eight RCTs) in people with asymptomatic HIV infection to AIDS.[133] It found no difference in protection against CMV disease between acyclovir compared with no treatment or placebo. However, acyclovir significantly reduced overall mortality (RR 0·81; $P = 0{\cdot}04$) and herpes simplex virus (HSV) and varicella zoster virus (VZV) infections ($P < 0{\cdot}001$ for both). One RCT (1227 CMV seropositive people with CD4 < 100/mm^3) compared valaciclovir, high-dose acyclovir, and low-dose acyclovir. It found increased mortality in the valaciclovir group, which did not reach statistical significance ($P = 0{\cdot}06$) and 1-year discontinuation rates of 51% for valaciclovir, 46% for high-dose acyclovir, and 41% for low-dose acyclovir.[134] The CMV rate was lower in the valaciclovir group than in the acyclovir groups (12% *v* 18%; $P = 0{\cdot}03$).

Stopping CMV prophylaxis

There are no randomized controlled trials or reviews. There are several small case series.[135–143] The study with the longest follow up (mean 20·4 months) found no relapses in 41 people discontinuing maintenance treatment.[135] However, another study with mean follow up of 14·5 months found five (29%) relapses among 17 participants who withdrew from maintenance; all of them occurred after the CD4 cell count had dropped again to < 50/mm^3 (8 days/10 months after this event).[138] In one observational series, 12/14 participants (86%) had evidence of immune reconstitution retinitis even before starting withdrawal of prophylaxis.[137] Worsening uveitis was associated with a substantial vision loss (> 3 lines) in three participants. It is difficult to conduct a RCT of adequate sample size to exclude modest differences in relapse rates. The observational evidence suggests that withdrawal of CMV maintenance treatment may be considered in selected people in whom CMV disease is in remission, CD4 > 100/mm^3, and HIV replication remains suppressed. We found no clear evidence on whether quantification of CMV viremia should be considered in the decision to withdraw from maintenance. One small case series found that relapses were associated with a drop in the CD4 cell count.[138] However, we found no randomized or other reliable evidence of when CMV maintenance treatment should be reinstituted.

Other Aids related illness

Non Hodgkin's lymphoma

Patients with AIDS-associated lymphoma/leukemia historically have a poor prognosis and were frequently treated with low-intensity therapy. There is one RCT comparing reduced therapy with standard dose: 198 HIV-seropositive patients with previously untreated, aggressive non-Hodgkin's lymphoma were randomly assigned to receive standard-dose therapy with methotrexate, bleomycin, doxorubicin, cyclophosphamide, vincristine, and dexamethasone (m-BACOD) along with granulocyte-macrophage colony-stimulating factor (GM-CSF; N = 94) or reduced-dose m-BACOD with GM-CSF administered only as indicated (N = 98).[144] A complete response was achieved in 39 of the 94 assessable patients assigned to low-dose therapy (41%) and in 42 of the 81 assessable patients assigned to standard-dose therapy (52%, $P = 0·56$). There were no significant differences in overall or disease-free survival; median survival times were 35 weeks for patients receiving low-dose therapy and 31 weeks for those receiving standard-dose therapy (RR for death in the standard-dose group = 1·17; 95% CI 0·84–1·63; $P = 0·25$). Toxic effects of chemotherapy rated grade 3 or higher occurred in 66 of 94 patients assigned to standard-dose therapy (70%) and 50 of 98 patients assigned to low-dose treatment (51%; $P = 0·008$). Hematologic toxicity accounted for the difference. The effect of HAART on treatment has yet to be established but results look more promising.

AIDS dementia complex

> **Case presentation 4 (continued)**
>
> The patient improves with amphotericin and is discharged home on oral fluconazole; however, he represents 3 months later with increasing confusion. CT scan shows no focal lesions and CSF obtained by lumbar puncture shows neither evidence of cryptococcal infection nor any white cells. You review the causes of confusion in late HIV disease.

A meta-analysis of 2411 patients in the ACTG 116A, ACTG116B/117, ACTG175, BMS010 and CTN002 trials had 21 documented cases of AIDS dementia complex (ADC) during the 15-month follow up period. The rates per 100 person-years of follow up were 0·70, 0·65, and 0·41 for the zidovudine, high-dose didanosine, and didanosine arms, respectively. There were no significant differences in risks of ADC between treatment arms (zidovudine *v* high-dose didanosine: $P = 0·30$; zidovudine *v* didanosine: $P = 0·97$; didanosine versus high-dose didanosine: $P = 0·41$).[145]

Progressive multifocal leukoencephalopathy

Progressive multifocal leukoencephalopathy (PMLE) affects about 4% of patients with AIDS, and survival after the diagnosis of leukoencephalopathy averages only about 3 months. JC virus PCR in blood has a poor positive predictive value (16%) but a good negative predictive value (96%) for PMLE.[146] However, in one study, PCR of CSF yielded sensitivity and specificity values of 100 and 90%, respectively.[147]

In observational studies no benefit has been found using cidofovir[148] nor cytarabine administered either intravenously or intrathecally.[149] A small observational study in 27 patients found the use of cidofovir was independently associated with a reduced risk of death (HR, 0·21; 95% CI 0·07–0·65; $P = 0·005$).[150]

> **Case presentation 4 (continued)**
>
> CSF samples are sent for JC virus PCR and this is positive. MRI scans show typical changes of PMLE. Lymph node biopsy does not show any evidence of lymphoma nor of *Mycobacterium avium-intracellulare*. He deteriorates further and dies in a hospice 2 months later.

Acknowledgments

The author is indebted to the work contained in the *Clinical Evidence in HIV* by Professor Margaret Johnson, Professor David Wilkinson, and Professor Andrew Phillips, published by BMJ Publishing Group Ltd, as a basis for this work.

References

1. Hecht FM, Busch MP, Rawal B *et al*. Use of laboratory tests and clinical symptoms for identification of primary HIV infection. *AIDS* 2002;**16**:1119-29.

2. Rosenberg ES, Altfeld M, Poon SH *et al.* Immune control of HIV-1 after early treatment of acute infection. *Nature* 2000;**407**:523–6.
3. Markowitz M, Vesanen M, Tenner-Racz K *et al.* The effect of commencing combination antiretroviral therapy soon after human immunodeficiency virus type 1 infection on viral replication and antiviral immune responses. *J Infect Dis* 1999;**179**:527–37.
4. Kinloch-De Loes S, Hirschel BJ, Hoen B *et al.* A controlled trial of zidovudine in primary human immunodeficiency virus infection. *N Engl J Med* 1995;**333**:408–13.
5. Darbyshire J, Foulkes M, Peto R *et al.* Immediate versus deferred zidovudine (AZT) in asymptomatic or mildly symptomatic HIV infected adults (Cochrane review). In: Cochrane Collaboration. *Cochrane Library.* Issue 3. Oxford: Update Software, 2002.
6. Ioannidis JP, Cappelleri JC, Lau J *et al.* Early or deferred zidovudine therapy in HIV-infected patients without an AIDS-defining illness. *Ann Intern Med* 1995;**122**:856–66.
7. Mellors JW, Munoz A, Giorgi JV *et al.* Plasma viral load and CD4+ lymphocytes as prognostic markers of HIV-1 infection. *Ann Intern Med* 1997;**126**:946–54.
8. Egger M, May M, Chene G *et al.* Prognosis of HIV-1-infected patients starting highly active antiretroviral therapy: a collaborative analysis of prospective studies. *Lancet* 2002;**360**:119–29.
9. British HIV Association (BHIVA) guidelines for the treatment of HIV-infected adults with antiretroviral therapy. *HIV Med* 2001;**2**:276–313.
10. Guidelines for using antiretroviral agents among HIV-infected adults and adolescents. Recommendations of the Panel on Clinical Practices for Treatment of HIV. *MMWR Recomm Rep* 2002;**51**(RR-7):1–55.
11. Dye C, Scheele S, Dolin P, Pathania V, Raviglione MC. Consensus statement. Global burden of TB: estimated incidence, prevalence, and mortality by country. WHO Global Surveillance and Monitoring Project. *JAMA* 1999;**282**:677–86.
12. UNAIDS. Report on the Global HIV/AIDS Epidemic 2002. In: *XIV International conference on AIDS.* Barcelona, 2002.
13. Cohen R, Muzaffar S, Capellan J, Azar H, Chinikamwala M. The validity of classic symptoms and chest radiographic configuration in predicting pulmonary TB. *Chest* 1996;**109**:420–3.
14. Long R, Scalcini M, Manfreda J, Jean-Baptiste M, Hershfield E. The impact of HIV on the usefulness of sputum smears for the diagnosis of TB. *Am J Public Health* 1991;**81**:1326–8.
15. Parry CM, Kamoto O, Harries AD *et al.* The use of sputum induction for establishing a diagnosis in patients with suspected pulmonary TB in Malawi. *Tuber Lung Dis* 1995;**76**:72–6.
16. Bruchfeld J, Aderaye G, Palme IB, Bjorvatn B, Kallenius G, Lindquist L. Sputum concentration improves diagnosis of TB in a setting with a high prevalence of HIV. *Trans R Soc Trop Med Hyg* 2000;**94**:677–80.
17. Perriens JH, St Louis ME, Mukadi YB *et al.* Pulmonary tuberculosis in HIV-infected patients in Zaire. A controlled trial of treatment for either 6 or 12 months. *N Engl J Med* 1995;**332**:779–84.
18. Selwyn PA, Hartel D, Lewis VA *et al.* A prospective study of the risk of tuberculosis among intravenous drug users with human immunodeficiency virus infection. *N Engl J Med* 1989;**320**:545–50.
19. Wilkinson D. Drugs for preventing tuberculosis in HIV infected persons. In: Cochrane Collaboration. *Cochrane Library.* Oxford: Update Software, 1999.
20. Bucher HC, Griffith LE, Guyatt GH *et al.* Isoniazid prophylaxis for tuberculosis in HIV infection: a meta-analysis of randomized controlled trials. *AIDS* 1999;**13**:501–7.
21. Kaplan JE, Hanson D, Dworkin M *et al.* Epidemiology of human immunodeficiency virus-associated opportunistic infections in the United States in the era of highly active antiretroviral therapy. *Clin Infect Dis* 2000;**30**(Suppl. 1):S5–14.
22. Kovacs JA, Hiemenz JW, Macher AM *et al.* *Pneumocystis carinii* pneumonia: a comparison between patients with the acquired immunodeficiency syndrome and patients with other immunodeficiencies. *Ann Intern Med* 1984;**100**:663–71.
23. Cregan P, Yamamoto A, Lum A, VanDerHeide T, MacDonald M, Pulliam L. Comparison of four methods for rapid detection of *Pneumocystis carinii* in respiratory specimens. *J Clin Microbiol* 1990;**28**:2432–6.
24. Ribes JA, Limper AH, Espy MJ, Smith TF. PCR detection of *Pneumocystis carinii* in bronchoalveolar lavage specimens: analysis of sensitivity and specificity. *J Clin Microbiol* 1997;**35**:830–5.

25. Miller RF, Kocjan G, Buckland J, Holton J, Malin A, Semple SJ. Sputum induction for the diagnosis of pulmonary disease in HIV positive patients. *J Infect* 1991;**23**:5–15.
26. Hughes WT, Feldman S, Chaudhary SC, Ossi MJ, Cox F, Sanyal SK. Comparison of pentamidine isethionate and trimethoprim-sulfamethoxazole in the treatment of *Pneumocystis carinii* pneumonia. *J Pediatr* 1978;**92**:285–91.
27. Sattler FR, Cowan R, Nielsen DM, Ruskin J. Trimethoprim-sulfamethoxazole compared with pentamidine for treatment of *Pneumocystis carinii* pneumonia in the acquired immunodeficiency syndrome. A prospective, noncrossover study. *Ann Intern Med* 1988;**109**:280–7.
28. MacFadden DK, Edelson JD, Hyland RH, Rodriguez CH, Inouye T, Rebuck AS. Corticosteroids as adjunctive therapy in treatment of *Pneumocystis carinii* pneumonia in patients with acquired immunodeficiency syndrome. *Lancet* 1987;**1**:1477–9.
29. Gagnon S, Boota AM, Fischl MA, Baier H, Kirksey OW, La Voie L. Corticosteroids as adjunctive therapy for severe *Pneumocystis carinii* pneumonia in the acquired immunodeficiency syndrome. A double-blind, placebo-controlled trial. *N Engl J Med* 1990;**323**:1444–50.
30. Bozzette SA, Sattler FR, Chiu J *et al.* A controlled trial of early adjunctive treatment with corticosteroids for *Pneumocystis carinii* pneumonia in the acquired immunodeficiency syndrome. California Collaborative Treatment Group. *N Engl J Med* 1990;**323**:1451–7.
31. Nielsen TL, Eeftinck Schattenkerk JK, Jensen BN. (Corticosteroid treatment of patients with AIDS and severe *Pneumocystis carinii* pneumonia. A European multicenter study. Danish-Dutch AIDS Study Group). *Ugeskr Laeger* 1993;**155**:2343–7.
32. Walmsley S, Levinton C, Brunton J *et al.* A multicenter randomized double-blind placebo-controlled trial of adjunctive corticosteroids in the treatment of *Pneumocystis carinii* pneumonia complicating the acquired immune deficiency syndrome. *J Acquir Immune Defic Syndr Hum Retrovirol* 1995;**8**:348–57.
33. Montaner JS, Guillemi S, Quieffin J *et al.* Oral corticosteroids in patients with mild *Pneumocystis carinii* pneumonia and the acquired immune deficiency syndrome (AIDS). *Tuber Lung Dis* 1993;**74**:173–9.
34. Smego RA, Jr., Nagar S, Maloba B, Popara M. A meta-analysis of salvage therapy for *Pneumocystis carinii* pneumonia. *Arch Intern Med* 2001;**161**:1529–33.
35. Jordan R, Gold L, Cummins C, Hyde C. Systematic review and meta-analysis of evidence for increasing numbers of drugs in antiretroviral combination therapy. *BMJ* 2002; **324**:757.
36. Robbins G, Shafer R, Smeaton L *et al.* Antiretroviral strategies in naive HIV+ subjects: comparison of sequential 3-drug regimens (ACTG 384). In: *XIV International AIDS conference*. Barcelona, 2002.
37. Bartlett JA, Johnson J, Herrera G, Sosa N, Rodriguez AE, Shaefer MS. Abacavir/Lamivudine (ABC/3TC) in combination with Efavirenz (NNRTI), Amprenavir/Ritonavir (PI) or Stavudine (NRTI): ESS40001(CLASS) preliminary 48 week results. In: *XIV International AIDS conference.* Barcelona, 2002.
38. Bersoff-Matcha SJ, Miller WC, Aberg JA *et al.* Sex differences in nevirapine rash. *Clin Infect Dis* 2001;**32**:124–9.
39. Mannheimer S, Friedland G, Matts J, Child C, Chesney M. The consistency of adherence to antiretroviral therapy predicts biologic outcomes for human immunodeficiency virus-infected persons in clinical trials. *Clin Infect Dis* 2002;**34**:1115–21.
40. Paterson DL, Swindells S, Mohr J *et al.* Adherence to protease inhibitor therapy and outcomes in patients with HIV infection. *Ann Intern Med* 2000;**133**:21–30.
41. Nieuwkerk PT, Sprangers MA, Burger DM *et al.* Limited patient adherence to highly active antiretroviral therapy for HIV-1 infection in an observational cohort study. *Arch Intern Med* 2001;**161**:1962–8.
42. Bangsberg D, Perry S, Charlesbois E. Adherence to HAART predicts progression to AIDS. In: *8th Conference on Retroviruses and Opportunistic Infections.* Chicago, 2001.
43. Fischl M, Rodriguez A, Scerpella E. Impact of directly observed therapy on outcomes in HIV clinical trials. In: *7th Conference on Retroviruses and Opportunistic Infections.* San Francisco, 2000.
44. Garcia de Olalla P, Knobel H, Carmona A, Guelar A, Lopez-Colomes JL, Cayla JA. Impact of adherence and highly active antiretroviral therapy on survival in HIV-infected patients. *J Acquir Immune Defic Syndr* 2002;**30**:105–10.
45. Claxton AJ, Cramer J, Pierce C. A systematic review of the associations between dose regimens and medication compliance. *Clin Ther* 2001;**23**:1296–310.

46. Bamberger JD, Unick J, Klein P, Fraser M, Chesney M, Katz MH. Helping the urban poor stay with antiretroviral HIV drug therapy. *Am J Public Health* 2000;**90**:699–701.
47. Nieuwkerk P, Gisolf E, Sprangers M, Danner S. Adherence over 48 weeks in an antiretroviral clinical trial: variable within patients, affected by toxicities and independently predictive of virological response. *Antivir Ther* 2001;**6**:97–103.
48. Chesney MA. Factors affecting adherence to antiretroviral therapy. *Clin Infect Dis* 2000;**30**(Suppl. 2):S171–6.
49. Tuldra A, Fumaz CR, Ferrer MJ *et al.* Prospective randomized two-arm controlled study to determine the efficacy of a specific intervention to improve long-term adherence to highly active antiretroviral therapy. *J Acquir Immune Defic Syndr* 2000;**25**:221–8.
50. Knobel H, Carmona A, Lopez JL *et al.* (Adherence to very active antiretroviral treatment: impact of individualized assessment). *Enferm Infecc Microbiol Clin* 1999;**17**: 78–81.
51. Gifford A, Bormann J, MJ Shively. Effects of group HIV patient education on adherence to antiretrovirals: a randomized controlled trial. In: *8th Conference on Retroviruses and Opportunistic Infections*. Chicago, 2001.
52. Goujard C, Peyramond D, Bernard N. Improved adherence to antiretroviral therapy at 6 months in HIV-1 infected individuals: impact of a face-to-face treatment education program: the Ciel Bleu study. In: *1st IAS Conference on HIV Pathogenesis and Treatment*. Buenos Aires, 2001.
53. Safren S, Hendriksen E, Boswell S. Twelve-week outcome of a cue-controlled paging system to increase ART adherence. In: *14th International AIDS Conference*. Barcelona, 2002.
54. Collier A, Ribaudo H, Feinberg J. Randomized study of telephone calls to improve adherence to antiretroviral therapy. In: *9th Conference on Retroviruses and Opportunistic Infections*. Seattle, 2002.
55. Rigsby MO, Rosen MI, Beauvais JE *et al.* Cue-dose training with monetary reinforcement: pilot study of an antiretroviral adherence intervention. *J Gen Intern Med* 2000;**15**:841–7.
56. Wall TL, Sorensen JL, Batki SL, Delucchi KL, London JA, Chesney MA. Adherence to zidovudine (AZT) among HIV-infected methadone patients: a pilot study of supervised therapy and dispensing compared with usual care. *Drug Alcohol Depend* 1995;**37**:261–9.
57. Samet J, Horton N, Dukes K. A randomized controlled trial of a multidimensional intervention to enhance adherence to antiretroviral therapy in HIV-infected patients with a history of alcohol problems. In: *14th International AIDS Conference*. Barcelona, 2002.
58. Gisolf EH, Dreezen C, Danner SA, Weel JL, Weverling GJ. Risk factors for hepatotoxicity in HIV-1-infected patients receiving ritonavir and saquinavir with or without stavudine. Prometheus Study Group. *Clin Infect Dis* 2000;**31**:1234–9.
59. Hernandez LV, Gilson I, Jacobson J, Affi A, Puetz TR, Dindzans VJ. Antiretroviral hepatotoxicity in human immunodeficiency virus-infected patients. *Aliment Pharmacol Ther* 2001;**15**:1627–32.
60. den Brinker M, Wit FW, Wertheim-van Dillen PM *et al.* Hepatitis B and C virus co-infection and the risk for hepatotoxicity of highly active antiretroviral therapy in HIV-1 infection. *AIDS* 2000;**14**:2895–902.
61. Greub G, Ledergerber B, Battegay M *et al.* Clinical progression, survival, and immune recovery during antiretroviral therapy in patients with HIV-1 and hepatitis C virus coinfection: the Swiss HIV Cohort Study. *Lancet* 2000;**356**:1800–5.
62. Graham CS, Baden LR, Yu E *et al.* Influence of human immunodeficiency virus infection on the course of hepatitis C virus infection: a meta-analysis. *Clin Infect Dis* 2001;**33**: 562–9.
63. Landau A, Batisse D, Piketty C *et al.* Long-term efficacy of combination therapy with interferon-alpha 2b and ribavirin for severe chronic hepatitis C in HIV-infected patients. *AIDS* 2001;**15**:2149–55.
64. Sauleda S, Juarez A, Esteban JI *et al.* Interferon and ribavirin combination therapy for chronic hepatitis C in human immunodeficiency virus-infected patients with congenital coagulation disorders. *Hepatology* 2001;**34**:1035–40.
65. Clarke S, Keenan E, Ryan M, Barry M, Mulcahy F. Directly observed antiretroviral therapy for injection drug users with HIV infection. *AIDS Read* 2002;**12**:305–7, 312–16.
66. Clarke SM, Mulcahy FM. Antiretroviral therapy for drug users. *Int J STD AIDS* 2000;**11**:627–31.
67. Gupta SB, Gilbert RL, Brady AR, Livingstone SJ, Evans BG. CD4 cell counts in adults with newly diagnosed HIV

infection: results of surveillance in England and Wales, 1990–1998. CD4 Surveillance Scheme Advisory Group. *AIDS* 2000;**14**:853–61.

68. Ioannidis JP, Cappelleri JC, Skolnik PR, Lau J, Sacks HS. A meta-analysis of the relative efficacy and toxicity of *Pneumocystis carinii* prophylactic regimens. *Arch Intern Med* 1996;**156**:177–88.
69. Bucher HC, Griffith L, Guyatt GH, Opravil M. Meta-analysis of prophylactic treatments against *Pneumocystis carinii* pneumonia and toxoplasma encephalitis in HIV-infected patients. *J Acquir Immune Defic Syndr Hum Retrovirol* 1997;**15**:104–14.
70. Anglaret X, Chene G, Attia A *et al.* Early chemoprophylaxis with trimethoprim-sulphamethoxazole for HIV-1-infected adults in Abidjan, Cote d'Ivoire: a randomized trial. Cotrimo-CI Study Group. *Lancet* 1999;**353**:1463–8.
71. El-Sadr WM, Luskin-Hawk R, Yurik TM *et al.* A randomized trial of daily and thrice-weekly trimethoprim-sulfamethoxazole for the prevention of *Pneumocystis carinii* pneumonia in human immunodeficiency virus-infected persons. Terry Beirn Community Programs for Clinical Research on AIDS (CPCRA). *Clin Infect Dis* 1999;**29**:775–83.
72. Para MF, Finkelstein D, Becker S, Dohn M, Walawander A, Black JR. Reduced toxicity with gradual initiation of trimethoprim-sulfamethoxazole as primary prophylaxis for *Pneumocystis carinii* pneumonia: AIDS Clinical Trials Group 268. *J Acquir Immune Defic Syndr* 2000;**24**:337–43.
73. Walmsley SL, Khorasheh S, Singer J, Djurdjev O. A randomized trial of N-acetylcysteine for prevention of trimethoprim-sulfamethoxazole hypersensitivity reactions in *Pneumocystis carinii* pneumonia prophylaxis (CTN 057). Canadian HIV Trials Network 057 Study Group. *J Acquir Immune Defic Syndr Hum Retrovirol* 1998;**19**:498–505.
74. Akerlund B, Tynell E, Bratt G, Bielenstein M, Lidman C. N-acetylcysteine treatment and the risk of toxic reactions to trimethoprim-sulphamethoxazole in primary *Pneumocystis carinii* prophylaxis in HIV-infected patients. *J Infect* 1997;**35**:143–7.
75. El-Sadr WM, Murphy RL, Yurik TM *et al.* Atovaquone compared with dapsone for the prevention of *Pneumocystis carinii* pneumonia in patients with HIV infection who cannot tolerate trimethoprim, sulfonamides, or both. Community Program for Clinical Research on AIDS and the AIDS Clinical Trials Group. *N Engl J Med* 1998;**339**:1889–95.
76. Chan C, Montaner J, Lefebvre EA *et al.* Atovaquone suspension compared with aerosolized pentamidine for prevention of *Pneumocystis carinii* pneumonia in human immunodeficiency virus-infected subjects intolerant of trimethoprim or sulfonamides. *J Infect Dis* 1999;**180**:369–76.
77. Dunne MW, Bozzette S, McCutchan JA *et al.* Efficacy of azithromycin in prevention of *Pneumocystis carinii* pneumonia: a randomized trial. California Collaborative Treatment Group. *Lancet* 1999;**354**:891–5.
78. Havlir DV, Dube MP, Sattler FR *et al.* Prophylaxis against disseminated *Mycobacterium avium* complex with weekly azithromycin, daily rifabutin, or both. California Collaborative Treatment Group. *N Engl J Med* 1996;**335**:392–8.
79. Saillourglenisson F, Chene G, Salmi LR, Hafner R, Salamon R. (Effect of dapsone on survival in HIV infected patients: a meta-analysis of finished trials). *Rev Epidemiol Sante Publ* 2000;**48**:17–30.
80. Detels R, Tarwater P, Phair JP, Margolick J, Riddler SA, Munoz A. Effectiveness of potent antiretroviral therapies on the incidence of opportunistic infections before and after AIDS diagnosis. *AIDS* 2001;**15**:347–55.
81. Gallant JE, Moore RD, Chaisson RE. Prophylaxis for opportunistic infections in patients with HIV infection. *Ann Intern Med* 1994;**120**:932–44.
82. Schacker T, Hu HL, Koelle DM *et al.* Famciclovir for the suppression of symptomatic and asymptomatic herpes simplex virus reactivation in HIV-infected persons. A double-blind, placebo-controlled trial. *Ann Intern Med* 1998;**128**:21–8.
83. Trikalinos TA, Ioannidis JP. Discontinuation of *Pneumocystis carinii* prophylaxis in patients infected with human immunodeficiency virus: a meta-analysis and decision analysis. *Clin Infect Dis* 2001;**33**:1901–9.
84. Lopez Bernaldo de Quiros JC, Miro JM *et al.* A randomized trial of the discontinuation of primary and secondary prophylaxis against *Pneumocystis carinii* pneumonia after highly active antiretroviral therapy in patients with HIV infection. Grupo de Estudio del SIDA 04/98. *N Engl J Med* 2001;**344**:159–67.
85. Mussini C, Pezzotti P, Govoni A *et al.* Discontinuation of primary prophylaxis for *Pneumocystis carinii* pneumonia and toxoplasmic encephalitis in human immunodeficiency virus type I-infected patients: the changes in opportunistic prophylaxis study. *J Infect Dis* 2000;**181**:1635–42.

86. Miro J, Lopez J, Podzamczer C *et al.* Discontinuation of toxoplasmic encephalitis prophylaxis is safe in HIV-1 and T. gondii co-infected patients after immunological recovery with HAART. Preliminary results of the GESIDA 04/98B study. In: Alexandria V, ed. *7th Conference on Retroviruses and Opportunistic Infections.* San Francisco: Foundation for Retrovirology and Human Health, 2000.
87. Tural C, Ruiz L, Holtzer C *et al.* Clinical utility of HIV-1 genotyping and expert advice: the Havana trial. *AIDS* 2002;**16**:209–18.
88. Durant J, Clevenbergh P, Halfon P *et al.* Drug-resistance genotyping in HIV-1 therapy: the VIRADAPT randomized controlled trial. *Lancet* 1999;**353**:2195–9.
89. Baxter JD, Mayers DL, Wentworth DN *et al.* A randomized study of antiretroviral management based on plasma genotypic antiretroviral resistance testing in patients failing therapy. CPCRA 046 Study Team for the Terry Beirn Community Programs for Clinical Research on AIDS. *AIDS* 2000;**14**:F83–93.
90. Kijak GH, Rubio AE, Pampuro SE *et al.* Discrepant results in the interpretation of HIV-1 drug resistance genotypic data among widely used algorithms. *HIV Med* 2003;**4**:72–8.
91. Cohen CJ, Hunt S, Sension M *et al.* A randomized trial assessing the impact of phenotypic resistance testing on antiretroviral therapy. *AIDS* 2002;**16**:579–88.
92. Durant J, Clevenbergh P, Garraffo R *et al.* Importance of protease inhibitor plasma levels in HIV-infected patients treated with genotypic-guided therapy: pharmacological data from the Viradapt Study. *AIDS* 2000;**14**:1333–9.
93. Ruiz L, Ribera E, Bonjoch A *et al.* Virological and immunological benefit of a salvage therapy that includes Kaletra plus Fortovase preceded or not by antiretroviral therapy interruption (TI) in advanced HIV-infected patients (6-month-follow up). In: *9th Conference on Retroviruses and Opportunistic Infections.* Seattle, 2002.
94. Katlama C, Dominguez S, Duvivier C *et al.* Benefits of Treatment Interruption (TI) in Patients with Multiple Therapy Failures, CD4 cells $< 200\ mm^{-3}$ and HIV RNA $> 50\,000$ cp/ml^{-1} (GIGHAART ANRS 097). In: *14th International AIDS Conference.* Barcelona, 2002.
95. Lundgren JD, Vella S, Paddam L *et al.* Interruption/Stopping Antiretroviral Therapy and the Risk of Clinical Disease: Results from the EuroSIDA Study. In: *9th Conference on Retroviruses and Opportunistic Infections.* Seattle, 2002.
96. van der Horst CM, Saag MS, Cloud GA *et al.* Treatment of cryptococcal meningitis associated with the acquired immunodeficiency syndrome. National Institute of Allergy and Infectious Diseases Mycoses Study Group and AIDS Clinical Trials Group. *N Engl J Med* 1997;**337**:15–21.
97. Leenders AC, Reiss P, Portegies P *et al.* Liposomal amphotericin B (AmBisome) compared with amphotericin B both followed by oral fluconazole in the treatment of AIDS-associated cryptococcal meningitis. *AIDS* 1997;**11**:1463–71.
98. Coker RJ, Viviani M, Gazzard BG *et al.* Treatment of cryptococcosis with liposomal amphotericin B (AmBisome) in 23 patients with AIDS. *AIDS* 1993;**7**: 829–35.
99. Larsen RA, Bozzette SA, Jones BE *et al.* Fluconazole combined with flucytosine for treatment of cryptococcal meningitis in patients with AIDS. *Clin Infect Dis* 1994;**19**:741–5.
100. Berry AJ, Rinaldi MG, Graybill JR. Use of high-dose fluconazole as salvage therapy for cryptococcal meningitis in patients with AIDS. *Antimicrob Agents Chemother* 1992;**36**:690–2.
101. Menichetti F, Fiorio M, Tosti A *et al.* High-dose fluconazole therapy for cryptococcal meningitis in patients with AIDS. *Clin Infect Dis* 1996;**22**:838–40.
102. Saag MS, Powderly WG, Cloud GA *et al.* Comparison of amphotericin B with fluconazole in the treatment of acute AIDS-associated cryptococcal meningitis. The NIAID Mycoses Study Group and the AIDS Clinical Trials Group. *N Engl J Med* 1992;**326**:83–9.
103. Mayanja-Kizza H, Oishi K, Mitarai S *et al.* Combination therapy with fluconazole and flucytosine for cryptococcal meningitis in Ugandan patients with AIDS. *Clin Infect Dis* 1998;**26**:1362–6.
104. de Gans J, Portegies P, Tiessens G *et al.* Itraconazole compared with amphotericin B plus flucytosine in AIDS patients with cryptococcal meningitis. *AIDS* 1992;**6**:185–90.
105. Graybill JR, Sobel J, Saag M *et al.* Diagnosis and management of increased intracranial pressure in patients with AIDS and cryptococcal meningitis. The NIAID Mycoses Study Group and AIDS Cooperative Treatment Groups. *Clin Infect Dis* 2000;**30**:47–54.
106. Fessler RD, Sobel J, Guyot L *et al.* Management of elevated intracranial pressure in patients with

Cryptococcal meningitis. *J Acquir Immune Defic Syndr Hum Retrovirol* 1998;**17**:137–42.

107. Schuman P, Capps L, Peng G *et al.* Weekly fluconazole for the prevention of mucosal candidiasis in women with HIV infection. A randomized, double-blind, placebo-controlled trial. Terry Beirn Community Programs for Clinical Research on AIDS. *Ann Intern Med* 1997;**126**:689–96.
108. McKinsey DS, Wheat LJ, Cloud GA *et al.* Itraconazole prophylaxis for fungal infections in patients with advanced human immunodeficiency virus infection: randomized, placebo-controlled, double-blind study. National Institute of Allergy and Infectious Diseases Mycoses Study Group. *Clin Infect Dis* 1999;**28**:1049–56.
109. Havlir DV, Dube MP, McCutchan JA *et al.* Prophylaxis with weekly versus daily fluconazole for fungal infections in patients with AIDS. *Clin Infect Dis* 1998;**27**:1369–75.
110. Powderly WG, Finkelstein D, Feinberg J *et al.* A randomized trial comparing fluconazole with clotrimazole troches for the prevention of fungal infections in patients with advanced human immunodeficiency virus infection. NIAID AIDS Clinical Trials Group. *N Engl J Med* 1995;**332**:700–5.
111. Smith D, Midgley J, Gazzard B. A randomized, double-blind study of itraconazole versus placebo in the treatment and prevention of oral or oesophageal candidosis in patients with HIV infection. *Int J Clin Pract* 1999;**53**:349–52.
112. Saag MS, Cloud GA, Graybill JR *et al.* A comparison of itraconazole versus fluconazole as maintenance therapy for AIDS-associated cryptococcal meningitis. National Institute of Allergy and Infectious Diseases Mycoses Study Group. *Clin Infect Dis* 1999;**28**:291–6.
113. Wheat J, Hafner R, Wulfsohn M *et al.* Prevention of relapse of histoplasmosis with itraconazole in patients with the acquired immunodeficiency syndrome. The National Institute of Allergy and Infectious Diseases Clinical Trials and Mycoses Study Group Collaborators. *Ann Intern Med* 1993;**118**:610–6.
114. Dunne M, Fessel J, Kumar P *et al.* A randomized, double-blind trial comparing azithromycin and clarithromycin in the treatment of disseminated *Mycobacterium avium* infection in patients with human immunodeficiency virus. *Clin Infect Dis* 2000;**31**:1245–52.
115. Cohn DL, Fisher EJ, Peng GT *et al.* A prospective randomized trial of four three-drug regimens in the treatment of disseminated *Mycobacterium avium* complex disease in AIDS patients: excess mortality associated with high-dose clarithromycin. Terry Beirn Community Programs for Clinical Research on AIDS. *Clin Infect Dis* 1999;**29**:125–33.
116. Singer J, Thorne A, Khorasheh S *et al.* Symptomatic and health status outcomes in the Canadian randomized MAC treatment trial (CTN010). Canadian HIV Trials Network Protocol 010 Study Group. Int J STD AIDS 2000;**11**:212–9.
117. Oldfield EC, 3rd, Fessel WJ, Dunne M *et al.* Once weekly azithromycin therapy for prevention of *Mycobacterium avium* complex infection in patients with AIDS: a randomized, double-blind, placebo-controlled multicenter trial. *Clin Infect Dis* 1998;**26**:611–9.
118. Faris MA, Raasch RH, Hopfer RL, Butts JD. Treatment and prophylaxis of disseminated *Mycobacterium avium* complex in HIV-infected individuals. *Ann Pharmacother* 1998;**32**:564–73.
119. Pierce M, Crampton S, Henry D *et al.* A randomized trial of clarithromycin as prophylaxis against disseminated *Mycobacterium avium* complex infection in patients with advanced acquired immunodeficiency syndrome. *N Engl J Med* 1996;**335**:384–91.
120. Benson CA, Williams PL, Cohn DL *et al.* Clarithromycin or rifabutin alone or in combination for primary prophylaxis of *Mycobacterium avium* complex disease in patients with AIDS: A randomized, double-blind, placebo-controlled trial. The AIDS Clinical Trials Group 196/Terry Beirn Community Programs for Clinical Research on AIDS 009 Protocol Team. *J Infect Dis* 2000;**181**:1289–97.
121. Tseng AL, Walmsley SL. Rifabutin-associated uveitis. *Ann Pharmacother* 1995;**29**:1149–55.
122. Dube MP, Sattler FR, Torriani FJ *et al.* A randomized evaluation of ethambutol for prevention of relapse and drug resistance during treatment of *Mycobacterium avium* complex bacteremia with clarithromycin-based combination therapy. California Collaborative Treatment Group. *J Infect Dis* 1997;**176**:1225–32.
123. Chaisson RE, Keiser P, Pierce M *et al.* Clarithromycin and ethambutol with or without clofazimine for the treatment of bacteremic *Mycobacterium avium* complex

disease in patients with HIV infection. *AIDS* 1997; **11**:311–17.

124. May T, Brel F, Beuscart C *et al.* Comparison of combination therapy regimens for treatment of human immunodeficiency virus-infected patients with disseminated bacteremia due to Mycobacterium avium. ANRS Trial 033 Curavium Group. Agence Nationale de Recherche sur le Sida. *Clin Infect Dis* 1997;**25**:621–9.
125. Gordin FM, Sullam PM, Shafran SD *et al.* A randomized, placebo-controlled study of rifabutin added to a regimen of clarithromycin and ethambutol for treatment of disseminated infection with *Mycobacterium avium* complex. *Clin Infect Dis* 1999;**28**:1080–5.
126. Chaisson RE, Benson CA, Dube MP *et al.* Clarithromycin therapy for bacteremic *Mycobacterium avium* complex disease. A randomized, double-blind, dose-ranging study in patients with AIDS. AIDS Clinical Trials Group Protocol 157 Study Team. *Ann Intern Med* 1994;**121**:905–11.
127. Currier JS, Williams PL, Koletar SL *et al.* Discontinuation of *Mycobacterium avium* complex prophylaxis in patients with antiretroviral therapy-induced increases in CD4+ cell count. A randomized, double-blind, placebo-controlled trial. AIDS Clinical Trials Group 362 Study Team. *Ann Intern Med* 2000;**133**:493–503.
128. El-Sadr WM, Burman WJ, Grant LB *et al.* Discontinuation of prophylaxis for *Mycobacterium avium* complex disease in HIV-infected patients who have a response to antiretroviral therapy. Terry Beirn Community Programs for Clinical Research on AIDS. *N Engl J Med* 2000;**342**:1085–92.
129. Moyle G, Harman C, Mitchell S, Mathalone B, Gazzard BG. Foscarnet and Ganciclovir in the treatment of CMV retinitis in AIDS patients: a randomized comparison. *J Infect* 1992;**25**:21–7.
130. Martin DF, Sierra-Madero J, Walmsley S *et al.* A controlled trial of valganciclovir as induction therapy for cytomegalovirus retinitis. *N Engl J Med* 2002;**346**: 1119–26.
131. Spector SA, McKinley GF, Lalezari JP *et al.* Oral ganciclovir for the prevention of cytomegalovirus disease in persons with AIDS. Roche Cooperative Oral Ganciclovir Study Group. *N Engl J Med* 1996;**334**: 1491–7.
132. Brosgart CL, Louis TA, Hillman DW *et al.* A randomized, placebo-controlled trial of the safety and efficacy of oral ganciclovir for prophylaxis of cytomegalovirus disease in HIV-infected individuals. Terry Beirn Community Programs for Clinical Research on AIDS. *AIDS* 1998;**12**:269–77.
133. Ioannidis JP, Collier AC, Cooper DA *et al.* Clinical efficacy of high-dose acyclovir in patients with human immunodeficiency virus infection: a meta-analysis of randomized individual patient data. *J Infect Dis* 1998;**178**:349–59.
134. Feinberg JE, Hurwitz S, Cooper D *et al.* A randomized, double-blind trial of valaciclovir prophylaxis for cytomegalovirus disease in patients with advanced human immunodeficiency virus infection. AIDS Clinical Trials Group Protocol 204/Glaxo Wellcome 123–014 International CMV Prophylaxis Study Group. *J Infect Dis* 1998;**177**:48–56.
135. Curi AL, Muralha A, Muralha L, Pavesio C. Suspension of anticytomegalovirus maintenance therapy following immune recovery due to highly active antiretroviral therapy. *Br J Ophthalmol* 2001;**85**:471–3.
136. Jouan M, Saves M, Tubiana R *et al.* Discontinuation of maintenance therapy for cytomegalovirus retinitis in HIV-infected patients receiving highly active antiretroviral therapy. *AIDS* 2001;**15**:23–31.
137. Whitcup SM, Fortin E, Lindblad AS *et al.* Discontinuation of anticytomegalovirus therapy in patients with HIV infection and cytomegalovirus retinitis. *JAMA* 1999;**282**:1633–7.
138. Torriani FJ, Freeman WR, Macdonald JC *et al.* CMV retinitis recurs after stopping treatment in virological and immunological failures of potent antiretroviral therapy. *AIDS* 2000;**14**:173–80.
139. Postelmans L, Gerard M, Sommereijns B, Caspers-Velu L. Discontinuation of maintenance therapy for CMV retinitis in AIDS patients on highly active antiretroviral therapy. *Ocul Immunol Inflamm* 1999;**7**:199–203.
140. Jabs DA, Bolton SG, Dunn JP, Palestine AG. Discontinuing anticytomegalovirus therapy in patients with immune reconstitution after combination antiretroviral therapy. *Am J Ophthalmol* 1998;**126**: 817–22.
141. Vrabec TR, Baldassano VF, Whitcup SM. Discontinuation of maintenance therapy in patients with quiescent cytomegalovirus retinitis and elevated CD4+ counts. *Ophthalmology* 1998;**105**:1259–64.

142. Macdonald JC, Torriani FJ, Morse LS, Karavellas MP, Reed JB, Freeman WR. Lack of reactivation of cytomegalovirus (CMV) retinitis after stopping CMV maintenance therapy in AIDS patients with sustained elevations in CD4 T cells in response to highly active antiretroviral therapy. *J Infect Dis* 1998;**177**:1182–7.
143. Tural C, Romeu J, Sirera G *et al.* Long-lasting remission of cytomegalovirus retinitis without maintenance therapy in human immunodeficiency virus-infected patients. *J Infect Dis* 1998;**177**:1080–3.
144. Kaplan LD, Straus DJ, Testa MA *et al.* Low-dose compared with standard-dose m-BACOD chemotherapy for non-Hodgkin's lymphoma associated with human immunodeficiency virus infection. National Institute of Allergy and Infectious Diseases AIDS Clinical Trials Group. *N Engl J Med* 1997;**336**:1641–8.
145. Raboud JM, Montaner JS, Rae S *et al.* Meta-analysis of five randomized controlled trials comparing continuation of zidovudine versus switching to didanosine in HIV-infected individuals. *Antivir Ther* 1997;**2**:237–47.
146. Andreoletti L, Lescieux A, Lambert V *et al.* Semiquantitative detection of JCV-DNA in peripheral blood leukocytes from HIV-1-infected patients with or without progressive multifocal leukoencephalopathy. *J Med Virol* 2002;**66**:1–7.
147. Garcia de Viedma D, Alonso R, Miralles P, Berenguer J, Rodriguez-Creixems M, Bouza E. Dual qualitative-quantitative nested PCR for detection of JC virus in cerebrospinal fluid: high potential for evaluation and monitoring of progressive multifocal leukoencephalopathy in AIDS patients receiving highly active antiretroviral therapy. *J Clin Microbiol* 1999;**37**:724–8.
148. Gasnault J, Kousignian P, Kahraman M *et al.* Cidofovir in AIDS-associated progressive multifocal leukoencephalopathy: a monocenter observational study with clinical and JC virus load monitoring. *J Neurovirol* 2001;**7**:375–81.
149. Hall CD, Dafni U, Simpson D *et al.* Failure of cytarabine in progressive multifocal leukoencephalopathy associated with human immunodeficiency virus infection. AIDS Clinical Trials Group 243 Team. *N Engl J Med* 1998;**338**:1345–51.
150. De Luca A, Giancola ML, Ammassari A *et al.* Potent anti-retroviral therapy with or without cidofovir for AIDS-associated progressive multifocal leukoencephalopathy: extended follow up of an observational study. *J Neurovirol* 2001;**7**:364–8.

Part 2
Special populations

12 Infection control

Eli Perencevich, Anthony Harris

Case presentation 1

Surgical site infections

A new chief of surgery, who happens to be a cardiothoracic surgeon, arrives at your hospital. She calls you and says that she is concerned that the risk-adjusted surgical site infection rates at her new hospital might be higher than the rates at her previous hospital. She wants to set up a meeting with you to discuss ways to minimize the risk of surgical site infection in her patients.

Burden of illness/relevance to clinical practice

Surgical site infections (SSIs) are defined as either incisional or organ/organ space infections. Incisional SSIs are then divided into superficial, involving the skin and subcutaneous tissue, and deep, involving the muscle and fascia.[1] Typically an infection is considered an SSI if it occurs within 30 days of the operation. SSI rates vary by procedure with rates being highest with cardiac surgery (2·5 infections per 100 patient discharges).[2] SSIs are the second most common cause of nosocomial infection after urinary tract infections, cause about 17% of all hospital-acquired infections,[3] and lead to increased costs and poorer patient outcomes in hospital inpatients.[4] Approximately 500 000 SSIs occur annually in the USA[5]; 77% of all those that died with an SSI were found to have the infection causally related to their deaths.[6] A UK study found that SSIs can result in a prolonged hospital stay of 8·2 days and added an average attributable cost of £1041.[7] In addition patients with an SSI recognized after hospital discharge can require more outpatient visits, ER visits, radiology services, re-admissions, and home health aid services and have over $3300 higher average total medical costs during the 8 weeks after discharge when compared with similar patients without SSI.[8] Costs and outcomes secondary to SSIs can vary by location and surgery type. Infections in cardiac surgery can add between $8200 (1982), and $42 000 (1985) to cost of care after adjusting for comorbidities, and these increased costs are likely attributable to excess hospital and intensive care unit (ICU) stays.[9–11] Overall, SSIs may result in $1–$10 billion in direct and indirect medical costs each year.[5,12]

Risk factors

The incidence of SSIs varies depending on the surgeon, the hospital, procedure type, and individual patient risk factors. The fact that confounding factors such as procedure type, duration of procedure, and baseline severity of illness of patients can impact surgical infection occurrence, necessitates the risk adjustment of SSI rates for fair comparison between surgeons and hospitals. Determination of risk factors is most useful when identified risk factors are modifiable. Therefore, factors such as specific hospital and procedure type may be interesting to note, but their identification as risk factors does not help surgeons, anesthesiologists and infection control personnel in preventing SSIs. In fact, duration of surgery, age, obesity, and underlying disease, are some of the most commonly noted risk factors for development of SSI, yet they are fixed parameters from the perspective of the infection control practitioner. While it may seem that identifying an individual surgeon as a risk factor could be more disruptive than helpful, it has been shown that one of the most successful ways to reduce SSIs is proper surveillance of infection rates and feedback of rates to individual surgeons.[13]

Throughout the rest of this section we will describe the evidence that supports specific risk factors for SSI with a particular focus on modifiable risk factors. It must be stated, however, that identifying a modifiable risk factor may or may not mean that an intervention that reduces or removes the risk factor will result in a benefit. For this we would need a randomized clinical trial.

Glucose control

Diabetes is known to increase the risk of developing a SSI. Unlike other comorbidities, such as obesity, there is a potential for lowering the risk of SSI through perioperative glucose control. Hyperglycemia (serum glucose > 220 mg/dL) during postoperative day 1 in diabetic patients was shown to be associated with an almost 3-fold increased risk of nosocomial infections.[14] In cardiothoracic surgery patients, a postoperative glucose level > 200 mg/dL within 48 hours after surgery was shown to increase the odds of developing an SSI by 86% in known diabetic patients and by 114% in patients with no history of diabetes, and these results were largely unchanged with multivariable analysis.[15]

Another group found that an elevated average blood glucose over the 48-hour postoperative period was the strongest predictor of deep sternal wound infection in diabetics undergoing open heart procedures.[16] Additionally, they performed a quasi-experimental trial in which historical controls, who had perioperative blood glucose controlled with subcutaneous insulin injections, were compared with a later group who had continuous insulin infusions, and they found that continuous insulin infusion was associated with a two-thirds reduction in the risk of deep sternal wound infection.[17] This is currently the best available evidence to support the efficacy of perioperative glucose control as a measure to prevent SSI. Trials that use historical controls, however, are limited by the fact that additional changes may occur through time, which cannot be controlled for in the quasi-experimental design, and could explain or partially explain the reduced infection rates.

Perioperative warming

Hypothermia is thought to increase a patient's risk of developing an SSI through thermoregulatory vasoconstriction and resultant reduced microbial killing and reduced tissue oxygen levels. Unwarmed patients in surgery lose heat until their core temperature falls about 2°C after which core temperature is stabilized by peripheral vasoconstriction and altered heat distribution.[18,19] In a randomized controlled trial in patients undergoing colorectal surgery, Kurz *et al.* demonstrated an approximately 3-fold reduction in SSI rates in patients actively warmed approximately 2°C to the desired temperature of 36·6°C by intravenous fluid warming and forced-air warming in the intraoperative period.[20] The same study also found that patients who were in the hypothermic arm of the study had 20% longer hospital stay.

A relatively small case–control study among patients who underwent cesarean section with 18 cases who developed SSI compared with 18 controls found intraoperative temperature not to be a significant risk factor for the development of SSI.[21] In a recent randomized controlled trial of patients undergoing breast, varicose vein, or hernia surgery, Melling *et al.* found that warming patients before surgery reduced postoperative SSIs. Patients were randomized to one of the following: systemic warming (whole-body warming by blanket and forced air in the 30-minute preoperative period), localized warming (30 minutes of preoperative warming localized to the planned wound area), and non-warming standard care.[22] The study found that both systemic warming (ARR 7·9%; 95% confidence interval. CI 1·0–14·8) and local warming (ARR 10·1%; 95% CI 3·6–16·6) were associated with reduced SSIs compared with standard non-warmed treatment. The study was not powered to find a difference between the systemic and local warming groups.

A broad recommendation across all types of surgery cannot be given, since patients who undergo certain procedures actually benefit from hypothermia. Mild hypothermia has a documented cerebroprotective effect in neurosurgery patients,[23] which would likely outweigh their very low risk of SSI.[24] In addition, core temperatures are lowered in cardiac surgery to protect the myocardium and central nervous system.[18]

Supplemental oxygen

Neutrophilic bactericidal activity is mediated by superoxide radical dependent oxidative killing, which is linked to the partial pressure of oxygen in the tissue.[25] A cohort study of patients at high risk for SSI found that the oxygen tension of the subcutaneous tissue measured perioperatively was a very strong predictor of subsequent development of SSI.[26] The infection rate was 43% (6 of 14 patients) in those with maximum oxygen tension between 40 and 50 mmHg and 0% (0 of 15 patients) in those with maximum oxygen tension > 90 mmHg. The wound hypoxia has been correlated with reduced leukocyte killing from depressed oxygen consumption and superoxide formation.[27]

A randomized controlled trial in patients undergoing colorectal surgery compared patients who received 30% inspired oxygen to those receiving 80% inspired oxygen.[25] The oxygen was given intraoperatively and in the 2 hours after surgery. Even though arterial oxygen saturation was normal in both groups, the subcutaneous partial pressure of oxygen was significantly higher in those that received 80% inspired oxygen. Importantly the infection rate was only 5·2% in the 80% inspired oxygen group compared with an infection rate of 11·2% in the 30% inspired oxygen group (ARR 6·0%; 95% CI 7·3–15·1). The duration of hospitalization was the same in both groups. The study was ended early because of the significant benefit from supplemental perioperative oxygen. A subgroup analysis found that higher oxygen was not associated with any additional risk for radiologically confirmed pulmonary atelectasis.[28] A smaller randomized study found improved tissue oxygenation in cervical spine surgical patients who received 36 hours of postoperative inspired oxygen of 28% compared with room air controls, but the study was not powered to assess infectious outcomes.[29] Supplemental perioperative oxygen is not yet widely adopted. This is perhaps due to the fact that its benefits have been tested in a randomized fashion in only a few types of surgical procedures and in only a small number of patients.

Hair removal

Hair shaving as part of the preparation of the surgical site has long been a practice of surgeons intent on preventing SSIs. However, it is now known that shaving changes the normal flora, removes the hair's natural protective effect and causes minor trauma, factors which, combined, increase the risk of infection.[30] Using a quasi-experimental study design, Sellick *et al.* found that switching from razor shaving to clipper removal of hair preoperatively reduced the rate of deep sternotomy SSIs from 1·2 to 0·2%, and reduced the rate of venectomy site SSI from 1·6 to 0·4%. They found no change in the superficial incisional infection rates after the change to perioperative clipper hair removal.[31] A randomized controlled trial of almost 2000 cardiac surgery patients found that electrically clipped patients had a one-third lower rate of mediastinitis than those who were manually shaved (odds ratio [OR] 3·25; 95% CI 1·11–9·32).[32] This study replicated an early randomized trial in elective surgeries, which showed reduced infections with hair clipping in the morning prior to surgery compared with shaving.[33]

A retrospective cohort study in intracranial surgical patients found that shaving of head hair prior to surgery did not reduce the rate of SSI compared with patients who had their hair spared.[30] The patients who had their hair spared all had their hair washed with shampoo and 4% chlorhexidine within 24 hours prior to surgery. These findings are similar to another study of neurosurgical patients that showed no change in SSI rates with the abandonment of preoperative hair shaving.[34] A prospective trial in pediatric neurosurgery patients found similar infection rates in children who had their hair shaved and those who did not.[35] It appears that hair removal should be limited to situations where it will impede the operation and, if necessary, hair should be removed as close to the operation as possible with clippers and not a razor.

Staphylococcus aureus elimination with mupirocin ointment

Staphylococcus aureus (*S. aureus*) is a frequent cause of SSIs. Mupirocin ointment may be successful in eliminating nasal carriage of *S. aureus*. A large cohort study of cardiothoracic surgery patients using both concurrent and historical controls found between a 4·5% and 5·8% reduction in SSIs in patients treated with nasal mupirocin ointment started on the day prior and continued for 4 days after surgery.[36] An analysis using this same data found that perioperative mupirocin was cost-effective and in most settings would be cost-saving.[37] In a recent large randomized controlled trial, surgical patients were randomly assigned to receive mupirocin or placebo in each anterior naris twice daily for up to 5 days before the operative procedure. The study was powered to detect a 50% reduction in *S. aureus* SSIs from 2·8% to 1·4%. The overall SSI rate was 7·9% in the mupirocin group and 8·5% in the placebo group. After the exclusion of patients with surgical-site infections whose wounds were not cultured, the rate of *S. aureus* infection at surgical sites was 2·3% (43 of 1892 patients) among mupirocin recipients and 2·4% (46 of 1894 patients) among placebo recipients. A subgroup analysis found that there was a lower rate of nosocomial *S. aureus* infections in *S. aureus* carriers treated with mupirocin (17 of 430 patients) compared with placebo (34 of 439 patients), (OR 4·9; 95% CI 0·25–0·92).

Perioperative antimicrobial prophylaxis

Not all surgeries require antibiotic prophylaxis. The initial step in deciding whether antimicrobial prophylaxis is indicated in a particular surgery is to determine which type of procedure will be performed. Box 12.1 lists the surgical wound classification scheme, which is by definition a postoperative assessment of intraoperative wound contamination, since breaks in sterile technique and other intraoperative findings cannot be predicted preoperatively. This classification allows the surgeon to estimate preoperatively the wound class of a given operation. Antimicrobial prophylaxis is indicated for clean-contaminated wounds (Class II), which is separate from the practice of bowel

Box 12.1 Surgical wound classification

Class I/clean
Uninfected operative wound with no inflammation and the respiratory, alimentary, genital, or uninfected urinary tract is not entered. Clean wounds are primarily closed and necessary drains are closed.

Class II/clean-contaminated
Operative wound with controlled entry into the respiratory, alimentary, genital, or urinary tract. Specifically, operations of the biliary tract, appendix, vagina, and oropharynx are included, if no evidence of infection or break in sterile technique.

Class III/contaminated
Open, fresh accidental wounds or ones with breaks in sterile technique, gastrointestinal spillage, or incisions in which non-purulent inflammation is encountered are contaminated.

Class IV/dirty-infected
Presence of old traumatic wounds with devitalized tissue or ones with existing clinical infection or perforated viscera suggesting pre-existing organisms prior to the operation.

Mangram *et al.*[38]

decontamination, and in clean wounds (Class I) if the SSI might be a clinical catastrophe, as would be the case in intravascular or joint prosthesis implantations.[38] Antimicrobial prophylaxis is not indicated in Class III or IV operations since these would involve specific antimicrobial treatment and would not be prophylaxis.

There are several issues surrounding the use of prophylactic antibiotics during the perioperative period including the timing of antibiotic initiation and the duration of dosing in the postoperative period. Classen *et al.* in a large prospective cohort study determined the effect of prophylactic antibiotic timing on the rate of SSI in 2847 patients who had clean (Class I) or clean-contaminated (Class II) operations.[39] Patients who received antibiotics preoperatively, defined as 0–2 hours prior to incision, had the lowest rate of SSI (0·6%). Higher rates of SSI were seen for perioperative administration, within 3 hours after incision (1·4%), and in those that received antibiotics more than 2 hours before (3·8%) and more than 3 hours after (3·3%) the incision. A logistic-regression analysis confirmed that timing of antimicrobial prophylaxis within 2 hours prior to incision was associated with the lowest odds of developing an SSI. The authors estimated that 27 SSIs would have been prevented in the 1-year study period if optimal timing of antimicrobial prophylaxis within 2 hours prior to incision was completely adhered to.[39]

It requires a great deal of institutional effort to ensure that antimicrobial prophylaxis is appropriately timed. At one medical center a random sample retrospective chart review found that, after the responsibility of antibiotic dosing had been shifted to the anesthesiologist with assistance of the pharmacy personnel in selecting patients for prophylaxis, the percentage of patients receiving antimicrobial prophylaxis within 1 hour prior to surgery rose from 38% to 88%.[40]

Antibiotic use is associated with the development of resistant organisms. In a retrospective cohort of all gastrointestinal surgeries over a 14-year period, a shift away from third-generation cephalosporins to first- and second-generation cephalosporins and a shift to intraoperative and not exclusively postoperative antibiotic use along with a shorter duration of antibiotics postoperatively was associated with a decline in the incidence of methicillin-resistant *Staphylococcus aureus* (MRSA).[41] This study is hard to interpret since the analysis was on the group and not on the individual level. The authors did not report if those patients that specifically received third-generation cephalosporins had higher levels of MRSA recovered from either surveillance or clinical isolates. In addition, no attempt to control for confounders in the development of MRSA was made, so which factor played the largest role in the development of MRSA is not known.

The duration of antimicrobial prophylaxis is controversial, despite accumulating data that does not support prolonged administration. Twenty-five years ago, Goldmann *et al.*, in a prospective double-blind trial compared a 6-day with a 2-day regimen of cephalothin prophylaxis in 200 patients undergoing prosthetic valve replacement. No cases of endocarditis in either group occurred, and SSI rates were similar in both groups suggesting that prolonged administration is not justified. A meta-analysis of 28 randomized trials with 9478 patients compared single versus multiple dose antimicrobial prophylaxis in a broad range of surgical procedure types and found no difference between the two groups; random effects model (OR 1·04; 95% CI 0·86–1·25).[42] Another meta-analysis of 25 randomized trials found that prophylactic antibiotics are effective in reducing SSIs in patients undergoing total hip and total knee replacement surgeries RR 0·24; 95% CI 0·14–0·43; NNT = 30), but found no benefit for prophylaxis extended beyond 1 day postoperatively.[43]

A recent cohort study of 2641 patients undergoing coronary artery bypass graft (CABG) surgery determined that prolonged antibiotic prophylaxis (> 48 hours after surgery) was not significantly associated with less risk of SSI compared with shorter duration (< 48 hours) antibiotic prophylaxis.[44] Interestingly, this study found that prolonged antibiotic prophylaxis beyond 48 hours after surgery was significantly associated with an increased risk of acquiring a clinical culture growing either cephalosporin-resistant Enterobacteriaceae and vancomycin-resistant enterococci when compared with shorter duration prophylaxis.

These findings support the current Centers for Disease Control and Prevention (CDC) guidelines for SSI prevention that suggest a full therapeutic dose of a bactericidal agent be given early enough so that peak levels are present at the time of the incision (for example, 1–2 g cefazolin no more than 30 minutes prior to incision) and that therapeutic levels be continued throughout the operation and for no more than a few hours after incisional closure.[38] Exceptions mentioned within these guidelines state that higher antibiotic doses should be used in obese patients and that initial doses of antibiotics in cesarean section should be given immediately after umbilical cord clamping.

Surveillance

The Study on the Efficacy of Nosocomial Infection Control (SENIC) suggested that an active surveillance program for nosocomial infections with subsequent feedback of the individual infection rates to surgeons could effectively reduce infection rates by about one-third.[45] However, this study was not a randomized controlled trial and the benefit was seen in only 8% of the hospitals recruited. A recent study using a quasi-experimental design that excluded SSIs recognized after discharge found that SSI surveillance with subsequent reporting of rates to individual surgeons led to a significant reduction in SSI rates after adjustment for confounding variables (RR = 0·62; 95% CI 0·44–0·86).[46] Benefits were also seen in reduced rates of urinary tract infections during the same surveillance and reporting period. A study using a similar methodology reported a 42% reduction in SSI rates after initiation of surveillance.[47]

With the current trends favoring shortened postoperative hospital stay and outpatient surgery, more SSIs are occurring after discharge from the hospital and, therefore, beyond the reach of most hospital infection control surveillance programs.[48] Seventy-five percent of surgeries are now estimated to occur in the outpatient or ambulatory setting, and, for those that do occur in the inpatient setting, postoperative length of stay is decreasing.[49] It is estimated that 47–84% of SSIs occur after discharge and that most of these are managed entirely in the outpatient setting.[48,50]

The difficult initial step in designing a surveillance program is to decide on the method of case finding. Many potential methods for SSI detection have been described and include routine direct wound examination by trained personnel, outpatient chart review, surgeon self-reporting, patient reporting, and the use of automated microbiological, pharmacy, and administrative data.[48,51,52] Each of these has weaknesses including universal acceptance, labor intensive direct or chart review methods, poor sensitivity of surgeon or patient reporting, and lack of availability of many automated database methods in many hospitals. Sands *et al.* reported that the sensitivity of patient and surgeon questionnaires to detect SSIs were 28% and 15%,[48] respectively, and developed highly sensitive and specific algorithms for the detection of SSIs using automated databases.[52] The choice of surveillance method should reflect the specific characteristics and resources available at each institution.

Ultimately, no single method should be used to reduce SSI rates. A comprehensive infection control program that uses many of the above strategies will have the greatest benefit through additive independent mechanisms and a combined effect. A 4-year observational study of a cardiothoracic surgery service after the initiation of a comprehensive infection control program that included surveillance, feedback to the surgeons, chlorhexidene showers the night before and morning of surgery, hair clipping if necessary, antibiotic prophylaxis in the holding area 30–120 minutes prior to surgery, and elimination of iced cardioplegia solution, along with other changes, found that the rate of SSIs was significantly reduced (OR = 0·37; 95% CI = 0·22–0·63). In addition there were trends toward reduced rates of deep chest infection and mortality.[2] A 24% reduction in mortality following CABG surgery was also achieved with the implementation of a multistate comprehensive quality improvement intervention.[53]

In conclusion, an optimal infection control program to limit SSIs in cardiac surgery patients should include surveillance for SSIs in the inpatient setting and if possible tracking of SSIs that manifest after hospital discharge. The SSI rates should be fed back to individual surgeons. In addition to surveillance, current practices and protocols for the perioperative period should be assessed and brought into line with current guidelines. Evidence supports the use of:

- perioperative glucose monitoring and control
- perioperative warming as feasible by procedure
- supplemental oxygen intraoperatively and for several hours after surgery
- hair removal if necessary by clipping
- perioperative antimicrobial prophylaxis with dosing that allows peak levels to be achieved prior to incision (cefazolin about 30 minutes prior and vancomycin about 1 hour prior) and repeat dosing if necessary to maintain levels during the procedure
- discontinuation of antibiotic prophylaxis within a few hours after completion of surgery.

Case presentation 2

Vancomycin-resistant bacteria

You are a physician in a 12-bed medical ICU and notice that your ICU seems to be having an increasing number of patients with vancomycin-resistant enterococcus (VRE) infections. An 80-year-old female is admitted to your medical ICU with a chronic obstructive pulmonary disease (COPD) exacerbation. She has had multiple admissions for COPD exacerbation in the past that have required antibiotic courses. In your 12-bed unit, you note that at present there are four patients on isolation precautions for VRE. In addition to treating her COPD exacerbation, you are concerned that she might be at risk for the following:

- already being colonized with VRE
- acquiring VRE from other patients
- spreading VRE to other patients.

Colonization and clinical presentation of VRE

Enterococci commonly cause urinary tract, wound, and bloodstream infections. They are part of the normal flora of the gastrointestinal tract. Enterococcal infections can be both endogenously acquired and acquired by patient-to-patient transmission. Endogenous acquisition arises when enterococcal isolates causing infection are identical to the patient's normal enterococcal flora.[54,55]

Glycopeptides interfere with cell wall synthesis by tightly binding to the D-alanine-D-alanine terminal dipeptide on the peptidoglycan precursor, sterically blocking the subsequent translycosylation and transpeptidation reactions. The vancomycin resistance mechanisms involve a series of reactions that ultimately result in the building of the cell wall by bypassing the D-alanine-D-alanine-containing pentapeptide intermediate structure, thereby eliminating the glycopeptide target.[56]

Since VRE are a form of enterococci, they are a cause of urinary tract, wound, and blood stream infections. However, colonization always precedes infection. Previous studies have suggested that VRE colonization rates exceed infection rates by 10:1–20:1.[57,58] This is the rationale for active surveillance interventions.

Colonization with VRE can last for an extended period with median time to clearance of VRE from the stool estimated to be 41–100 days after initial colonization with the organism.[58,59] Several patients in these studies were colonized with the same organism for greater than 1 year.[58,60] A study among hemodialysis patients found that 25% of VRE colonized patients developed infection versus a 1% infection rate in uncolonized patients.[61]

Burden of illness of VRE

The Centers for Disease Control and Prevention's (CDC) National Nosocomial Infections Surveillance (NNIS) system found that in 1999 compared with a period of 1994–1998, the percentage of nosocomial infections caused by vancomycin-resistant enterococci isolated in ICUs increased by 43% (http://www.cdc.gov/ncidod/hip/nniss/ar_surv99.pdf). Among 1579 enterococci isolates tested in 1999, 25·2% of isolates were vancomycin resistant.

Enterococci are generally thought to be organisms with low pathogenicity.[62] However, VRE infections occur in seriously ill hospitalized patients including those in specific geographically isolated locations such as ICUs or hemodialysis centers and in unique hospitalized populations, such as oncology patients or solid-organ transplant patients.[63] The recognition that vancomycin resistance is mediated by genes on conjugative and transposable elements raised the alarm that resistance could be transferred to other pathogenic organisms, as has been demonstrated experimentally to occur in

Staphylococcus aureus.[64] Recently, two clinical cases have occurred of vancomycin-resistant *Staphylococcus aureus*. Both organisms contained the *mecA* and *vanA* genes mediating methicillin and oxacillin resistance respectively.[65,66]

A matched study comparing patients with VRE bacteremia to those without bacteremia found that the mortality specifically related to VRE bacteremia and not underlying illness was 37%.[67] Presence of vancomycin resistance in enterococcal bacteremia is associated with 2–3-fold increase in the odds of death when compared with bacteremia in patients of similar age, sex, and severity of illness with enterococcal bacteremia lacking vancomycin resistance.[68,69] VRE-infected patients are more likely to have recurrent bacteremia compared with VSE (vancomycin-susceptible enterococci)-infected patients.[70]

Enterococcal bacteremia was associated with an additional 21 days of hospitalization with added costs of $7880/episode if the bacteremia occurred in the ICU and $4856/episode if it occurred on the general medical/surgical wards, compared with matched patients without enterococcal bacteremia.[71]

Risk factors for VRE

The relative causal component of risk factors for VRE is still uncertain. In general, it is felt that VRE incidence increases owing to antibiotic use both on a patient level and hospital level and owing to patient-to-patient transmission.

Risk factors for VRE include:

- antibiotic use
- length of stay in the hospital or time at risk prior to the event of interest, namely acquisition of the antibiotic-resistant bacteria
- comorbid illnesses
- severity of illness
- breaks to our normal anatomic physical barriers, such as Foley catheters, ET tubes, and central lines.[72,73]

Numerous studies have demonstrated these categories as risk factors but unfortunately very few have concurred on common risk factors. Differences have arisen because of differences in study design/epidemiological methodology.[74–76] Molecular typing studies, such as pulse-field gel electropheresis and ribotyping, have differed in their conclusions based on whether VRE is endemic or epidemic.[72,77]

Although it is clear that antibiotic use and patient-to-patient transmission are important modifiable risk factors for VRE, it is unclear what level of resistance is attributable to them as individual or combined risk factors. Future studies need to address these issues.

Preventive measures aimed at decreasing VRE

Glove and gown use

There are no randomized controlled trials that have assessed the use of gowns or gloves for reducing transmission of VRE. A quasi-experimental study by Slaughter *et al.* was done to assess the effect of universal use of gloves and gowns with that of glove use alone on the acquisition of vancomycin-resistant enterococci in a medical ICU. It was determined that all hospital employees would always use gloves and gowns when attending eight particular beds in the medical ICU and would always use gloves alone when attending others. Compliance with precautions was monitored weekly. The primary outcome was the number of patients acquiring VRE. A secondary outcome was compliance with the precautions. One hundred and eighty-one patients were admitted to the ICU during the study period: 24 patients (25·8%) in the glove-and-gown group and 21 (23·9%) in the glove-only group acquired VRE ($P > 0{\cdot}05$).

Compliance with precautions was 79% (1864 of 2363 handwashing opportunities) in glove-and-gown rooms and 62% (1243 of 2001 handwashing opportunities) in glove-only rooms ($P < 0{\cdot}001$).[78] Therefore the benefit of gowns may be due to enhanced compliance with precautions. There is microbiologic evidence to support the use of gloves when patients are being cared for with VRE. Tenorio *et al.* cultured the hands of healthcare workers before entering the rooms of patients with VRE, upon leaving the room while wearing gloves, and after removing gloves. The study revealed that gloves reduced the acquisition of VRE on the healthcare workers' hands by 71% (12 of 17) subjects.[79]

Active versus passive surveillance

One of the most controversial infection control areas is the use of so-called active surveillance for preventing hospital transmission of VRE. Active surveillance can be defined as the periodic screening of patients at risk for VRE colonization using perirectal or rectal cultures. This includes the isolation of patients found to be colonized with VRE in single rooms or cohorted in rooms with other colonized patients. This allows immediate implementation of infection-control measures to prevent patient-to-patient transmission of VRE.[80]

There are no randomized trials of active surveillance for VRE. Methodologically designing such a trial would be extremely challenging. Evidence to support this practice is based on microbiologic detection rates, quasi-experimental before–after studies, and outbreak investigations. Evidence exists that active surveillance can detect a large number of unrecognized patients colonized with VRE that otherwise would remain a reservoir for continued transmission.[59,77,81] This is based on the assumption that successful containment of VRE by infection control measures is most likely to succeed if VRE colonized patients can be isolated geographically before VRE spreads to multiple wards within the hospital.[80]

Passive surveillance can be defined as isolating patients found to be infected with VRE on clinical cultures or those who have a history of previous VRE infection from a previous stay and excludes the use of additional cultures to look for colonization. The strategy of passive surveillance would be expected to miss the 90% of patients who are colonized with VRE but do not manifest infection.[82,83]

Studies that have examined active surveillance have largely been quasi-experimental before–after designs. In a study by Ostrowksy *et al.*, active surveillance has been shown to be effective in reducing VRE colonization in a geographic area of Iowa.[84] Thirty healthcare facilities in Iowa participated in implementing the CDC's guidelines for decreasing the transmission of VRE. Implementation of the guidelines included active surveillance, recommendations for infection control, and education. The overall prevalence of VRE decreased in the 3 years of the study from 2·2% to 1·4 to 0·5%.

Another study compared the incidence rate of new clinical cultures for VRE in the entire hospital in periods before active surveillance was instituted and during a 15-month interruption of active surveillance to the periods when active surveillance was in effect in two ICUs.[85] They found that despite only 58% compliance in obtaining active surveillance cultures, the incidence rate of new clinical cultures for VRE in the entire hospital was reduced by an average of 48% with the use of active surveillance in two separate ICUs. Although this study looked at infections with VRE and not colonization, it did demonstrate the ability of active surveillance for VRE in a geographically isolated unit to have effects beyond the area of intervention. Active surveillance with isolation of colonized patients in combination with reduced antibiotic prescriptions was found to decrease VRE transmission and VRE infections in an oncology unit that had endemic VRE.[86] In addition, active surveillance in a community hospital[87] was found effective. It is important to note that before–after studies are a very limited design, being subject to a number of important biases including co-interventions, temporal ambiguity, and lack of a proper comparison group. Also lacking is evidence for specific indications for the implementation of active surveillance such as the optimal institutional or ward/unit VRE prevalence under which it should be used. These studies make no mention of the cost-effectiveness of active surveillance and make no attempt to separate its effect from that of antibiotic control programs. Also, they do not address other important confounding variables or clustering.

Decreasing antibiotic use

It is clear that antibiotic use is associated with increasing VRE incidence.[77,82,88,89] However, it is still unclear which antibiotics are the most important causal risk factors and what the relative importance of each individual antibiotic is. Antibiotic control programs aimed at decreasing VRE have generally focused their efforts on decreasing the use of vancomycin, cephalosporins, and antianaerobic antimicrobial agents. Studies have lacked a definite causality between decreasing antibiotic use and decreased VRE incidence. There have been no randomized clinical trials. Most studies have used quasi-experimental before–after designs. However, in light of the clear association between antibiotic use and bacterial resistance in general, it seems wise to use antibiotics prudently in patients at risk for VRE.

Most studies that have led to decreased rates of VRE have combined multiple interventions that have made it difficult to determine which component of the interventions was successful. For example, in an endemic setting of VRE, the following interventions were done: patient surveillance cultures were taken, patients were assigned to geographic cohorts, nurses were assigned to patient cohorts, gowns and gloves were worn on room entry, compliance with infection-control procedures was monitored, patients were educated about VRE transmission, patients taking antimicrobial agents were evaluated by an infectious disease specialist, and environmental surveillance was performed. During use of the above interventions, the incidence of VRE bloodstream infections decreased significantly from 2·1 patients per 1000 patient-days to 0·45 patients per 1000 patient-days.[86]

Hand disinfection

VRE is believed to be transmitted from patient to patient. Thus efforts aimed at improving hand disinfection compliance should lead to decreases in VRE. To this date, no studies have shown an effect on increased hand disinfection as a single intervention in decreasing VRE. It is believed that products such as alcohol-based disinfectants that may lead to sustained increased hand disinfection compliance may have an impact on VRE but to date no studies have shown this effect.

In 1995 the Subcommittee on the Prevention and Control of Antimicrobial-Resistant Microorganisms in Hospitals of the CDC's Hospital Infection Control Practices Advisory Committee (HICPAC) published recommendations to control the spread of vancomycin resistance.[80] These guidelines included recommendations for:

- prudent vancomycin use
- education of hospital staff as to the current state of understanding with regard to VRE
- efforts a microbiology lab might take in identifying enterococci and vancomycin resistance
- prevention and control of nosocomial transmission of VRE
- detection and reporting vancomycin resistance in *Staphylococcus aureus* and in *Staphylococcus epidermidis*.

The panel stated from the outset that "the data are limited and considerable research will be required to elucidate fully the epidemiology of VRE and determine cost-effective control strategies."[80]

Case presentation 2

Methicillin-resistant bacteria

A 45-year-old male with type 1 diabetes is admitted with a soft-tissue infection of the left foot. You are called by the patient's attending physician when wound cultures are positive for MRSA and *Pseudomonas aeruginosa*. The patient is being treated with vancomycin and piperacillin-tazobactam. The current plan for the patient is a course of antibiotics. No immediate surgery is planned although the patient may require arterial bypass surgery at some point. The attending physician asks you the following questions:

- What should I do to prevent other patients from acquiring this patient's MRSA?
- What is this patient's risk in terms of morbidity and mortality?
- What is the role for decolonization in this patient?

As hospital epidemiologist, you decide to put the patient on contact precautions involving the use of gloves and gowns. You explain to the physician that the patient is at risk for an increased hospital length of stay. The patient is also at risk of increased mortality if he develops a MRSA bacteremia. You advise against decolonization in this patient and in this setting.

Colonization and clinical presentation of MRSA

MRSA

Staphylococcus aureus are gram-positive bacteria that commonly cause wound, respiratory, and bloodstream infections. MRSA are bacteria that have acquired the *mecA* gene, a gene that alters *PBP 2a* rendering MRSA resistant to β-lactam antibiotics.[90,91] The nasal vestibule is the most consistent carrier site of MRSA. Other important sites of carriage include wounds and the perineal area.[92]

Similar to VRE, colonization with MRSA usually precedes infection with the organism. In one study of nasal carriers of MRSA, 38% subsequently developed MRSA bacteremia.[93] Studies suggest that colonization rates exceed infection rates by a ratio of 3:1.[92,94] The mean number of days between colonization and bacteremia was 11 days. Among patients colonized with MRSA, long-term carriage rate seems to vary between 30–60% depending upon the patient population.[95]

Burden of illness of MRSA

The CDC's NNIS system found that in 1999 compared with a period of 1994 to 1998, the percentage of nosocomial infections caused by MRSA isolated in ICUs increased by 37% (http://www.cdc.gov/ncidod/hip/nniss/ar_surv99.pdf). Among 2106 *S. aureus* isolates tested in 1999, 52·3% of isolates were methicillin-resistant.

Death rates attributable to MRSA infections have been estimated to be 2·5 times higher than that attributable to methicillin-sensitive *Staphylococcus aureus*.[96] In a recent study, mean cost attributable to MRSA infection was $9275.[97] MRSA infections have been shown to increase hospital length of stay by 4 days.[97]

A meta-analysis was performed to assess the impact of methicillin resistance on mortality in *S. aureus* bacteremia: 31 cohort studies were included; 24 found no significant difference in mortality and seven found a significant difference. When results were pooled using a random-effects model, a significant increase in mortality owing to MRSA bacteremia was evident (OR 1·93; 95% CI 1·54–2·42; $P < 0{\cdot}001$). It should be noted that significant statistical heterogeneity existed among the studies.[98]

Risk factors for MRSA

The relative causal component of risk factors for MRSA is still uncertain. In general, it is felt that MRSA incidence increases owing to antibiotic use both on a patient level and hospital level and because of patient to patient transmission.

Risk factors include antibiotic use, length of stay in the hospital or time at risk prior to the event of interest (namely acquisition of the antibiotic-resistant bacteria) comorbid illness, severity of illness, and breaks to normal anatomic physical barriers such as Foley catheters, ET tubes, and central lines.[92,99,100] Numerous studies have demonstrated these categories as risk factors but, unfortunately, very few have concurred on common risk factors. Differences have arisen owing to differences in study design/ epidemiological methodology.[75]

Although it is clear that antibiotic use and patient-to-patient transmission are important risk factors for MRSA, it is unclear what level of resistance is attributable to them as individual or combined risk factors. Future studies need to address these issues.

Preventive measures aimed at decreasing MRSA incidence

Hand disinfection

In contrast to VRE, there are data suggesting that increased compliance with hand disinfection can decrease MRSA. A study by Pittet *et al.* demonstrated that, following institution of a whole-hand hygiene program that included the institution of an alcohol-based hand disinfectant, compliance with hand disinfection increased from 48% to 66% and was associated with a decrease in the incidence of MRSA infections from 2·16 to 0·93 episodes per 10 000 patient days. A limitation of this study is that it was a multifaceted intervention that included active surveillance, implementation of prevention guidelines, and the use of an alcohol-based hand disinfectant, so it was difficult to determine the magnitude of benefit that was directly attributable to hand disinfection alone.[101] This is a common problem in quasi-experimental before–after study designs in the infection control literature.

Active surveillance

For reasons similar to those given above for VRE, active surveillance for MRSA should be effective in decreasing MRSA rates. In contrast to VRE, which involves active surveillance using perirectal or rectal cultures, active surveillance for MRSA should involve the use of nasal cultures. If more than one site is cultured, wound cultures and perineal cultures can be considered to increase the sensitivity of the active surveillance. [92]

An important study that showed the effect of active surveillance and its positive effect on reducing MRSA was done by Girou *et al.*[94] The intervention involved active surveillance that led to a decrease in MRSA acquisition rates from 5·8% to 1·4% while the rate of initial MRSA positivity remained at 4%, suggesting that the intervention was responsible for the decreased acquisition rates.[94] A confounding variable that could have altered the results of this study was that decolonization routines were being used in addition to active surveillance.

Decolonization

Many decolonization regimens have been used for MRSA. They have included both topical and systemic agents, including mupirocin, rifampin, and chlorhexidine baths. A Cochrane review on eradication of MRSA has recently been published.[102] Six randomized trials have been done to assess decolonization[103–108] The percentage of subjects with nasal MRSA colonization alone was reported in six studies and ranged from 26% to 100%. Eradication on day 14 post treatment was the most frequently reported outcome. In all six clinical trials, no statistically significant differences in MRSA eradication was noted. However, most of the studies were small and underpowered to detect differences. The confidence intervals generally are wide and do not rule out clinically important effects. In addition, the results of many trials are conflicting owing to differences in study design, presence of confounding variables, or the co-implementation of other infection control interventions.

In summary, active surveillance for VRE or MRSA may help reduce transmission; however, data are limited. Improving adherence to hand disinfection and reducing antibiotic use are worthwhile strategies. Currently, clinical trial evidence does not support routine decolonization of MRSA.

References

1. Horan TC, Gaynes RP, Martone WJ, Jarvis WR, Emori TG. CDC definitions of nosocomial surgical site infections, 1992: a modification of CDC definitions of surgical wound infections. *Infect Control Hosp Epidemiol* 1992;**13**:606–8.
2. McConkey SJ, L'Ecuyer PB, Murphy DM, Leet TL, Sundt TM, Fraser VJ. Results of a comprehensive infection control program for reducing surgical-site infections in coronary artery bypass surgery. *Infect Control Hosp Epidemiol* 1999;**20**:533–8.
3. National Nosocomial Infections Surveillance (NNIS) report, data summary from October 1986–April 1996, issued May 1996. A report from the National Nosocomial Infections Surveillance (NNIS) System. *Am J Infect Control* 1996;**24**:380–8.
4. Brachman PS, Dan BB, Haley RW, Hooton TM, Garner JS, Allen JR. Nosocomial surgical infections: incidence and cost. *Surg Clin North Am* 1980;**60**:15–25.
5. Wong ES. Surgical site infections. In: Mayhall CG, ed. *Hospital Epidemiology and Infection Control, 2nd ed.* Philadelphia: Lippincott, 1999.
6. Smyth ET, Emmerson AM. Surgical site infection surveillance. *J Hosp Infect* 2000;**45**:173–84.
7. Coello R, Glenister H, Fereres J *et al.* The cost of infection in surgical patients: a case-control study. *J Hosp Infect* 1993;**25**:239–50.
8. Perencevich E, Sands K, Cosgrove S, Guadagnoli E, Meara E, Platt R. The Health and Economic Impact of Surgical Site Infections Diagnosed after Hospital Discharge. *Emerg Infect Dis* 2003;**9**:196–203.
9. Nelson RM, Dries DJ. The economic implications of infection in cardiac surgery. *Ann Thorac Surg* 1986;**42**:240–6.
10. Taylor GJ, Mikell FL, Moses HW *et al.* Determinants of hospital charges for coronary artery bypass surgery: the economic consequences of postoperative complications. *Am J Cardiol* 1990;**65**:309–13.
11. Hall RE, Ash AS, Ghali WA, Moskowitz MA. Hospital cost of complications associated with coronary artery bypass graft surgery. *Am J Cardiol* 1997;**79**:1680–2.
12. Holtz TH, Wenzel RP. Postdischarge surveillance for nosocomial wound infection: a brief review and commentary. *Am J Infect Control* 1992;**20**:206–13.
13. Gaynes RP, Culver DH, Horan TC, Edwards JR, Richards C, Tolson JS. Surgical site infection (ssi) rates in the united states, 1992–1998: the national nosocomial infections surveillance system basic ssi risk index. *Clin Infect Dis* 2001;**33**(Suppl. 2):S69–77.
14. Pomposelli JJ, Baxter JK, III, Babineau TJ *et al.* Early postoperative glucose control predicts nosocomial infection rate in diabetic patients. *J Parenter Enteral Nutr* 1998;**22**:77–81.
15. Latham R, Lancaster AD, Covington JF, Pirolo JS, Thomas CS. The association of diabetes and glucose control with surgical-site infections among cardiothoracic surgery patients. *Infect Control Hosp Epidemiol* 2001;**22**:607–12.
16. Zerr KJ, Furnary AP, Grunkemeier GL, Bookin S, Kanhere V, Starr A. Glucose control lowers the risk of wound infection in diabetics after open heart operations. *Ann Thorac Surg* 1997;**63**:356–61.
17. Furnary AP, Zerr KJ, Grunkemeier GL, Starr A. Continuous intravenous insulin infusion reduces the incidence of deep sternal wound infection in diabetic patients after cardiac surgical procedures. *Ann Thorac Surg* 1999;**67**:352–62.
18. Sessler DI. Mild perioperative hypothermia. *N Engl J Med* 1997;**336**:1730–7.
19. Kurz A, Sessler DI, Christensen R, Dechert M. Heat balance and distribution during the core-temperature plateau in anesthetized humans. *Anesthesiology* 1995;**83**:491–9.

20. Kurz A, Sessler DI, Lenhardt R. Perioperative normothermia to reduce the incidence of surgical-wound infection and shorten hospitalization. Study of Wound Infection and Temperature Group. *N Engl J Med* 1996;**334**:1209–15.
21. Munn MB, Rouse DJ, Owen J. Intraoperative hypothermia and post-cesarean wound infection. *Obst Gynecol* 1998;**91**:582–4.
22. Melling AC, Ali B, Scott EM, Leaper DJ. Effects of preoperative warming on the incidence of wound infection after clean surgery: a randomized controlled trial. *Lancet* 2001;**358**:876–80.
23. Ginsberg MD, Sternau LL, Globus MY, Dietrich WD, Busto R. Therapeutic modulation of brain temperature: relevance to ischemic brain injury. *Cerebrovasc Brain Metab Rev* 1992;**4**:189–225.
24. Winfree CH, Baker KZ, Connollly ES. Perioperative normothermia and surgical-wound infection. *N Engl J Med* 1996;**335**:749–50.
25. Greif R, Akca O, Horn EP, Kurz A, Sessler DI. Supplemental perioperative oxygen to reduce the incidence of surgical-wound infection. Outcomes Research Group. *N Engl J Med* 2000;**342**:161–7.
26. Hopf HW, Hunt TK, West JM *et al.* Wound tissue oxygen tension predicts the risk of wound infection in surgical patients. *Arch Surg* 1997;**132**:997–1005.
27. Allen DB, Maguire JJ, Mahdavian M *et al.* Wound hypoxia and acidosis limit neutrophil bacterial killing mechanisms. *Arch Surg* 1997;**132**:991–6.
28. Akca O, Podolsky A, Eisenhuber E *et al.* Comparable postoperative pulmonary atelectasis in patients given 30% or 80% oxygen during and 2 hours after colon resection. *Anesthesiology* 1999;**91**:991–8.
29. Whitney JD, Heiner S, Mygrant BI, Wood C. Tissue and wound healing effects of short duration postoperative oxygen therapy. *Biol Res Nurs* 2001;**2**:206–15.
30. Bekar A, Korfali E, Dogan S, Yilmazlar S, Baskan Z, Aksoy K. The effect of hair on infection after cranial surgery. *Acta Neurochir* 2001;**143**:533–6.
31. Sellick JA, Jr., Stelmach M, Mylotte JM. Surveillance of surgical wound infections following open heart surgery. *Infect Control Hosp Epidemiol* 1991;**12**:591–6.
32. Ko W, Lazenby WD, Zelano JA, Isom OW, Krieger KH. Effects of shaving methods and intraoperative irrigation on suppurative mediastinitis after bypass operations. *Ann Thorac Surg* 1992;**53**:301–5.
33. Alexander JW, Fischer JE, Boyajian M, Palmquist J, Morris MJ. The influence of hair-removal methods on wound infections. *Arch Surg* 1983;**118**:347–52.
34. Miller JJ, Weber PC, Patel S, Ramey J. Intracranial surgery: to shave or not to shave? *Otol Neurotol* 2001; **22**:908–11.
35. Tang K, Yeh JS, Sgouros S. The influence of hair shave on the infection rate in neurosurgery. A prospective study. *Pediatr Neurosurg* 2001;**35**:13–17.
36. Kluytmans JA, Mouton JW, VandenBergh MF *et al.* Reduction of surgical-site infections in cardiothoracic surgery by elimination of nasal carriage of *Staphylococcus aureus*. *Infect Control Hosp Epidemiol* 1996;**17**:780–5.
37. VandenBergh MF, Kluytmans JA, van Hout BA *et al.* Cost-effectiveness of perioperative mupirocin nasal ointment in cardiothoracic surgery. *Infect Control Hosp Epidemiol* 1996;**17**:786–92.
38. Mangram AJ, Horan TC, Pearson ML, Silver LC, Jarvis WR. Guideline for Prevention of Surgical Site Infection, 1999. Centers for Disease Control and Prevention (CDC) Hospital Infection Control Practices Advisory Committee. *Am J Infect Control* 1999;**27**:97–134.
39. Classen DC, Evans RS, Pestotnik SL, Horn SD, Menlove RL, Burke JP. The timing of prophylactic administration of antibiotics and the risk of surgical-wound infection. *N Engl J Med* 1992;**326**:281–6.
40. Matuschka PR, Cheadle WG, Burke JD, Garrison RN. A new standard of care: administration of preoperative antibiotics in the operating room. *Am Surg* 1997;**63**:500–3.
41. Fukatsu K, Saito H, Matsuda T, Ikeda S, Furukawa S, Muto T. Influences of type and duration of antimicrobial prophylaxis on an outbreak of methicillin-resistant *Staphylococcus aureus* and on the incidence of wound infection. *Arch Surg* 1997;**132**:1320–5.
42. McDonald M, Grabsch E, Marshall C, Forbes A. Single-versus multiple-dose antimicrobial prophylaxis for major surgery: a systematic review. *Aust NZ J Surg* 1998;**68**: 388–96.
43. Glenny A, Song F. Antimicrobial prophylaxis in total hip replacement: a systematic review. *Health Technol Assess* 1999;**3**:1–57.
44. Harbarth S, Samore MH, Lichtenberg D, Carmeli Y. Prolonged antibiotic prophylaxis after cardiovascular surgery and its effect on surgical site infections and antimicrobial resistance. *Circulation* 2000;**101**:2916–21.

45. Haley RW, Culver DH, White JW *et al.* The efficacy of infection surveillance and control programs in preventing nosocomial infections in US hospitals. *Am J Epidemiol* 1985;**121**:182–205.
46. Delgado-Rodriguež M, Gomez-Ortega A, Sillero-Arenas M, Martinez-Gallego G, Medina-Cuadros M, Llorca J. Efficacy of surveillance in nosocomial infection control in a surgical service. *Am J Infect Control* 2001;**29**: 289–94.
47. Mead PB, Pories SE, Hall P, Vacek PM, Davis JH, Jr., Gamelli RL. Decreasing the incidence of surgical wound infections. Validation of a surveillance-notification program. *Arch Surg* 1986;**121**:458–61.
48. Sands K, Vineyard G, Platt R. Surgical site infections occurring after hospital discharge. *J Infect Dis* 1996;**173**:963–70.
49. Hecht AD. Creating greater efficiency in ambulatory surgery. *J Clin Anesth* 1995;**7**:581–4.
50. Brown RB, Bradley S, Opitz E, Cipriani D, Pieczarka R, Sands M. Surgical wound infections documented after hospital discharge. *Am J Infect Control* 1987;**15**:54–8.
51. Manian FA. Surveillance of surgical site infections in alternative settings: exploring the current options. *Am J Infect Control* 1997;**25**:102–5.
52. Sands K, Vineyard G, Livingston J, Christiansen C, Platt R. Efficient identification of postdischarge surgical site infections: use of automated pharmacy dispensing information, administrative data, and medical record information. *J Infect Dis* 1999;**179**:434–41.
53. O'Connor GT, Plume SK, Olmstead EM *et al.* A regional intervention to improve the hospital mortality associated with coronary artery bypass graft surgery. The Northern New England Cardiovascular Disease Study Group. *JAMA* 1996;**275**:841–6.
54. Zervos MJ, Kauffman CA, Therasse PM, Bergman AG, Mikesell TS, Schaberg DR. Nosocomial infection by gentamicin-resistant *Streptococcus faecalis*. An epidemiologic study. *Ann Intern Med* 1987;**106**:687–91.
55. Murray BE, Singh KV, Markowitz SM *et al.* Evidence for clonal spread of a single strain of β-lactamase-producing *Enterococcus* (*Streptococcus*) *faecalis* to six hospitals in five states. *J Infect Dis* 1991;**163**:780–5.
56. Arthur M, Courvalin P. Genetics and mechanisms of glycopeptide resistance in enterococci. *Antimicrob Agents Chemother* 1993;**37**:1563–71.
57. Lam S, Singer C, Tucci V, Morthland VH, Pfaller MA, Isenberg HD. The challenge of vancomycin-resistant enterococci: a clinical and epidemiologic study. *Am J Infect Control* 1995;**23**:170–80.
58. Montecalvo MA, de Lencastre H, Carraher M *et al.* Natural history of colonization with vancomycin-resistant *Enterococcus faecium. Infect Control Hosp Epidemiol* 1995;**16**:680–5.
59. Goetz AM, Rihs JD, Wagener MM, Muder RR. Infection and colonization with vancomycin-resistant *Enterococcus faecium* in an acute care Veterans Affairs Medical Center: a 2-year survey. *Am J Infect Control* 1998;**26**:558–62.
60. Roghmann MC, Qaiyumi S, Johnson JA, Schwalbe R, Morris JG, Jr. Recurrent vancomycin-resistant *Enterococcus faecium* bacteremia in a leukemia patient who was persistently colonized with vancomycin-resistant enterococci for two years. *Clin Infect Dis* 1997;**24**:514–15.
61. Roghmann MC, Fink JC, Polish L *et al.* Colonization with vancomycin-resistant enterococci in chronic hemodialysis patients. *Am J Kidney Dis* 1998;**32**:254–7.
62. Moellering RC, Jr. Emergence of Enterococcus as a significant pathogen. *Clin Infect Dis* 1992;**14**:1173–6.
63. Cetinkaya Y, Falk P, Mayhall CG. Vancomycin-resistant enterococci. *Clin Microbiol Rev* 2000;**13**:686–707.
64. Noble WC, Virani Z, Cree RG. Co-transfer of vancomycin and other resistance genes from *Enterococcus faecalis* NCTC 12201 to *Staphylococcus aureus. FEMS Microbiol Lett* 1992;**72**:195–8.
65. Public Health Dispatch: Vancomycin-Resistant *Staphylococcus aureus* – Pennsylvania, 2002. *MMWR Morb Mortal Wkly Rep* 2002;**51**:902.
66. National Nosocomial Infections Surveillance (NNIS) system report, data summary from January 1992–April 2000, issued June 2000. *Am J Infect Control* 2000;**28**:429–48.
67. Edmond MB, Ober JF, Dawson JD, Weinbaum DL, Wenzel RP. Vancomycin-resistant enterococcal bacteremia: natural history and attributable mortality. *Clin Infect Dis* 1996;**23**:1234–9.
68. Shay DK, Maloney SA, Montecalvo M *et al.* Epidemiology and mortality risk of vancomycin-resistant enterococcal bloodstream infections. *J Infect Dis* 1995;**172**:993–1000.
69. Vergis EN, Hayden MK, Chow JW *et al.* Determinants of vancomycin resistance and mortality rates in enterococcal bacteremia. a prospective multicenter study. *Ann Intern Med* 2001;**135**:484–92.

70. Linden PK, Pasculle AW, Manez R *et al.* Differences in outcomes for patients with bacteremia due to vancomycin-resistant *Enterococcus faecium* or vancomycin-susceptible *E. faecium*. *Clin Infect Dis* 1996;**22**:663–70.
71. Caballero-Granado FJ, Becerril B, Cuberos L, Bernabeu M, Cisneros JM, Pachon J. Attributable mortality rate and duration of hospital stay associated with enterococcal bacteremia. *Clin Infect Dis* 2001;**32**:587–94.
72. Hayden MK. Insights into the epidemiology and control of infection with vancomycin-resistant enterococci. *Clin Infect Dis* 2000;**31**:1058–65.
73. Kaye KS, Fraimow HS, Abrutyn E. Pathogens resistant to antimicrobial agents. Epidemiology, molecular mechanisms, and clinical management. *Infect Dis Clin North Am* 2000;**14**:293–319.
74. Harris AD, Samore MH, Carmeli Y. Control group selection is an important but neglected issue in studies of antibiotic resistance. *Ann Intern Med* 2000;**133**:159.
75. Harris AD, Karchmer TB, Carmeli Y, Samore MH. Methodological principles of case-control studies that analyzed risk factors for antibiotic resistance: a systematic review. *Clin Infect Dis* 2001;**32**:1055–61.
76. Harris AD, Samore MH, Lipsitch M, Kaye KS, Perencevich E, Carmeli Y. Control-group selection importance in studies of antimicrobial resistance: examples applied to *Pseudomonas aeruginosa*, Enterococci, and *Escherichia coli*. *Clin Infect Dis* 2002;**34**:1558–63.
77. Morris JG, Jr., Shay DK, Hebden JN *et al.* Enterococci resistant to multiple antimicrobial agents, including vancomycin. Establishment of endemicity in a university medical center. *Ann Intern Med* 1995;**123**:250–9.
78. Slaughter S, Hayden MK, Nathan C *et al.* A comparison of the effect of universal use of gloves and gowns with that of glove use alone on acquisition of vancomycin-resistant enterococci in a medical intensive care unit. *Ann Intern Med* 1996;**125**:448–56.
79. Tenorio AR, Badri SM, Sahgal NB *et al.* Effectiveness of gloves in the prevention of hand carriage of vancomycin-resistant enterococcus species by health care workers after patient care. *Clin Infect Dis* 2001;**32**:826–9.
80. Recommendations for preventing the spread of vancomycin resistance. Hospital Infection Control Practices Advisory Committee (HICPAC) [published erratum appears in *Infect Control Hosp Epidemiol* 1995;**16**:498] *Infect Control Hosp Epidemiol* 1995;**16**:105–13.
81. Weinstein JW, Roe M, Towns M *et al.* Resistant enterococci: a prospective study of prevalence, incidence, and factors associated with colonization in a university hospital. *Infect Control Hosp Epidemiol* 1996;**17**:36–41.
82. Ostrowsky BE, Venkataraman L, D'Agata EM, Gold HS, DeGirolami PC, Samore MH. Vancomycin-resistant enterococci in intensive care units: high frequency of stool carriage during a non-outbreak period. *Arch Intern Med* 1999;**159**:1467–72.
83. Boyce JM. Vancomycin-resistant enterococcus. Detection, epidemiology, and control measures. *Infect Dis Clin North Am* 1997;**11**:367–84.
84. Ostrowsky BE, Trick WE, Sohn AH *et al.* Control of vancomycin-resistant enterococcus in health care facilities in a region. *N Engl J Med* 2001;**344**:1427–33.
85. Siddiqui AH, Harris AD, Hebden JN, Wilson PD, Morris JG, Jr., Roghmann MC. The effect of active surveillance for vancomycin-resistant enterococci in high-risk units on vancomycin resistance hospital-wide. *Am J Infect Control* 2002;**30**:40–3.
86. Montecalvo MA, Jarvis WR, Uman J *et al.* Infection-control measures reduce transmission of vancomycin-resistant enterococci in an endemic setting. *Ann Intern Med* 1999;**131**:269–72.
87. Jochimsen EM, Fish L, Manning K *et al.* Control of vancomycin-resistant enterococci at a community hospital: efficacy of patient and staff cohorting. *Infect Control Hosp Epidemiol* 1999;**20**:106–9.
88. Rao GG, Ojo F, Kolokithas D. Vancomycin-resistant gram-positive cocci: risk factors for faecal carriage. *J Hosp Infect* 1997;**35**:63–9.
89. Tornieporth NG, Roberts RB, John J, Hafner A, Riley LW. Risk factors associated with vancomycin-resistant *Enterococcus faecium* infection or colonization in 145 matched case patients and control patients. *Clin Infect Dis* 1996;**23**:767–72.
90. Neu HC. The crisis in antibiotic resistance. *Science* 1992;**257**:1064–73.
91. Spratt BG. Resistance to antibiotics mediated by target alterations. *Science* 1994;**264**:388–93.
92. Solberg CO. Spread of *Staphylococcus aureus* in hospitals: causes and prevention. *Scand J Infect Dis* 2000;**32**:587–95.
93. Pujol M, Pena C, Pallares R *et al.* Nosocomial *Staphylococcus aureus* bacteremia among nasal carriers

of methicillin-resistant and methicillin-susceptible strains. *Am J Med* 1996;**100**:509–16.

94. Girou E, Pujade G, Legrand P, Cizeau F, Brun-Buisson C. Selective screening of carriers for control of methicillin-resistant *Staphylococcus aureus* (MRSA) in high-risk hospital areas with a high level of endemic MRSA. *Clin Infect Dis* 1998;**27**:543–50.
95. Rampling A, Wiseman S, Davis L *et al.* Evidence that hospital hygiene is important in the control of methicillin-resistant *Staphylococcus aureus*. *J Hosp Infect* 2001;**49**:109–16.
96. Rubin RJ, Harrington CA, Poon A, Dietrich K, Greene JA, Moiduddin A. The economic impact of *Staphylococcus aureus* infection in New York City hospitals. *Emerg Infect Dis* 1999;**5**:9–17.
97. Chaix C, Durand-Zaleski I, Alberti C, Brun-Buisson C. Control of endemic methicillin-resistant *Staphylococcus aureus*: a cost-benefit analysis in an intensive care unit. *JAMA* 1999;**282**:1745–51.
98. Cosgrove SE, Sakoulas G, Perencevich EN, Schwaber MJ, Karchmer AW, Carmeli Y. Comparison of mortality associated with methicillin-resistant and methicillin-susceptible *Staphylococcus aureus* bacteremia: a meta-analysis. *Clin Infect Dis* 2003;**36**:53–9.
99. Graffunder EM, Venezia RA. Risk factors associated with nosocomial methicillin-resistant *Staphylococcus aureus* (MRSA) infection including previous use of antimicrobials. *J Antimicrob Chemother* 2002;**49**:999–1005.
100. Herwaldt LA. Control of methicillin-resistant *Staphylococcus aureus* in the hospital setting. *Am J Med* 1999;**106**:11S–18S, 48S–52S.
101. Pittet D, Hugonnet S, Harbarth S *et al.* Effectiveness of a hospital-wide program to improve compliance with hand hygiene. Infection Control Program. *Lancet* 2000;**356**: 1307–12.
102. Loeb M, Main C, Walker-Dilks C, Eady A. Antimicrobial drugs for treating methicillin-resistant *Staphylococcus aureus* colonizations. Cochrane Database Systematic Review 2003;(4):CD003340.
103. Muder RR, Boldin M, Brennen C *et al.* A controlled trial of rifampicin, minocycline, and rifampicin plus minocycline for eradication of methicillin-resistant *Staphylococcus aureus* in long-term care patients. *J Antimicrob Chemother* 1994;**34**:189–90.
104. Harbarth S, Dharan S, Liassine N, Herrault P, Auckenthaler R, Pittet D. Randomized, placebo-controlled, double-blind trial to evaluate the efficacy of mupirocin for eradicating carriage of methicillin-resistant *Staphylococcus aureus*. *Antimicrob Agents Chemother* 1999;**43**:1412–16.
105. Parras F, Guerrero MC, Bouza E *et al.* Comparative study of mupirocin and oral co-trimoxazole plus topical fusidic acid in eradication of nasal carriage of methicillin-resistant *Staphylococcus aureus*. *Antimicrob Agents Chemother* 1995;**39**:175–9.
106. Chang SC, Hsieh SM, Chen ML, Sheng WH, Chen YC. Oral fusidic acid fails to eradicate methicillin-resistant *Staphylococcus aureus* colonization and results in emergence of fusidic acid-resistant strains. *Diagn Microbiol Infect Dis* 2000;**36**:131–6.
107. Walsh TJ, Standiford HC, Reboli AC *et al.* Randomized double-blinded trial of rifampin with either novobiocin or trimethoprim-sulfamethoxazole (TMP-SMX) against methicillin-resistant *Staphylococcus aureus* colonization: prevention of antimicrobial resistance and effect of host factors on outcome. *Antimicrob Agents Chemother* 1993;**37**:1334–42.
108. Peterson LR, Quick JN, Jensen B *et al.* Emergence of ciprofloxacin resistance in nosocomial methicillin-resistant *Staphylococcus aureus* isolates. Resistance during ciprofloxacin plus rifampin therapy for methicillin-resistant *S. aureus* colonization. *Arch Intern Med* 1990;**150**:2151–5.

13
Infections in neutropenic hosts

Stuart J Rosser, Eric J Bow

Case presentation

A 34-year-old male was admitted complaining of fever, generalized malaise, and increasing fatigue over the preceding 4 weeks. On examination, he was pale; his blood pressure was 122/78 mmHg; oral temperature, 38·2°C, and pulse, 110 per minute. His liver had a 14-cm span in the mid-clavicular line and the spleen tip was 10 cm below the left costal margin. Petechiae were present in the skin of the lower limbs. A complete blood count revealed a total leukocyte count of 35×10^9/liter, an absolute neutrophil count (ANC) of $0{\cdot}824 \times 10^9$/liter, an absolute lymphocyte count (ALC) of $0{\cdot}4 \times 10^9$/liter, an absolute monocyte count (AMC) of $0{\cdot}2 \times 10^9$/liter, and a circulating blast count of 33×10^9/liter. His serum uric acid was elevated at 590 micromol/liter and his serum lactate dehydrogenase was 1890 IU/liter. A chest roentgenogram was normal. A bone marrow examination revealed a hypercellular marrow specimen 90% infiltrated by blast cells, some of which contained Auer rods. Acute myeloid leukemia (AML) (French–American–British classification, M2) was diagnosed.

A typical AML remission-induction regimen was administered, consisting of a 7-day continuous infusion of cytarabine plus an anthracycline, idarubicin, administered daily on days 1, 2, and 3. Beginning on day + 1 of cytotoxic therapy, ciprofloxacin 500 mg every 12 hours and oral acyclovir 800 mg every 12 hours were administered to prevent aerobic gram-negative bacterial infections, and reactivation of herpes simplex virus mucositis, respectively. Oral fluconazole 400 mg daily was administered to prevent superficial and invasive fungal infection due to *Candida albicans*. The blood cultures obtained at the time of hospital admission remained sterile, and the fever resolved as the cytotoxic therapy was administered. The ANC fell to $< 0{\cdot}5 \times 10^9$/liter on day + 3 of induction therapy and to $< 0{\cdot}1 \times 10^9$/liter on day + 5.

Acute leukemia is a rapidly progressive disease. In the untreated patient, it results in early death owing to hemorrhage or infection – the consequences, respectively, of thrombocytopenia and neutropenia from marrow failure. Historically, infection has been the major contributor to mortality and has been designated as the primary cause of death in over one-third of acute leukemia cases. Notwithstanding advances in cytotoxic chemotherapy for the underlying malignancy and in the use of marrow-stimulating growth factors and antimicrobials to support individuals through their disease- and treatment-related marrow insufficiency, infection remains the major contributor to 66% of deaths in patients treated for acute myeloid leukemia (AML).[1] The early recognition and appropriate treatment of infection remains a priority in the care of these profoundly immunocompromised individuals.

Case presentation continued

A detailed physical examination as well as diagnostic and microbiological testing suggested no obvious infection and the fever was subsequently felt to be disease-related.

Neutrophils are the principal mediators of non-specific (innate) cellular immunity. A deficiency in either the number or function of neutrophils can predispose an individual to infection. Diminished numbers of neutrophils, as opposed to qualitative defects in granulocyte function, are the more common cause of granulocytic immunodeficiency. While a total neutrophil count of $< 1{\cdot}0 \times 10^9$/liter of blood defines neutropenia, the risk of bacterial and fungal sepsis rises exponentially below a level of $0{\cdot}5 \times 10^9$/liter. This profound degree of neutropenia occasionally arises from an underlying inflammatory, infectious or malignant condition, but is more often a consequence of the treatment of these diseases. In particular, the treatment of hematological and other malignancies with certain cytotoxic regimens will reliably induce profound and protracted neutropenia. Much of the data regarding the epidemiology, microbiology, diagnosis, and treatment of neutropenic sepsis is derived from studies of leukemia and bone marrow transplant patients. While there may be subtle differences in the characteristics of neutropenia-related sepsis arising from one disease state to the next, most of what we have learned from the hematology and oncology studies can be generalized to other conditions producing neutropenia of similar magnitude and duration.

The febrile neutropenic episode

Chemotherapy for acute myeloid leukemia will predictably result in neutropenia, with absolute neutrophil counts of $< 0{\cdot}5 \times 10^9$/liter for 10–14 days, or longer. While a patient may become febrile at any point during the course of treatment, the median time to fever is typically 9–10 days from the first chemotherapy day, or about 3 days following the onset of neutropenia.[2] The designation of a "febrile neutropenic episode" (FNE) applies when a neutropenic patient's oral temperature exceeds 38°C for at least 1 hour. The fever itself arises from the production of pro-inflammatory cytokines (interleukin-1α, IL-1β, IL-4, IL-6, and tumor necrosis factor-α),[3] most often in response to either infection- or therapy-related cell membrane damage.[4–8] While fever is generally the first, and frequently the only sign of infection in these individuals, not all febrile episodes will be the direct result of infection. The Infectious Diseases Society of America (IDSA) defines fever due to an infection as an episode associated with an oral temperature above 38·3°C (101°F) in the absence of non-infectious causes.[9] Some of the common non-infectious causes of fever in populations being treated for malignancies are outlined in Box 13.1. Febrile neutropenic episodes associated with infection may be further classified as microbiologically documented (either bacteremic or non-bacteremic) or clinically documented, where a site of infection is identified without a pathogen or where fever occurs without an alternate explanation. Accumulating experience with the etiology of febrile neutropenic events has resulted in as few as 8% of episodes being classified as "unexplained".[10]

Box 13.1 Fever in the neutropenic cancer patient: non-infectious causes

- Underlying malignancy
- Infusion of blood products
- Drugs: cytarabine, cyclophosphamide, hydroxyurea, polyenes (e.g. amphotericin B deoxycholate)
- Non-infectious inflammatory conditions: phlebitis, hematomas, thromboembolic disease

Measures to prevent infection in the neutropenic host

Protective isolation

Non-antimicrobial measures aimed at preventing infections in patients with established or anticipated neutropenia have included: the placement of patients in a single room; the use of gowns, gloves, and masks by hospital personnel when entering patients' rooms; positive pressure ventilation in patients' rooms; and high efficiency particulate air (HEPA) filtration, with or without laminar (unidirectional) flow. Prospective randomized studies have not supported the routine use any of these measures to reduce the rate of invasive bacterial infections.[11,12] HEPA-filtered air supplies with laminar flow may protect patients from invasive pulmonary aspergillosis and from death owing to fungal infections,[13] particularly when those patients are cared for in close proximity to hospital construction and maintenance projects.[14] As part of routine care, however, placement of patients in a single room and diligent hand washing on the part of healthcare workers and visitors are encouraged, while other protective measures (HEPA filtration, with or without laminar flow) are reserved for high-risk patients (see "Risk assessment" below).

Prophylactic antimicrobials

The pathogens most commonly implicated in neutropenic sepsis are bacteria derived from colonized skin and mucosal surfaces.[15,16] With this in mind, investigators have sought to prevent infections by reducing the burden of potential pathogens with antimicrobials. Initial efforts with oral, non-absorbable agents had equivocal effects on infection-related outcomes in the neutropenic host,[17–24] and had several economic and logistical drawbacks. Early studies using trimethoprim-sulfamethoxazole (TMP-SMX) showed reductions in bloodstream,[25,26] microbiologically documented,[26,27] and overall infections.[27] However, subsequent meta-analyses of studies that compared fluoroquinolone-based prophylaxis with TMP-SMX or with no prophylaxis implied that the risk of infection-related morbidity and mortality in TMP-SMX-treated populations was not significantly lower than for the groups receiving no prophylactic agent.[28] The latter finding may have been related to an increasing prevalence over the past two decades of TMP-SMX resistance in aerobic gram-negative bacteria causing neutropenic sepsis.[29,30]

Meta-analyses of studies where fluoroquinolones (for example, ciprofloxacin, norfloxacin, enoxacin, ofloxacin, and perfloxacin) were used as prophylaxis have shown consistent reductions in the risk of infection with gram-negative bacilli or *Staphylococcus aureus*.[28,31,32] On the surface, fluoroquinolone prophylaxis, when compared with TMP-SMX or to no prophylaxis, appeared also to reduce the incidence of febrile neutropenic episodes: however, subsequent analyses restricted to the blinded studies suggested no such benefit,[28] and the aggregate data showed no effect on the use of systemic antimicrobials or overall mortality. Nonetheless, fluoroquinolone prophylaxis has been associated with a reduced risk of infection-related mortality. The latter finding may derive from a declining incidence of invasive gram-negative bacterial infections in the fluoroquinolone-treated patients, and a proportional increase in fluoroquinolone-resistant gram-positive infections, which are themselves associated with a lower infection-related mortality.

Recommendations regarding the use of fluoroquinolone prophylaxis in neutropenic patients will vary from institution to institution. In general, prophylaxis is reserved for those individuals whose duration of neutropenia is anticipated to be > 10 days; for those whose neutropenia is expected to be profound (ANC $< 0{\cdot}1 \times 10^9$/liter), and for persons treated at institutions where the prevalence of quinolone-resistance among facultatively anaerobic gram-negative bacilli is < 5–10%. In practice, the majority of these patients will be undergoing treatment for hematological malignancies.

Studies of antifungal chemoprophylaxis have focused on high-risk patients (see discussion of "Risk assessment" below), and on the prevention of infections due to yeasts. Filamentous fungi such as *Aspergillus* spp. are generally acquired through inhalation of conidia, which subsequently germinate to produce tissue-invasive disease. As such, they are more suitable targets for environmental control measures (see discussion of "Protective isolation" above) than for antimicrobial prophylaxis. Yeasts, on the other hand, colonize the mucosal surfaces of chemotherapy-treated patients, and are more prone to translocate across damaged epithelium, subsequently causing invasive fungal infections in the neutropenic host. These characteristics make yeasts a more appealing target for orally administered prophylactic antifungals. A recent meta-analysis of the randomized controlled trials of systemic antifungal prophylaxis[33] noted improved outcomes in the prophylaxis groups with regard to the subsequent requirement for empirical intravenous systemic antifungal therapy with amphotericin B deoxycholate, the incidence of superficial fungal infection or proven invasive fungal infection, and fungal infection-related mortality. In this analysis, an overall mortality benefit could be documented only for patients undergoing allogeneic hematopoietic stem cell transplant, or for those experiencing profound and prolonged neutropenia (ANC $< 0{\cdot}5 \times 10^9$/liter for more than 14 days). The effects were most pronounced with the use of the azole antifungals, fluconazole, and itraconazole, specifically in the groups undergoing allogeneic hematopoietic stem cell transplantation[33] and remission-induction therapy for AML.[34] Fluconazole has several pharmacokinetic advantages over itraconazole, and its use as a prophylactic agent is currently supported for patients undergoing stem cell transplantation.[35–37]

Case presentation (continued)

By day + 9, the patient complained of pain with swallowing. On day + 12, he complained of chills, muscle aches, headache, and abdominal discomfort. His oral temperature was 39·2°C, respiratory rate 26 per minute, pulse 100 per minute, and blood pressure 122/72 mmHg lying down and 98/60 mmHg standing. The oropharynx was diffusely erythematous with ulcerations over the hard palate and right buccal margin. There was no lymphadenopathy. The chest examination revealed inspiratory râles over the right medial basal segment. The abdominal examination revealed normal bowel sounds, but focal tenderness over the right lower quadrant was noted with light palpation. The ANC and AMC were 0, the ALC $0{\cdot}3 \times 10^9$/liter, and the platelet count was 12×10^9/liter. A chest roentgenogram was unremarkable.

Blood cultures were obtained from each lumen of the central venous catheter and from a peripheral site. Intravenous fluids and empirical antibacterial therapy with a third-generation cephalosporin, ceftazidime, were administered; 24 hours later the blood cultures from all catheter lumens were reported as growing gram-positive cocci in chains. The patient remained febrile. Further blood cultures were obtained and vancomycin was empirically added to the ceftazidime.

Assessment and management of the febrile neutropenic episode

When a patient with an absolute neutrophil count of $< 0{\cdot}5 \times 10^9$/liter meets the temperature criteria for a febrile neutropenic episode, vigorous attempts to document a source and/or to isolate a potential pathogen must be made. This requires a focused physical examination, and a minimum laboratory evaluation consisting of a full blood count, creatinine, liver enzyme tests, a chest *x* ray film; cultures of urine and sputum if urinary or respiratory symptoms are present; and cultures of blood drawn from each lumen of any indwelling venous catheter, as well as blood from one peripheral site (if possible). The latter recommendation derives from a study of neutropenic cancer patients,[38] in which a negative culture from either a central or peripheral site had a predictive value for the absence of "true bacteremia" of 98–99%. A positive culture at either site had a predictive value for the presence of "true bacteremia" that was substantially lower (63% for the central venous catheter, 73% for the peripheral site). Overall, single negative cultures from the central or peripheral sites are more helpful in ruling out a true bacteremia, than single positive cultures are at ruling it in. The high negative predictive values were not sensitive to changes in overall prevalence of true bloodstream infection.

If infection is suspected, empirical therapy with broad-spectrum antimicrobial agents should be instituted. Consensus recommendations also advise that any neutropenic individual with a clinically suspected infection should receive treatment, even in the absence of fever.[9] The choice of empiric therapy will be influenced by the results of the physical examination and key laboratory tests, by whether or not the individual's circumstances suggest a low risk for serious infection (see below), and by an understanding of which endogenous microflora cause infections most often in this population.

Physical examination

The salient features of a focused history and physical examination, as they pertain to the evaluation of a febrile neutropenic patient, are summarized in Table 13.1. The classic signs of inflammation associated with pyogenic infection in an immunocompetent individual may be absent or diminished in the context of absolute neutropenia. A seminal descriptive analysis of presenting signs and symptoms for neutropenic versus non-neutropenic hosts showed that, with regard to skin and soft-tissue infections, edema was reduced in neutropenic patients (73% of neutropenic versus 100% of non-neutropenic individuals, $P = 0{\cdot}02$), while fluctuance and exudation were for the most part absent (5% *v* 50%; $P = 0{\cdot}003$; and 5% *v* 92%; $P < 0{\cdot}001$, respectively).[39] Where pneumonia was ultimately diagnosed, cough and sputum production were less frequent among neutropenic patients (67% *v* 93%; $P = 0{\cdot}002$; and 58% *v* 85%; $P = 0{\cdot}003$, respectively), but bacteremia was more common (55% *v* 17%; $P < 0{\cdot}001$).[39] This effect of neutropenia on the presentation of bacterial sepsis must be taken into account in the evaluation of the patient.

Risk assessment

An individual's risk of developing serious complications related to infection during a febrile neutropenic episode will have a bearing on the type of empiric antimicrobial therapy that is recommended and the setting in which it is administered. The concept of infection risk in this population has been more extensively reviewed elsewhere.[40,41] Patients may be conveniently divided into low-, intermediate- and high-risk groups.

Low-risk individuals are those for whom the duration of neutropenia is expected to be short (3–5 days), who are clinically stable and without significant co-morbidities, and who are ambulatory. These individuals may be treated empirically with oral antibacterial agents during their febrile neutropenic episodes, where the following circumstances apply:

- the individual is judged to be compliant
- immediate access to medical care is available in the event of deterioration
- a caretaker is present to monitor the patient.

Intermediate-risk patients are those with solid tumors or lymphoproliferative malignancies who are undergoing stem cell transplantation and who may therefore be expected to have a more prolonged period of neutropenia (8–13 days). By definition they should have minimal comorbidity and be clinically stable. They are treated initially with inpatient intravenous therapy and, if an early

Table 13.1 Physical examination of the febrile neutropenic patient

Region	Examine for
Head and neck	
fundi	Retinal hemorrhages (bleeding diatheses)
	Retinal exudates(disseminated fungal infection)
auditory canals/tympanic membranes	Erythema (otitis externa/media; viral upper respiratory infection)
	Vesicles (herpetic infection)
anterior nasal mucosa	Ulcerations/vesicular lesions (fungal disease, herpetic infection)
oropharynx	Mucositis (predisposition to bacteremias/fungemias)
	Ulcerative gingivo-stomatitis (anaerobic bacteria)
	Pseudomembranous pharyngitis (thrush, a risk for candidemia)
Chest	Râles (more consistent than cough/sputum in diagnosis of pneumonia)
	Edema, pain, erythema around central venous catheter tunnel and exit sites
Abdomen	Localized tenderness (right lower quadrant: typhlitis; right upper quadrant: hepatobiliary infection; perianal tissues [not a digital rectal examination]: cellulitis, abscess or fistula)
Skin	Tenderness, erythema, swelling around intravenous sites
	Ulcerative or necrotic lesions (*Pseudomonas aeruginosa, Staphylococcus aureus, Aspergillus* spp.)
	Diffuse pustular/erythematous lesions (metastatic seeding with *Candida* spp.)
	Vesicular lesions (Herpes simplex/zoster)
	Hypersensitivity reactions

response is achieved, they may be "stepped down" to complete a course of further intravenous or oral therapy as an outpatient. High-risk patients are those receiving treatment for hematological malignancies (cytotoxic chemotherapy and/or stem cell allografting) for whom the duration of severe neutropenia will be protracted (> 14 days), who may have significant comorbidities, or who are unstable (hemodynamically). These patients are much more likely to develop medical complications or to die,[42] and should be treated as inpatients with intravenous antibiotics until their febrile neutropenic episode resolves.

The dichotomization of febrile neutropenic patients into only low-risk and high-risk categories with regard to recommendations for empiric antimicrobial therapy has also been advocated.[9] Here, the assessment of risk relies on a validated scoring system developed by a multinational collaborative group, in which treatment for a solid tumor, young age, outpatient status, and the absence of hypotension, symptoms, or significant comorbidity result in higher point-scores: achieving a higher total point score (≥ 21) defines an individual as being at "low risk" for complications, and warrants the management outlined above for low-risk patients.[43]

Spectrum of bacterial infections in neutropenic cancer patients

In previous decades more than 75% of the systemic infections in patients dying with acute leukemia were due to enterobacteriaceae (*Escherichia coli, Klebsiella pneumoniae*), *Pseudomonas aeruginosa* or *Staphylococcus aureus*.[44,45] More recently, gram-positive organisms have come to predominate as the etiologic agents of bacteremic infections. This shift may be related to several factors, including:

- the widespread use of central venous access catheters,[46] which predictably results in a greater incidence of bacteremia with gram-positive skin colonizers such as the coagulase-negative staphylococci
- more intensive chemotherapeutic regimens, with greater toxicity to the gastrointestinal mucosa,[47–49] and easier access to the bloodstream for viridans group streptococci and enterococci
- fluoroquinolone chemoprophylaxis, which suppresses the aerobic gram-negative bacilli colonizing the gut epithelium, but not the coexistent microaerophilic streptococci or coagulase-negative staphylococci.

It is therefore prudent to ensure adequate coverage for gram-positive pathogens in any empiric antibacterial regimen, particularly if the individual has received fluoroquinolone chemoprophylaxis. However, the risk of infection-related mortality is still highest for aerobic gram-negative bacteremic infections, particularly when *P. aeruginosa* is the causative agent[50] and all recommended empiric antibacterial regimens must include specific coverage for the latter organism.

Choice and duration of empirical antibacterial therapy

Table 13.2 lists a range of single-agent and combination antimicrobial regimens that have been used successfully in the management of fever from suspected infection in the neutropenic host. Low-risk patients for whom oral therapy is deemed appropriate may be treated with ciprofloxacin and amoxicillin-clavulanate, if the former drug has not been administered as part of a prophylactic regimen. Vancomycin may be added to an empiric regimen at the start of treatment if infection of an intravascular device is suspected (and coagulase-negative staphylococci are therefore implicated), or if the individual is known to be colonized with a penicillin-resistant gram-positive pathogen,[51] such as methicillin-resistant *S. aureus*. Alternatively, it may be added to a regimen between days 3 and 5 of antimicrobial treatment, if the patient remains febrile, and if the chosen empirical regimen is judged to have suboptimal coverage for *S. aureus* and streptococci (for example, ceftazidime monotherapy). However, given that 40% of patients with gram-positive bacteremias may respond to these regimens (i.e. ceftazidime alone),[52–54] and given that vancomycin use has been associated with an increased risk of colonization and infection with glycopeptide-resistant enterococci,[55–57] the routine use of vancomycin in empiric regimens is not recommended. In general, while individual patient factors (renal impairment, allergy) may influence the choice of antibacterial agents, the selection of any particular regimen depends more on institutional practice and local antimicrobial resistance patterns than on a proven survival benefit for any single drug or combination therapy.

Patients who are profoundly neutropenic, who remain febrile (without a documented source of infection) despite 5–7 days of empirical antibacterial therapy, and for whom neutrophil counts are not expected to recover in the short term are at high risk (approximately 20%) for invasive fungal infections.[9,58] Empirical antifungal therapy – generally with amphotericin B deoxycholate at doses of 0·5–0·7 mg/kg per day – is felt to reduce the risk of invasive fungal infection in these patients by anywhere from 50–80%, and to reduce mortality from fungal infections by 23–45%.[52–54] Of the two early,

Table 13.2 Empirical antibacterial regimens for the management of febrile neutropenic episodes

Regimen type	Antimicrobial type	Examples
Monotherapy	Anti-pseudomonal penicillin + β-lactamase inhibitor	Piperacillin/tazobactam, ticarcillin/clavulanate
	Carbapenem	Imipenem/cilastatin, meropenem
	Fluoroquinolone	Ciprofloxacin, levofloxacin
	3rd or 4th generation cephalosporin	Ceftazidime, cefipime, ceftriaxone,* cefixime*
Combination therapy	Antipseudomonal β-lactam +	Piperacillin, carbapenem, or antipseudomonal cephalosporin
	Aminoglycoside	Gentamicin, tobramycin, amikacin, netilmicin
	or	
	Fluoroquinolone	Ciprofloxacin, levofloxacin

*Outpatient therapy

suggestive studies of empiric amphotericin B therapy in febrile neutropenic cancer patients – where amphotericin B was added to background antibacterial therapy – one used a cohort design with historical controls,[52] and the other was a small, non-blinded, randomized study that was underpowered to show statistically significant differences in overall mortality or deaths attributable to fungal infection.[53] A larger randomized trial undertaken in the late 1980s suggested the trend towards reduced morbidity and mortality attributable to fungal infections, particularly in the highest-risk subgroups.[54] Overall, the available data have justified a BII recommendation (B – should usually be offered; II – based on clinical trials, with [at least] laboratory endpoints; United States Public Health Service/Infectious Diseases Society of America rating scheme) for the use of any antifungal agent in the neutropenic patient who remains febrile on broad-spectrum antibacterials for > 3 days, if the neutrophil counts are not expected to recover in the ensuing 5–7 days. While newer antifungal agents, such as the lipid-based formulations of amphotericin B,[59–62] intravenous itraconazole,[63] and voriconazole,[64] appear to have equivalent efficacy to amphotericin B deoxycholate as empirical antifungal therapy in neutropenic hosts, the latter medication remains the mainstay of therapy in this population.

The decision to modify or discontinue empirical antibacterial or antifungal therapy will be influenced by several factors. If a specific microbe is isolated and implicated as the cause of the febrile episode, the spectrum of antimicrobial therapy can be narrowed to cover that organism (or group of organisms), and an appropriate course of therapy should then be undertaken for the organism and anatomic site involved. Other decisions regarding continued antimicrobial therapy will depend on the resolution of the febrile episode, and the recovery of the neutrophil count to $> 0{\cdot}5 \times 10^9$/liter.

The median time to defervescence for low-risk patients is 2–3 days,[65,66] while for high-risk patients it is 4–6 days.[53,67–69] Given these parameters, and in the absence of a positive culture, a documented source of infection, or clinical deterioration, changes to the empirical regimen are generally not warranted for the first 5 days of the febrile episode. Otherwise, expert opinion suggests the following guidelines.[9]

- Patients who defervesce within the first 5 days of empirical therapy should have their treatment continued for a total of at least 7 days; low-risk patients may step down to oral therapy; high-risk patients should continue on their intravenous medications.

- Patients who remain febrile, in the absence of an identifiable source of infection, should have their antimicrobial agents continued until 4 or 5 days after their neutrophil counts rise to > 0·5 × 10⁹/liter, or, if the counts do not recover, to a total of 2 weeks' treatment; the patient must be in stable condition prior to stopping the antimicrobials, and the need for further antimicrobials should be assessed on an ongoing basis, until the neutrophil count recovers.

Case presentation (continued)

The patient remained febrile over the first 5 days of antibacterial therapy. The gram-positive organism in the blood cultures was identified as a viridans group *Streptococcus* (*S. mitis*). By day + 17 of induction therapy (day + 5 of antibacterial therapy), the patient remained febrile with oral temperatures peaking daily between 38·5°C and 39°C and continued to complain of right lower quadrant pain, now associated with diarrhea and signs of peritoneal irritation. Stool cultures grew no pathogenic bacteria or yeasts, and a test for *Clostridium difficile* toxin A and B in the liquid stool was negative. Repeated blood cultures and chest roentgenogram were ultimately non-diagnostic. A computerized tomographic examination of the abdomen identified cecal and ascending colonic wall thickening, with additional thickening of the ileal wall and the sigmoid colonic wall, consistent with neutropenic enterocolitis. The patient was treated with metronidazole intravenously. Over the course of the next 72 hours (until day + 20 of induction), the fever persisted; however, the patient's condition stabilized. The volume of diarrhea decreased and the abdominal pain, while still present, began to subside. The ANC and AMC were 0·001 and 0·2 × 10⁹/liter, respectively. By day + 22, the ANC, AMC, and platelet count were 0·186, 0·8 and 37 × 10⁹/liter, respectively, consistent with marrow regeneration. The fever had abated, and the diarrhea resolved.

Selected infectious problems in the neutropenic host

Some infections in the neutropenic host may be anticipated. For example, in the clinical example above, a viridans streptococcal bacteremia in the context of mucositis with ciprofloxacin prophylaxis and empiric therapy with ceftazidime – neither of which affords reliable coverage for gram-positive organisms – is not unexpected. Certain other infectious syndromes are relatively common in the neutropenic host, and deserve specific attention.

Neutropenic enterocolitis

Neutropenic enterocolitis presents with a clinical triad of persistent fever, abdominal pain, and diarrhea. The spectrum of pathology ranges from mild mucosal inflammation to transmural necrosis. Its true incidence is not known, but is probably related to the intensity of the chemotherapeutic regimen.[70] Onset of the first sign of neutropenic enterocolitis, diarrhea, occurs at a median of 10 days from the start of chemotherapy, and the syndrome is diagnosed at a median of 15 days from the start of chemotherapy.[71] The condition must be differentiated from other common causes of diarrhea in neutropenic cancer patients, including *Clostridium difficile* toxin-mediated diarrhea, and the direct effects of antimicrobial and cytotoxic agents. Abdominal computed tomography typically shows thickening of the bowel mucosa,[71,72] with more frequent involvement of the cecum. The condition is associated with a high risk for translocation of, and subsequent bloodstream infection with, bacteria and yeasts.

Treatment is supportive, with fluids, blood products, analgesics, parenteral nutrition, and broad-spectrum antimicrobial therapy, including specific coverage for anaerobic bacteria and for yeasts. It is not uncommon for the fever associated with this condition to persist until resolution of the neutropenic episode, as in the case above: the addition of empirical amphotericin B therapy to the patient's antimicrobial regimen in the context of continued fever on broad-spectrum antibacterials was not considered necessary, given the diagnosis of neutropenic enterocolitis. Surgery is reserved for cases with perforation or refractory bleeding, and most patients can be managed medically.[72]

Infections of intravascular devices

Central venous catheters are commonly implanted in patients undergoing protracted courses of chemotherapy, both for the administration of medications and for blood sampling. These catheters have up to a 20-fold increased risk of infection compared with peripheral devices.[73] Infection may occur at any point along the length of the device and, epidemiologically, these infections may be categorized[74] as:

- exit site infections, with < 2 cm of inflammation at the site where the catheter leaves the skin
- tunnel infections, with > 2 cm of inflammation, extending proximally from the exit site
- port pocket infections, where inflammation with or without fluctuance overlies the buried access bulb of an completely-implanted system
- a catheter-related bloodstream infection, where blood cultures drawn from the device lumen(s) are positive.

Tunnel infections account for up to 50% of line-related infections; exit sites for 25%; febrile bacteremias (bloodstream infection) for 19%; and septic thrombophlebitis for 6%.[75] A bloodstream infection is generally attributed to an intravenous catheter if positive blood cultures are obtained from the catheter port or lumen, and no other source of infection (for example, pneumonia, translocation of bowel microflora) is suspected. Quantitative blood cultures showing higher colony counts from a catheter lumen than from peripheral sites, or isolation of > 15 colony forming units on the tip of a removed catheter by the semiquantitative roll-plate technique[76] would also implicate an intravascular device as the source of bacteremia.

Central venous line removal is not required for all cases of catheter-associated bacteremia. Infections due to coagulase-negative staphylococci can be treated with the catheter left in place,[77,78] although there is a greater potential for bacteremic relapse with this practice (20% *v* 3% with catheter removal).[79,80] The majority of exit site infections not due to *Pseudomonas* spp. may also be treated with the catheter *in situ*.[78] In other circumstances where the intravenous device is implicated in the febrile neutropenic episode, it should be removed.

Most febrile neutropenic episodes and bacteremias, for which a source other than the intravascular device itself is suspected, can be managed without catheter removal.[81] If blood cultures remain persistently positive after 48 hours of effective therapy, removal of the catheter may be warranted.[77]

Case presentation (continued)

On day +32, just prior to planned hospital discharge, the patient was noted to have a low-grade fever (oral temperature 38°C) and to be complaining of right upper quadrant discomfort. An examination revealed a liver span of 14 cm. A liver function profile demonstrated a total bilirubin of 24 micromol/liter, an aspartate transaminase (AST) of 34 IU/liter, alanine transferase (ALT) of 54 IU/liter, lactate dehydrogenase (LDH) of 203 IU/liter, alkaline phosphatase (ALP) of 267 IU/liter, and gamma glutamyl transferase (GGT) of

376 IU/liter consistent with a cholestatic enzymopathy. A repeat infused CT scan of the abdomen demonstrated multiple radiolucencies present in the parenchyma of the liver and the spleen. Surveillance cultures from the rectum obtained on day + 15 and day + 20 had previously yielded a heavy growth of *Candida glabrata*. A diagnosis of hepatosplenic fungal infection was suspected. Further blood cultures grew no pathogens and a chest CT demonstrated no evidence of nodular lesions or consolidation. Culture of an open biopsy of the liver failed to grow any micro-organisms; however, a silver methenamine-stained preparation demonstrated the presence of budding yeasts consistent with invasive candidiasis. On the basis of this information, a diagnosis of hepatosplenic fungal infection – presumed to have developed while the patient was receiving fluconazole antifungal prophylaxis – was established.

Hepatosplenic fungal disease

Hepatosplenic fungal disease manifests as a persistent or recrudescent febrile illness in an individual who has received broad-spectrum antibacterial therapy for a febrile neutropenic episode, and whose neutrophil count has recovered.[82–85] Colonization of the gastrointestinal tract by yeasts,[7,34,86] and chemotherapy with high-dose cytarabine[84,87] are risk factors. There is often an associated fungemic episode, the median time to which is day + 15; the median time to recognition of the hepatosplenic infection is day + 40, at which time the neutrophil counts have recovered.[7] The pathogenesis is presumed to involve translocation of opportunistic yeasts across a damaged gut epithelium,[7,87] with fungemic seeding of the liver and spleen. Most of the cases are accounted for by *Candida* spp.

The presenting signs and symptoms of hepatosplenic fungal disease include fever in 85% and abdominal pain in over 50% of cases, with a cholestatic enzymopathy (elevated serum ALP and GGT). The total bilirubin may also be elevated. A CT scan showing multiple hypodense lesions in the liver and spleen, some of which may have a "bull's eye" appearance,[88] reinforces the presumptive diagnosis. Histopathologic examination of a liver biopsy will show typical granulomatous changes, with fungal elements on methenamine silver or PAS staining. Cultures of the biopsy specimen are most often negative (in one study, none of 28 laparoscopic biopsies was culture positive[89]), but the combination of an appropriate history with suggestive laboratory, imaging, and histology results should be sufficient to make the diagnosis.

There are no prospective studies comparing response rates among the different regimens used to treat hepatosplenic fungal disease. Amphotericin B deoxycholate, at a dose of 0·6 mg/kg per day, is considered the mainstay of therapy. Approximately half of the members of an expert panel recommended adding flucytosine to the amphotericin B regimen[90] for the treatment of patients who are acutely ill with their hepatosplenic fungal disease. Based on case-report and case-series data[91–93] it has been suggested[58] that patients who are stable, and who have not been heavily colonized or fungemic with a fluconazole-resistant species of *Candida* (*C. glabrata, C. krusei*), can be treated successfully with this triazole antifungal at doses of 6 mg/kg per day (approximately 400 mg per day in an average sized adult). The lipid-based formulations of amphotericin B have also shown promise in the treatment of hepatosplenic fungal disease.[94] It is recommended that any treatment be continued until symptoms, laboratory and imaging markers have resolved, or the lesions have calcified, and that patients continue to receive antifungal therapy during subsequent antileukemic therapy.[95] For individuals with refractory disease, adjunctive therapy with gamma-interferon and granulocyte-macrophage colony stimulating factor may be of some benefit.[96]

References

1. Hann I, Viscoli C, Paesmans M, Gaya H, Glauser M. A comparison of outcome from febrile neutropenic episodes in children compared with adults: results from four EORTC studies. *Br J Haematol* 1997;**99**:580–8.
2. Laverdière M, Rotstein C, Bow EJ *et al.* Impact of fluconazole prophylaxis on fungal colonization and infection rates in neutropenic patients. *J Antimicrob Chemother* 2000;**46**:1001–8.
3. Mackowiak PA, Bartlett JG, Bordon BC *et al.* Concepts of fever: recent advances and lingering dogma. *Clin Infect Dis* 1997;**35**:119–38.
4. Antin JH, Ferrara JL. Cytokine dysregulation and acute graft-versus-host disease. *Blood* 1992;**80**:2964–8.
5. Ferrara JL. Cytokines other than growth factors in bone marrow transplantation. *Curr Opin Oncol* 1994;**6**:127–34.
6. Krenger W, Ferrara JL. Graft-vs-host disease and the Th1/Th2 paradigm. *Immunol Res* 1996;**15**:50–73.
7. Bow EJ, Loewen R, Cheang MS, Shore TB, Rubinger M, Schacter B. Cytotoxic therapy-induced D-xylose malabsorption and invasive fungal infection during remission-induction therapy for acute myeloid leukemia in adults. *J Clin Oncol* 1997;**15**:2254–61.
8. Sonis ST. Mucositis as a biological process: a new hypothesis for the development of chemotherapy-induced stomatotoxicity. *Oral Oncol* 1998;**34**:39–43.
9. Hughes WT, Armstrong D, Bodey GP, *el al.* 2002 guidelines for the use of antimicrobial agents in neutropenic patients with cancer. *Clin Infect Dis* 2002;**34**:730–51.
10. Peacock JE, Herrington DA, Wade JC *et al.* Ciprofloxacin plus piperacillin compared with tobramycin plus piperacillin as empirical therapy in febrile neutropenic patients. A randomized, double-blind trial. *Ann Intern Med* 2002;**137**:77–87.
11. Schimpff SC, Hahn DM, Brouillet MD, Young VM, Fortner CL, Wiernik PH. Comparison of basic infection prevention techniques, with standard room reverse isolation or with reverse isolation plus added air filtration. *Leuk Res* 1978;**2**:231–40.
12. Nauseef WM, Maki DG. A study of the value of simple protective isolation in patients with granulocytopenia. *N Engl J Med* 1981;**304**:448–53.
13. Sherertz RJ, Belani A, Kramer BS *et al.* Imact of air filtration on nosocomial aspergillus infections. Unique risk of bone marrow transplant recipients. *Am J Med* 1987;**83**:709–18.
14. Loo VG, Bertrand C, Dixon C *et al.* Control of construction-associated nosocomial aspergillosis in an antiquated haematology unit. *Infect Control Hosp Epidemiol* 1996;**17**:360–4.
15. Bodey GP, Rodriguez V, Chang H-Y, Narboni G. Fever and infection in leukemic patients–a study of 492 consecutive patients. *Cancer* 1978;**41**:1610–22.
16. Schimpff SC, Young VM, Greene WH. Origin of infection in acute nonlymphocytic leukemia: significance of hospital aquisition of potential pathogens. *Ann Intern Med* 1972;**77**:707–14.
17. Levi JA, Vincent PC, Jennis F, Lind DE, Gunz FW. Prophylactic oral antibiotics in the management of acute leukemia. *Med J Aust* 1973;**1**:1025–9.
18. Levine AS, Siegel SE, Schreiber AD *et al.* Protected environments and prophylactic antibiotics. A prospective controlled study of their utility in acute leukemia. *N Engl J Med* 1973;**288**:477–87.
19. Preisler HD, Goldstein IM, Henderson ES. Gastrointestinal "sterilization" in the treatment of patients with acute leukemia. *Cancer* 1970;**26**:1076–81.
20. Yates JW, Holland JF. A controlled study of isolation and endogenous microbial suppression in acute myelocytic leukemia patients. *Cancer* 1973;**32**:1490–8.
21. Schimpff SC, Greene WH, Young VM *et al.* Infection prevention in acute nonlymphocytic leukemia–laminar air flow room reverse isolation with oral nonabsorbable antibiotic prophylaxis. *Ann Intern Med* 1975;**82**: 351–8.
22. Rodriguez V, Bodey GP, Freireich EJ *et al.* Randomized trial of protected environment-prophylactic antibiotics in 145 adults with acute leukemia. *Medicine* 1978;**57**: 253–66.
23. Dietrich M, Rasch H, Rommel K. Antimicrobial therapy as part of the decontamination procedure for patients with acute leukemia. *Eur J Cancer* 1973;**9**:443–4.
24. Dietrich M, Gaus W, Vossen J, van der Waaij D, Wendt F, EORTC International Antimicrobial Therapy Cooperative Project Group. Protective isolation and antimicrobial

decontamination in patients with high susceptibility to infection: a prospective cooperative study of gnotobiotic care in acute leukemia patients. 1. Clinical results. *Infection* 1977;**5**:107–14.

25. Gurwith MJ, Brunton JL, Lank BA, Harding GKM, Ronald AR. A prospective controlled investigation of prophylactic trimethoprim/sulfamethoxazole in hospitalized granulocytopenic patients. *Am J Med* 1979;**66**:248–56.
26. Gualtieri RJ, Donowitz GR, Kaiser DL, Hess CE, Sande MA. Double-blind randomized study of prophylactic trimethoprim-sulfamethoxazole in granulocytopenic patients with hematologic malignancies. *Am J Med* 1983;**74**: 934–40.
27. Dekker AW, Rozenberg-Arska M, Sixma JJ *et al.* Prevention of infection by trimethoprim-sulfamethoxazole plus amphotericin B in patients with acute nonlymphocytic leukemia. *Ann Intern Med* 1981;**95**: 555–9.
28. Engels EA, Lau J, Barza M. Efficacy of quinolone prophylaxis in neutropenic cancer patients: a meta-analysis. *J Clin Oncol* 1998;**16**:1179–87.
29. Bow EJ, Rayner E, Louie TJ. Comparison of norfloxacin with cotrimoxazole for infection prophylaxis in acute leukemia. The trade-off for reduced gram-negative sepsis. *Am J Med* 1988;**84**:847–54.
30. Lew MA, Kehoe K, Ritz J *et al.* Ciprofloxacin versus trimethoprim/sulfamethoxazole for prophylaxis of bacterial infections in bone marrow transplant recipients: a randomized, controlled trial. *J Clin Oncol* 1995;**13**: 239–50.
31. Cruciani M, Rampazzo R, Malena M *et al.* Prophylaxis with fluoroquinolones for bacterial infections in neutropenic patients: a meta-analysis. *Clin Infect Dis* 1996;**23**: 795–805.
32. Rotstein C, Mandell L, Goldberg N. Fluoroquinolone prophylaxis for profoundly neutropenic cancer patients: a meta-analysis. *Curr Oncol* 1997;**4**(Suppl. 2):S2–S7.
33. Bow EJ, Laverdiere M, Lussier N, Rotstein C, Cheang MS, Ioannou S. Antifungal prophylaxis for severely neutropenic chemotherapy recipients: a meta analysis of randomized-controlled clinical trials. *Cancer* 2002;**94**: 3230–46.
34. Rotstein C, Bow EJ, Laverdière M, Ioannou S, Carr D, Moghaddam N. Randomized placebo-controlled trial of fluconazole prophylaxis for neutropenic cancer patients: benefit based upon purpose and intensity of cytotoxic therapy. *Clin Infect Dis* 1999;**28**:331–40.
35. Dykewicz CA, Jaffe HA, Kaplan JE. Guidelines for preventing opportunistic infections among haematopoietic stem cell transplant recipients – Recommendations of CDC, the Infectious Diseases Society of America, and the American Society of Blood and Marrow Transplantation. *Biol Blood Marrow Transplant* 2000;**6**:659–727.
36. Dykewicz CA. Hospital infection control in haematopoietic stem cell transplant recipients. *Emerg Infect Dis* 2001;**7**:263–7.
37. Dykewicz CA. Summary of the guidelines for preventing opportunistic infections among hematopoietic stem cell transplant recipients. *Clin Infect Dis* 2001;**33**:139–44.
38. DesJardin JA, Falagas ME, Ruthazer R, and *et al.* Clinical utility of blood cultures drawn from indwelling venous catheters in hospitalized patients with cancer. *Ann Intern Med* 199;**131**:641–7.
39. Sickles EA, Greene WH, Wiernik PH. Clinical presentation of infection in granulocytopenic patients. *Arch Intern Med* 1975;**135**:715–19.
40. Rolston KVI, Rubenstein EB, Freifeld A. Early empirical antibiotic therapy for febrile patients at low risk. *Infect Dis Clinic N Amer* 1996;**10**:223.
41. Rolston KVI. New trends in patient management: Risk-based therapy for febrile patients with neutropenia. *Clin Infect Dis* 1999;**29**:515–21.
42. Talcott JA, Siegal RD, Finberg R, Goldman L. Risk assessment in cancer patients with fever and neutropenia: a prospective, two-center validation of a prediction rule. *J Clin Oncol* 1992;**10**:316.
43. Klastersky J, Paesmans M, Rubenstein EB *et al.* The Multinational Association for Supportive Care in Cancer risk index: A multinational scoring system for identifying low-risk febrile neutropenic cancer patients. *J Clin Oncol* 2000;**18**:3038–51.
44. Hersh EM, Bodey GP, Nies BA, Freireich EJ. Causes of death in acute leukemia–a ten-year study of 414 patients from 1954–1963. *JAMA 1965*;**193**:105–9.
45. Chang HY, Rodriguez V, Narboni G, Bodey GP, Luna MA, Freireich EJ. Causes of death in adults with acute leukemia. *Medicine* 1976;**55**:259–68.
46. Lowder JN, Lazarus HM, Herzig RH. Bacteremias and fungemias in oncologic patients with central venous catheters. *Arch Intern Med* 1982;**142**:1456–9.

47. Weisman SJ, Scoopo FJ, Johnson G, Altman AJ, Quinn JJ. Septicemia in pediatric oncology patients: the significance of viridans streptococcal infections. *J Clin Oncol* 1990;**8**:453–9.
48. Bishop JF, Lowenthal RM, Joshua D *et al.* Etoposide in acute nonlymphocytic leukemia. *Blood* 1990;**75**:27–32.
49. Bochud P-Y, Eggiman P, Calandra T, Van Melle G, Saghafi L, Francioli P. Bacteremia due to viridans streptococcus in neutropenic patients with cancer: clinical spectrum and risk factors. *Clin Infect Dis* 1994;**18**:25–31.
50. Schimpff SC, Satterlee W, Young VM, Serpick A. Empiric therapy with carbenicillin and gentamicin for febrile patients with cancer and granulocytopenia. *N Engl J Med* 1971;**284**:1061–5.
51. Feld R. Vancomycin as part of initial empirical antibiotic therapy for febrile neutropenia in patients with cancer: pros and cons. *Clin Infect Dis* 1999;**29**:503–7.
52. EORTC International Antimicrobial Therapy Cooperative Project Group. Ceftazidime combined with a short or long course of amikacin for empirical therapy of gram-negative bacteremia in cancer patients with granulocytopenia. *N Engl J Med* 1987;**317**:1692–8.
53. EORTC International Antimicrobial Therapy Cooperative Project Group, National Cancer Institute of Canada – Clinical Trials Group. Vancomycin added to empirical combination antibiotic therapy for fever in granulocytopenic patients. *J Infec Dis* 1991;**163**:951–8.
54. EORTC International Antimicrobial Therapy Cooperative Project Group. Efficacy and toxicity of single daily doses of amikacin and ceftriaxone versus multiple daily doses of amikacin and ceftazidime for infection in patients with cancer and granulocytopenia. *Ann Intern Med* 1993;**119**:584–93.
55. Shay DK, Maloney SA, Montecalvo M *et al.* Epidemiology and mortality risk of vancomycin-resistant enterococcal bloodstream infections. *J Infec Dis* 1995;**172**:993–1000.
56. Morris JG, Shay DK, Hebden JN *et al.* Enterococci resistant to multiple antimicrobial agents, including vancomycin. *Ann Intern Med* 1995;**123**:250–9.
57. Edmond MB, Ober JF, Weinbaum DL *et al.* Vancomycin-resistant Enterococcus faecium bacteremia: risk factors for infection. *Clin Infect Dis* 1995;**20**:1126–33.
58. Rex JH, Walsh TJ, Sobel JD *et al.* Practice guidelines for the treatment of candidiasis. *Clin Infect Dis* 2000;**30**:662–78.
59. Prentice HG, Hann IM, Herbrecht R *et al.* A randomized comparison of liposomal versus conventional amphotericin B for the treatment of pyrexia of unknown origin in neutropenic patients. *Br J Haematol* 1997;**98**:711–8.
60. White MH, Bowden RA, Sandler ES *et al.* Randomized, double-blind clinical trial of amphotericin B colloidal dispersion vs amphotericin B in the empirical treatment of fever and neutropenia. *Clin Infect Dis* 1998;**27**:296–302.
61. Leenders ACAP, Daenen S, Jansen RLH *et al.* Liposomal amphotericin B compared with amphotericin B deoxycholate in the treatment of documanted and suspected neutropenia-associated invasive fungal infection. *Br J Haematol* 1998;**103**:205–12.
62. Walsh TJ, Finberg RW, Arndt C *et al.* Liposomal amphotericin B for empirical therapy in patients with persistent fever and neutropenia. *N Engl J Med* 1999;**340**:764–71.
63. Boogaerts M, Winston DJ, Bow EJ *et al.* Intravenous and oral itraconazole versus intravenous amphotericin B deoxycholate as empirical antifungal therapy for persistent fever in neutropenic patients with cancer who are receiving broad-spectrum antibacterial therapy. A randomized, controlled trial. *Ann Intern Med* 2001;**135**:412–22.
64. Walsh TJ, Pappas P, Winston DJ *et al.* Voriconazole compared with liposomal amphotericin B for empirical antifungal therapy in patients with neutropenia and persistent fever. *N Engl J Med* 2002;**346**:225–34.
65. Maher DW, Lieschke GJ, Green M *et al.* Filgrastim in patients with chemotherapy-induced febrile neutropenia – a double-blind, placebo-controlled trial. *Ann Intern Med* 1994;**121**:492–501.
66. Kern WV, Cometta A, de Bock R *et al.* Oral versus intravenous empirical antimicrobial therapy for fever in patients with granulocytopenia who are receiving cancer chemotherapy. *N Engl J Med* 1999;**341**:312–18.
67. de Pauw BE, Deresinski SC, Feld R, Lane-Allman EF, Donnelly JP. Ceftazidime compared with piperacillin and tobramycin for the empiric treatment of fever in neutropenic patients with cancer. *Ann Intern Med* 1994;**120**:834–44.

68. Cometta A, Calandra T, Gaya H *et al.* Monotherapy with meropenem versus combination therapy with ceftazidime plus amikacin as empirical therapy for fever in granulocytopenic patients with cancer. *Antimicrob Agents Chemother* 1996;**40**:1108–15.
69. Peacock JE, Herrington DA, Wade JC *et al.* Ciprofloxacin plus piperacillin compared with tobramycin plus piperacillin as empirical therapy in febrile neutropenic patients – A randomized, double-blind trial. *Ann Intern Med* 2002;**137**:77–86.
70. Yates J, Glidewell O, Wiernik P *et al.* Cytosine arabinoside with daunorubicin or adriamycin for therapy of acute myeloid leukemia: a CALGB study. *Blood* 1982;**60**:454–62.
71. Kasper K Loewen R, Bow E. Neutropenic enterocolitis (NEC) in adult leukemia (AL) patients (pts) in Manitoba. *Clin Infect Dis* 1996;**23**:866.
72. Gomez L, Martino R, Rolston KV. Neutropenic enterocolitis: spectrum of the disease and comparison of definite and possible cases. *Clin Infect Dis* 1998;**27**:695–9.
73. Maki DG. Reactions associated with midline catheters for intravenous access. *Ann Intern Med* 1995;**123**:884–6.
74. Greene JN. Catheter-related complications of cancer therapy. *Infect Dis Clinic N Amer* 1996;**10**:255–95.
75. Press OW, Ramsey PG, Larson EB, Fefer A, Hickman RO. Hickman catheter infections in patients with malignancies. *Medicine* 1984;**63**:189–200.
76. Maki DG, Weise CE, and Sarafin HW. A semiquantitative culture method for identifying intravenous-catheter-related infection. *N Engl J Med* 1977;**296:**1305–9.
77. Hiemenz J, Skelton J, and Pizzo PA. Perspective on the management of catheter-related infections in cancer patients. *Pediat Infect Dis J* 1986;**5**:6–11.
78. Benezra D, Kiehn TE, Gold GWM, Brown AE, Turnbull ADM, Armstrong D. Prospective study of infections in indwelling central venous catheters using quantitative blood cultures. *Am J Med* 1988;**85**:495–8.
79. Raad I, Davis S, Khan A, Tarrand J, Bodey GP. Catheter removal affects recurrence of catheter-related coagulase-negative staphylococcal bacteremia (CRCNSB). *Infect Control Hosp Epidemiol* 1992;**13**:215–21.
80. Raad II and Bodey GP. Infectious complications of indwelling vascular catheters. *Clin Infect Dis* 1992;**15**:197–210.
81. Raaf JH. Results from use of 826 vascular access devices in cancer patients. *Cancer* 1985;**55**:1312.
82. Ong ST, Kuch YK. Hepatic candidiasis: persistent pyrexia in a patient with acute myeloid leukemia after recovery from consolidation therapy-induced neutropenia. *Ann Acad Med* 1993;**22**:257–60.
83. Fleece DM, Faerber E, de Chadarévian J-P. Pathological case of the month. *Arch Pediat Adolesc Med* 1998;**152**:1033–4.
84. Woolley I, Curtis D, Szer J *et al.* High dose cytosine arabinoside is a major risk factor for the development of hepatosplenic candidiasis in patients with leukemia. *Leukemia Lymphoma* 1997;**27**:469–74.
85. Verdeguer A, Fernandez JM, Esquembre C, Ferris J, Ruiz JG, Castel V. Hepatosplenic candidiasis in children with acute leukemia. *Cancer* 1990;**65**:874–7.
86. Chubachi A, Miura I, Ohshima A *et al.* Risk factors for hepatosplenic abscesses in patients with acute leukemia receiving empiric azole treatment. *Am J Med Sci* 1994;**308**:309–12.
87. Bow EJ, Loewen R, Cheang MS, Schacter B. Invasive fungal disease in adults undergoing remission-induction therapy for acute myeloid leukemia: the pathogenetic role of the antileukemic regimen. *Clin Infect Dis* 1995;**21**:361–9.
88. van Eiff M, Fahrenkamp A, Roos N, Fegler W, van de Loo J. Hepatosplenic candidosis – a late manifestation of candida septicemia. *Mycoses* 1990;**33**:283–90.
89. Antilla V-J, Ruutu P, Bondestam S *et al.* Hepatosplenic yeast infection in patients with acute leukemia: a diagnostic problem. *Clin Infect Dis* 1994;**18**:979–81.
90. Edwards JE, Bodey GP, Bowden RA *et al.* International conference for the development of a consensus on the management and prevention of severe candidal infections. *Clin Infect Dis* 1997;**25**:43–59.
91. Kauffman CA, Bradley SF, Ross SC, Weber DR. Hepatosplenic candidiasis: successful treatment with fluconazole. *Am J Med* 1991;**91**:137–41.
92. Anaissie EJ, Bodey GP, Kantarjian H *et al.* Flucaonazole therapy for chronic disseminated candidiasis in patients with prior amphotericin B therapy. *Am J Med* 1991;**91**:142–50.
93. Flannery MT, Simmons DB, Saba H, Altus P, Wallach PM, Adelman HM. Fluconazole in the treatment of

hepatosplenic candidiasis. *Arch Intern Med* 1992;**152**:406–8.

94. Sharland M, Hay RJ, Davies EG. Liposomal amphotericin B in hepatic candidosis. Archives of Diseases of Children 1994;**70**:546–7.
95. Walsh TJ, Whitcomb PO, Revankar SG, Pizzo PA. Successful treatment of hepatosplenic candidiasis through repeated cycles of chemotherapy and neutropenia. *Cancer* 1995;**76**:2357–62.
96. Poynton CH, Barnes RA, Rees J. Interferon γ and granulocyte-macrophage colony-stimulating factor for the treatment of hepatosplenic candidosis in patients with acute leukemia. *Clin Infect Dis* 1998;**26**:239–40.

14
Infections in general surgery

Christine H Lee

Surgical site infections

Case presentation 1

A previously healthy 17-year-old male underwent emergency appendectomy for perforated appendicitis. Perioperatively, he received intravenous gentamicin and metronidazole. Within 24 hours of surgery, he developed progressively severe, generalized abdominal and right flank pain. This was associated with nausea, anorexia, and diaphoresis. On examination, he appeared flushed. His heart rate was 140 per minute, blood pressure 100/40 mmHg, respiratory rate 26 per minute, and temperature of 39.4°C. His abdomen was diffusely tender. Examination of the surgical site revealed areas of dusky discoloration, purulent discharge and foul odor.

Postoperative surgical site soft tissue infections

It is estimated that more than 40 million surgeries are performed each year in the USA.[1] Surgical site infections (SSI), previously called surgical wound infections, are one of the most common types of infections among surgical patients and occur following 1–10% of operations.[2,3] This, however, is likely to be an underestimation as the postoperative length of hospital stay has decreased significantly over the past decade and several studies indicate that over 50% of SSIs occur after hospital discharge.[4–6] Currently, there is no established method for performing routine outpatient SSI surveillance.

SSIs are subclassified into superficial incisional, involving the skin and subcutaneous tissues; deep incisional, affecting the fascial and muscle layers of the incision, and organ space, which describes infections in any part of the organs or spaces other than the incision that was exposed during the procedure. Organ space infections include postoperative intra-abdominal abscesses, empyema, or mediastinitis.[7] Management of organ space infections is predominantly surgical and is beyond the scope of this review. The SSI risk factors, burden on healthcare costs, associated morbidity, mortality and preventative measures are well described in Chapter 12 of this book.

Evaluation of postoperative patients with suspected infection

Fever is the most common symptom of postoperative infection. Fever occurs in approximately 30–40% of patients after a major operative procedure.[8,9] Fever during the first 3 days of the postoperative period is often due to a non-infectious cause: medications, atelectasis, deep vein thrombosis, or injury to tissue.[10] In a retrospective review of patients undergoing major gynecologic surgery, Fanning *et al.* identified that 84% of patients, who were discharged within 3 days despite experiencing fever of ≥ 38·0°C, did not have a documented infectious etiology for the fever.[8] Presence of fever alone is not an indication for initiation of antibiotic therapy.

A postoperative patient with fever requires a systematic, complete evaluation. This includes careful, repeat history, complete physical examination, along with supportive laboratory tests, if indicated: complete blood count with differential, urinalysis, bacteriologic cultures of blood, tissue/aspirated fluid from surgical site. Selective imaging studies, particularly computed tomography of the abdomen and pelvis, may be useful in evaluating a patient with late onset, postoperative fever, after abdominal surgery, without an apparent source, in localizing occult infection or intra-abdominal abscess. The common causes of non-surgical site-related, postoperative infections and fever, which include urinary, respiratory tracts and catheter-related infections, may be delineated by meticulous assessment of the patient. The majority of SSIs occur 5 or more days after surgery but necrotizing soft tissue infections, particularly due to clostridial species or Group A streptococci can manifest within 36 hours of an operation.[11]

If the clinical assessment establishes the diagnosis of surgical site infection, as indicated by presence of purulent discharge from the wound, then the treatment is to open the wound for drainage. No RCTs have been identified which have compared drainage to conservative management. The next step is to determine whether further operative intervention is necessary. SSIs, with the exception of uncomplicated cellulitis, require mechanical procedures to open an infected wound, drain abscesses and remove devitalized tissues. An empiric antibiotic therapy is warranted along with exploration of the wound if there is painful spreading erythema over the surgical incision site, suggestive of cellulitis, or accompanying fever of ≥ 38·0°C, tenderness, edema and an extending margin of erythema at or around the surgical incision site.

A number of factors will influence the choice of empiric antimicrobial agent(s). These include patient-associated factors, such as host immunity, presence of diabetes mellitus, and length of preoperative hospital stay; procedure-associated factors, such as the type and duration of perioperative antimicrobial prophylaxis, and the duration of operation and class of surgical site;[12] and institution-specific factors such as the hospital's microbial antibiogram (antibiotic susceptibility profile). Many SSIs are polymicrobial, often including microbes resistant to antibiotics. *Staphylococcus aureus* is the most commonly isolated organism from SSIs, followed by *S. pyogenes*, *Escherichia coli*, other Enterobacteriaceae, and anaerobes.[13,14] Based on these data, the responsible pathogens and the antibiotic susceptibility can be postulated and appropriate antibiotic can be instituted until the culture results are available.

Diagnostic work-up recommendations include obtaining aerobic and anaerobic cultures from the site of infection prior to initiating antibiotic treatment. The rationale for obtaining culture is to identify the bacteria involved in the infection and to institute appropriate antibiotic therapy.[15] Cultures should be transported at room temperature to the laboratory in appropriate aerobic and anaerobic transport media within 2 hours of specimen collection. Deep aspirates or tissue cultures are superior to swab samples in providing clinically relevant results.[16] The results of culture and antibiotic susceptibility can aid in modifying the antibiotic regimen as treatment failure can occur in the presence of resistant organisms.[17,18]

Postoperative necrotizing fasciitis

Case presentation 1 (continued)

The surgical site was completely exposed and packed with sterile dressings. The infectious diseases service was consulted who recommended surgical exploration of the wound to rule out possible necrotizing fasciitis and the addition of intravenous cefazolin to the existing antibiotic regimen of gentamicin and metronidazole. Surgical exploration revealed infection tracking into transversalis fascia and internal oblique. Portions of the transversalis fascia were necrotic. Infected and necrotic materials were completely evacuated. A drain was placed in the pelvis. Histopathology confirmed the diagnosis of necrotizing fasciitis. Culture of the tissue grew mixed facultative anaerobic and anaerobic intestinal organisms.

Necrotizing fasciitis is a rare but potentially life-threatening, soft tissue infection and it encompasses two types based on the bacteriologic entities.[19] Type I is caused by anaerobic species, especially *Bacteroides fragilis* in combination with one or more facultative anaerobic organisms other than Group A streptococci. Type II is caused by Group A streptococci, alone or in combination with other bacteria, most commonly *S. aureus*. It is useful to distinguish the two types of necrotizing fasciitis as the medical management of type II differs from type I, although there is no difference in surgical management between the two types. Postoperative necrotizing fasciitis, as with other necrotizing fasciitis, is usually an acute, rapidly extensive inflammatory process.[20] The affected area is initially exquisitely painful and tender and this is associated with rapidly progressive erythema, and poorly demarcated edema. The course is followed by fever, hemodynamic instability, skin discoloration from erythema to violaceous-grey, bullae formation, and crepitation may be present. By day 4 and 5 of onset, frank cutaneous gangrene develops. Owing to associated morbidity and mortality with delay in diagnosis and management, it is paramount to recognize and institute immediate operative intervention when necrotizing fasciitis is clinically suspected.[21,22]

During the early stage, it may be difficult to clinically distinguish necrotizing fasciitis from cellulitis as the local features of the affected area may be non-specific. Presence of severe systemic toxicity and fever, despite an innocuous cutaneous appearance, should alert the clinician to possible underlying necrotizing fasciitis. The diagnosis of necrotizing fasciitis is made at surgery and it is essential to extensively excise the affected skin and subcutaneous tissues beyond healthy fascia.[20,22] Post debridement, a patient with necrotizing fasciitis usually requires critical care support and at times repeated debridement.

Empiric antibiotic therapy and intravenous fluid must be promptly administered as soon as the diagnosis of invasive soft tissue infection is considered. Initially, the antimicrobial therapy should consist of a regimen, which reliably targets streptococci, *S. aureus*, Enterobacteriaceae, and anaerobic organisms. For type I necrotizing fasciitis, broad-spectrum antibiotic is continued as the infection is due to mixed organisms. In Type II necrotizing fasciitis, confirmed by detection of Group A streptococci, a combination of high-dose intravenous penicillin G and clindamycin is the treatment of choice.[23–25] Necrotizing fasciitis may be accompanied by streptococcal toxic shock syndrome (STSS), as evidenced by a blood pressure of 90 mmHg systolic or below and evidence of end-organ damage, including renal, liver, pulmonary (adult respiratory distress syndrome) impairment in addition to rash or necrosis. A comparative observational study by Kaul *et al.*[26] showed that intravenous immunoglobulin (IVIG) administration for STSS was associated with increase in 30-day survival. Others have also described the successful use of IVIG in patients with STSS.[27–28]

In summary, despite advances in surgical techniques and infection control practices, SSIs continue to be common nosocomial infections.

The basic principle of management of SSIs is to open the infected site and allow it to drain. Antibiotics have an adjunct role only when there is invasive infection. There are no randomized controlled trials that have specifically addressed the duration of antibiotic therapy for SSIs, after its initiation. The patient's overall clinical response to surgical and adjunct pharmacological interventions should guide the duration and the route of antibiotic administration.

Mesh infections post-incisional hernia repair

Case presentation 2

A 59-year-old woman presented with a 4-day history of purulent discharge from a previous abdominal surgical site, fever, and malaise. One month prior to this, she had undergone abdominal wall sarcoma resection, followed by insertion of polytetrafluoroethylene mesh and reconstruction of the abdominal wall. She had a temperature of 37·6°C, a blood pressure of 128/82 mmHg, a respiratory rate of 20 breaths per minute, a heart rate of 90 beats per minute, and oxygen saturation of 96% while breathing ambient air. Abdominal examination revealed erythema and induration over the right, lateral aspect of the abdomen. There were three small areas of opening with thick, purulent yellow secretion at the right lateral corner of the graft. The white blood cell count was $14{\cdot}3 \times 10^9$/liter. The skin and subcutaneous tissues were opened and the mesh exposed. The patient was managed with surgical debridement and irrigation of the wound.

The culture of the wound grew *S. aureus*, sensitive to methicillin. Intravenous cloxacillin 2 g was started and the surgeon sought your advice for further management of this patient.

Following an elective laparotomy, between 10 and 20% of patients develop incisional hernia.[29] Without prompt reduction and repair, there may be serious complications, such as incarceration and strangulation of the small bowel.[29–31] The major risk factors for developing incisional hernia are obesity, malnutrition, wound infection, and reopened incisions.[32] After a primary repair, several studies have found high rates of recurrent hernia, from 24 to 54%. A number of studies,[33,34] including a multicenter randomized trial,[29] indicated reduced relapse rates using prosthetic biomaterials compared with suture repair of the hernia.

Evidence to guide management of mesh infections is based on biological principles and animal studies, as there are no cohort or randomized controlled trials. Polypropylene (Marlex, Bard Inc.) and polytetrafluoroethylene (Gore-Tex, WL Gore and Assoc. Inc.) are the most commonly used prosthetic biomaterials for ventral hernia repairs.[34] Compared with polypropylene mesh (PPM), polytetrafluoroethylene (PTFE) possesses significantly superior mechanical properties, which facilitate incorporation of the mesh into fibrocollagenous tissue and at the same time prevent permeation of water. PPM has been shown to cause extensive visceral adhesions and erosion of the skin or intestines with long-term use.[35–37] Two small animal studies addressed the role of PPM and PTFE use in repair of contaminated abdominal wall defects. Bleichrodt *et al.*[35] from the Netherlands studied 42 rats; PTFE patch were used on 21 rats to repair abdominal wall defects contaminated with bacteria and, similarly, 21 other rats received PPM mesh. Wound infection occurred in 16/21 rats in the PTFE and in 14/21 rats in the PPM group. Two rats in each group died as a result of ileus (1/4) or peritonitis (3/4). In contrast, Brown *et al.*[36] reported significantly fewer number of bacteria ($P < 0{\cdot}05$) adhered to PTFE compared to PPM, among 100 guinea pigs with simulated abdominal wall defects in the presence of *S. aureus*-related intra-abdominal infection. Based on the above results and paucity of human studies, it appears that there is a lack of distinction between the two prosthetic biomaterials in repair of contaminated abdominal wall defects.

Contrary to common perception, there are no data to suggest that infection occurs more commonly in use of mesh insertion, compared with conventional suture repair. The reported incidence of infection related to mesh use is 0·03–0·8%, and that of suture repair is 1–1·2%.[38–41]

The immediate host response to mesh implantation is recruitment and infiltration of inflammatory cells. In an ideal milieu, acute inflammation is replaced by fibroblasts and multinucleated giant cells, leading to complete incorporation of deposited mesh into the neighbouring tissues and induction of collagen synthesis.[42,43] When the inserted mesh is not properly taken up, complications such as accumulation of seromas (an excellent medium for bacterial growth), chronic sinus formation, fecal fistula or mesh extrusion may occur.[32,44–47] In a study by Amid *et al.*[48] the majority of these complications were attributable to errors in surgical techniques, for example improper positioning of the mesh, inadequate fixation and use of non-absorbable sutures.

Surgical site infections occurring early in the postoperative phase are usually independent of mesh utilization. These infections are primarily limited to the skin or subcutaneous layers and do not appear to interfere with proper mesh incorporation into host tissues.[32,43] With administration of appropriate antibiotics, proper drainage and debridement, it is rarely necessary to remove the mesh to eradicate the infection.[40]

Deep prosthetic-related infections, on the other hand, usually occur several weeks to months post surgery and occur infrequently at a rate of 0·03–0·8%.[38] Mesh-related infections result in cardinal symptoms of inflammation with a wide spectrum of severity. The factors that determine clinical presentation include: the virulence of the infecting pathogen; the nature of the host tissue and its ability to support microbial growth, and the host response to the presence of these pathogens. Most patients present with a subacute to indolent course, characterized by progressive, crescendo wound pain, occasionally accompanied by cutaneous draining sinuses. Fever, soft tissue swelling, and erythema may be absent. Rarely, some may present with acute, fulminant sepsis with high-grade fever, severe pain over the surgical site, and soft tissue swelling, erythema, and exudates. The infecting organism in this acute form is typically virulent, such as *S. aureus*, and it can elicit more systemic inflammatory responses compared to innocuous organisms, for example coagulase-negative staphylococci, Bacillus and *Corynebacteria* spp. beta-hemolytic streptococci, and aerobic, enteric Gram-negative bacilli are also capable of causing mesh-related infections, and these pathogens can incite severe inflammatory reactions similar to *S. aureus*.

Case presentation 2 (continued)

During the 2 weeks of local surgical site care and intravenous antibiotic therapy, the patient's signs and symptoms of systemic infection resolved. The abdominal surgical site was left open and she was discharged home with an intravenous antibiotic and daily surgical site care by a visiting home-care nurse. One month following the hospital discharge, the patient presented with purulent, foul smelling green suppuration from the abdominal wound and the exposed mesh. She was afebrile and hemodynamically stable. The surgical site culture grew *Pseudomonas aeruginosa*. At this time, you recommended removal of the infected mesh but the surgeon was reluctant to do so.

Based on the results from the combined European and American groups' observations, which included 12 374 cases of hernia repair using mesh, only eight patients developed mesh infection; five of the eight patients required removal of the mesh.[49,50] In a case report series consisting of three patients, the infections were completely eradicated in all the patients after the removal of the infected mesh.[50] Hence, based on these limited observational findings, it appears that patients who experience refractory infections despite repetitive drainage, lavage, and appropriate systemic antibiotic therapy may improve following removal of the prosthetic material. It is improbable that an adequately powered, prospective, randomized trial of conservative therapy versus surgical management for mesh infection will ever take place, given the very low rate of infectious complications and significant risks and morbidity associated with reoperation.

When a patient presents with infection, the decision and the timing of the mesh removal should be tailored to each patient, while considering the benefit and risks associated with repeat surgery in the individual patient. For patients who display evidence of persistent sepsis, while infected with virulent organisms, such as *S. aureus*, or aerobic, enteric Gram-negative bacilli, immediate removal of the mesh is likely necessary.

In conclusion, although mesh-related wound infection is rare, it is a clinically important complication. The risk of infection can be minimized with strict adherence to aseptic techniques during mesh preparation and implantation, while conforming to current perioperative recommended guidelines for SSI prevention.

Acute diverticulitis

Case presentation 3

A 62-year-old woman with a history of diverticulosis and hypertension presented with a 3-day history of left lower quadrant pain, anorexia, low-grade fever, and chills. There was associated dysuria, urinary urgency, and frequency. On physical examination, blood pressure was 116/62 mm Hg; heart rate, 110 beats per minute; temperature 38·2°C. The jugular venous pressure was 2 cm below the sternal angle and the mucous membranes were dry. There were normal bowel sounds, moderate tenderness and rigidity in the left lower quadrant and suprapubic area. There was no costovertebral angle tenderness.
The white blood cell count was $16{\cdot}7 \times 10^9$/liter; hemoglobin 104 g/liter; platelets 407 $\times 10^9$/liter. Routine biochemical tests and urinalysis were normal. A clinical diagnosis of diverticulitis was made. You admitted the patient for intravenous hydration and for consultation with a general surgeon. You searched the literature to determine optimal evidence-based diagnosis of diverticulitis.

Epidemiology

Acquired colonic diverticular disease is common in industrialized countries, where it is estimated to affect approximately 5–10% of individuals over 45 years of age and nearly 80% of the elderly over 85.[51] There is a growing evidence that the overall prevalence is increasing and the incidence in patients under 40 years of age is 2–5%.[52,53] The increase in prevalence in younger patients seems to be without regard to a particular socioeconomic or ethnic group.[54] There is a male preponderance for younger patients compared to both sexes being equally affected in the elderly population.[54]

Prior to a few decades ago, diverticular disease was exceedingly rare in developing countries and Japan, attributed largely to sufficient dietary fibre consumption.[55] Recent studies indicate its increasing incidence in Africa and Japan with the introduction of the westernized diet, which is high in refined carbohydrate and low in fibre.[55,56]

Diverticulitis refers to inflammation of diverticulosis and approximately 15–20% of patients with diverticulosis will develop diverticulitis.[57] Up to 20% of patients with diverticulitis are younger than 50 years old. There is no clear evidence that younger patients have more severe diverticulitis, as previously thought, although there may be delay in diagnosis owing to the atypical age of presentation and subsequent development of complications.[54]

Pathogenesis

Colonic diverticulosis occurs due to elevated intraluminal pressure and thinning of the colonic wall.[58] The weakening of the bowel leads to herniation of mucosa and submucosa. Diets high in refined carbohydrate and low in dietary fibre lead to diminished stool bulk, an increase in gastrointestinal transit time, and subsequent increases in intraluminal pressure.[59] Diverticulitis ensues when faecal material or undigested food particles lodge in a diverticulum, which can cause obstruction of the diverticulum neck. This results in accumulation of mucus, bacterial overgrowth, and loss of blood supply to already distended diverticulum. In the majority of cases, the outcome is a microscopic perforation and localized inflammatory process. Hinchey *et al.* created a useful method to classify inflammatory conditions associated with diverticulitis.[60] Stage I is defined as small, confined pericolonic abscesses, which can to lead larger paracolic abscesses (stage II). Stage III depicts generalized suppurative peritonitis and stage IV is fecal peritonitis. With recurrent episodes of inflammation, fibrosis, and stricture of the colonic wall may emerge.[61]

Diagnosis of acute diverticulitis

Clinical features

The most common symptom of acute diverticulitis is a gradual onset of constant lower abdominal pain, particularly in the left lower quadrant, as the descending and sigmoid colons are involved in 90% of the cases.[62,63] There may be associated changes in bowel habits, especially in the setting of partial bowel obstruction. Non-specific symptoms such as anorexia, nausea, and vomiting may accompany abdominal pain. When there is involvement of the bowel segment near the bladder or presence of colovesical fistula then urinary urgency, frequency, or dysuria may occur.[59] No studies were identified that specifically addressed the diagnostic accuracy of the clinical examination for diverticulitis.

Profuse rectal bleeding is unusual in acute diverticulitis but microscopic faecal blood may be present. Often, low-grade fever, mild leukocytosis, and localised lower quadrant abdominal tenderness are found. Presence of peritonitis reflects perforation of peridiverticular abscess or diverticulum. Patients receiving corticosteroids may not reveal evidence of peritonitis despite extensive colonic inflammation or perforation.

Case presentation 3 (continued)

After reviewing the literature with regard to the role of diagnostic imaging studies in the acute setting of suspected diverticulitis, you decided that your patient required a computed tomography (CT). The CT of the abdomen and pelvis with water-soluble contrast revealed pericolic fat inflammation, multiple diverticula, thickening of the bowel wall. There was also a 3 cm pelvic abscess.

Imaging studies

Since up to 12% of patients with acute diverticulitis may have free intraperitoneal air, it is important to include chest and abdominal radiographs in the initial management of patients presenting with a significant abdominal pain and possible underlying diverticulitis.[64]

Helical CT scans with water-soluble colonic contrast materials have been shown to be very useful in ascertaining the presence of acute diverticulitis, with a positive predictive value of 100% and a negative predictive value of 98%.[62,63,65,66] Owing to high risk of perforation, colonoscopy and barium enema should be avoided in acute diverticulitis. CT scanning, on the other hand, appears safe and can be performed even in critically ill patients.

The modern multislice CT scans, which provide speed and high-resolution imaging, when performed with rectal, oral (water-soluble), and intravenous contrasts have shown to accurately delineate intraperitoneal and colonic diseases.[67,68] Ambrosetti *et al.*[69] prospectively evaluated 542 consecutive patients presenting with acute left colonic diverticulitis with high resolution CT scans and contrast enema. The authors found the sensitivity of CT to be 98%, compared with contrast enema at 92% ($P < 0.01$), using a reference standard which included either test being positive, or pathological evidence of diverticulitis in resected surgical tissue. In addition to superior performance compared to contrast enema (CE) in terms of sensitivity, CT, also correlated with CE, was found to have better capacity to grade the severity of the inflammation with statistically significant differences ($P < 0.02$). This and several studies support the use of CT in evaluating patients in acute presentation compatible with underlying diverticulitis, requiring hospitalization to confirm the diagnosis, assess the severity of the inflammation, and to further direct patient management.[63,66,69,70]

Case presentation 3 (continued)

On day 3 of the admission, the patient developed sudden onset of diffuse abdominal pain and vomiting. On examination, she was pale and diaphoretic. There was generalized abdominal guarding and rebound tenderness. A plain film of the abdomen showed increased gas in small and large intestines.

Treatment of acute diverticulitis

Medical management

Approximately 85% of patients with a first attack of acute diverticulitis will respond to conservative management, which consists of intravenous fluid administration, bowel rest, and broad-spectrum antibiotic therapy for 7–10 days.[52,71] No RCTs were identified that have assessed the individual efficacy of these components. Patients with a mild, first episode of acute diverticulitis, who are able to maintain oral hydration, can be treated as outpatients given oral antibiotics effective against intestinal bacteria, for example ciprofloxacin and metronidazole.[51]

The majority of patients admitted to hospital with initial onset of acute diverticulitis will improve within 2–4 days with bowel rest, appropriate intravenous antibiotic, and fluid therapy. The antibiotic therapy should consist of a regimen that reliably targets colonic Gram-negative and anaerobic organisms. Several randomized trials demonstrated no statistically significant difference in overall outcomes between various collated antibiotic regimens for intra-abdominal infections: ciprofloxacin and metronidazole versus imipenem/cilastatin[72]; piperacillin/tazobactam versus cefotaxime and metronidazole[73]; ertapenem versus ceftriaxone and metronidazole[74]; cefoxitin versus gentamicin and clindamycin[75]; piperacillin/tazobactam versus clindamycin and gentamicin.[76]

After the resolution of the initial acute attack, patients should be counselled to consume dietary fibre regularly and be advised to undergo colonoscopy to rule out underlying colonic cancer. Approximately 5–15% of the patients treated with medical management will experience recurrent diverticulitis within 2 years.[77]

Surgical management

Fifteen per cent of patients presenting with acute diverticulitis will require either percutaneous drainage or surgical intervention.[71] Small abscesses (< 5 cm in diameter) usually drain spontaneously because of the development of fistulae between the colon and the abscess and they generally resolve with antibiotic treatment alone.[78] Abscesses that are 5–15 cm in diameter can be drained percutaneously under radiological guidance. With the administration of appropriate antibiotic therapy and adequate percutaneous drainage, patients in this group frequently improve within 72 hours, as indicated by a reduction in pain and normalization of leukocytosis.[61,79] Some of the advantages of percutaneous drainage are rapid control of sepsis and avoidance of general anesthesia, and drainage may obviate the need for a second operation to restore the contiguity of the colon.

Laparotomy is required when abscesses cannot be drained percutaneously because of inaccessibility, mulitiloculation, or lack of clinical response. Resection with primary anastomosis is the operative procedure of choice in such situations, as well as for patients who require definitive surgery even after a successful medical management, unless there are prohibiting factors such as edematous intestinal ends or inadequate bowel preparation.[51,61]

The absolute indications for immediate colonic resection are uncontrolled sepsis, visceral perforation, generalized peritonitis or colonic obstruction.[61] A review of practices and a recent prospective randomized study by Zeitoun *et al.*[80] determined that primary resection was superior to secondary resection in the treatment of generalized peritonitis related to diverticulitis in terms of immediate mortality and morbidity. In the latter study, 105 patients with sigmoid diverticulitis and generalized peritonitis were randomized to undergo primary or secondary colonic resection. Primary resection resulted in fewer re-operations (2 of 55 *v* 9 of 48, $P = 0{\cdot}02$) and shorter hospital stay (median 15 *v* 24 days, $P < 0{\cdot}05$).

References

1. Perl TM, Cullen JJ, Wenzel RP, *et al.* Intranasal mupirocin to prevent postoperative Staphylococcus aureus infections. *N Engl J Med* 2002;**346**:1871–7.
2. Horan T, Culver D, Gaynes R, *et al.* Nosocomial infections in surgical patients in the United States, January 1986-June 1992. *Infect Control Hosp Epidemiol* 1993;**14**:73–80.
3. Campos ML, Cipriano ZM, Freitas PF. Suitability of the NNIS index for estimating surgical-site infection risk at a small university hospital in Brazil. *Infect Control Hosp Epidemiol* 2001;**22**:268–72.
4. Sands K, Vineyard G, Platt R. Surgical site infections occurring after hospital discharge. *J Infect Dis* 1996;**173**:963–70.
5. Reimer K, Gleed C, Nicolle LE. The impact of postdischarge infection on surgical wound infection rates. *Infect Control* 1987;**8**:237–40.
6. Burns SJ, Dippe SE. Postoperative wound infections detected during hospitalization and after discharge in a community hospital. *Am J Infect Control* 1982;**10**:60
7. Horan TC, Gaynes RP, Martone WJ, *et al.* CDC definitions of nosocomial surgical site infections, 1992: A modification of CDC definitions of surgical wound infections. *Am J Infect Control* 1992;**20**:271–4.
8. Fanning J, Brewer J. Delay of hospital discharge secondary to postoperative fever – is it necessary? *J Am Osteopath Assoc* 2002;**102**:660–1.
9. Kossoff EH, Vining EP, Pyzik PL, *et al.* The postoperative course and management of 106 hemidecortications. *Pediatr Neurosurg* 2002;**37**:298–303.
10. Hager WD. Postoperative infections: prevention and management. In: Rock JA, Thompson JD, eds. *TeLinde's Operative Gynecology, 8th edn.* Philadelphia: Lippincott-Raven, 1997.
11. Dellinger PE. Surgical infections and choice of antibiotics. In Townsend CM Jr, ed. *Sabioston Textbook of Surgery, the Biological Basis of Modern Surgical Practice, 16th edn.* Illinois: Saunders Company, 2001.
12. Mangram AJ, Horan TC, Pearson ML, Silver LC, Jarvis WR. Guideline for prevention of surgical site infection, 1999. Centers for Disease Control and Prevention, Hospital Infection Control Practices Advisory Committee. *Am J Infect Control* 1999;**27**:97–132.

13. Jjuuko G, Moodley J. Abdominal wound sepsis associated with gynaecological surgery at King Edward VIII Hospital, Durban. *S African J Surg* 2002;**40**:11–14.
14. Jonkers D, Elenbaas T, Terporten P, Nieman F, Stobberringh E. Prevalence of 90-days postoperative wound infections after cardiac surgery. *Eur J Cardiothorac Surg* 2003;**23**:97–102.
15. Bowler PG, Duerden BI, Armstrong DG. Wound microbiology and associated approaches to wound management. *Clin Microbiol Rev* 2001;**14**:244–69.
16. Miller MJ, Holmes HT. Specimen collection, transport and storage. In: Murray PR, Baron EJ, Pfaller MA, Tenover FC, Yolken RH, eds. *Manual of Clincial Microbiology, 7th edn.* Washington, DC: ASM Press, 1999.
17. Sayek I. The role of beta-lactam/beta-lactamase inhibitor combinations in surgical infections. *Surg Infect* 2001;**2**(Suppl. 1):23–32.
18. Elsakr R, Johnson DA, Younes Z, Oldfield EC III. Antimicrobial treatment of intra-abdominal infections. *Dig Dis* 1998;**16**:47–60.
19. Giuliana A, Lewis F Jr, Hadley K, Blaisdell FW. Bacteriology of necrotizing fasciitis. *Am J Surg* 1977;**134**:52–7.
20. Casali RE, Tucker WE, Petrino RA, *et al.* Postoperative necrotizing fasciitis of the abdominal wall. *Am J Surg* 1980;**140**:787.
21. Stamenkovic I, Lew PD. Early recognition of potentially fatal necrotizing fasciitis: use of frozen-section biopsy. *N Engl J Med* 1984;**310**:1689.
22. Tamussino K. Postoperative infection. *Clin Obstet Gynecol* 2002;**45**:562–73.
23. Stevens DL, Yan S, Bryant AE. Penicillin-binding protein expression at different growth stages determines penicillin efficacy in vitro and in vivo: an explanation for the inoculum effect. *J Infect Dis* 1993;**167**:1401–5.
24. Stevens DL, Bryant AE, Hackett SP. Antibiotic effects on bacterial viability, toxin production and host response. *Clin Infect Dis* 1995;**20**:S154–S157.
25. Stevens DL, Madaras-Kelly KJ, Richards DM. In vitro antimicrobial effects of various combinations of penicillin and clindamycin against four strains of *Streptococcus pyogenes. Antimicrob Agents Chemother* 1998;**42**:1266–8.
26. Kaul R, McGeer A, Norrby-Teglund A, *et al.* Intravenous immunoglobulin therapy for streptococcal toxic shock syndrome – A comparative observational study. *Clin Infect Dis* 1999;**28**:800–7.
27. Barry W, Hudgins L, Donta ST, Pesanti EL. Intravenous immunoglobulin therapy for toxic shock syndrome. *JAMA* 1992;**267**:3315–16.
28. Lamothe F, D'Amico P, Ghosn P, *et al.* Clinical usefulness of intravenous human immunoglobulin in invasive group A streptococcal infections: Case report and review. *Clin Infect Dis* 1995;**21**:1469–70.
29. Luijendijk RW, Hop WC, van den Tol P, *et al.* A comparison of suture repair with mesh repair for incisional hernia. *N Engl J Med* 2000;**343**:392–8.
30. Read RC, Yoder G. Recent trends in the management of incisional herniation. *Arch Surg* 1989;**124**:485–8.
31. Manninen MJ, Lavonius M, Perhoniemi VJ. Results of incisional hernia repair: a retrospective study of 172 unselected hernioplasties. *Eur J Surg* 1991;**157**:29–31.
32. Birolini C, Utiyama EM, Rodrigues Jr. AJ, Birolini D. Elective colonic operation and prosthetic repair of incisional hernia: does contamination contraindicate abdominal wall prosthesis use? *J Am Coll Surg* 2000;**191**:366–72.
33. Anthony T, Bergen PC, Kim L, *et al* Factors affecting recurrence following incisional herniorrhaphy. *World J Surg* 2000;**24**:95–101.
34. Kercher KW, Sing RF, Lohr C, Matthews BD, Heniford BT. Feature: Successful salvage of infected polytetrafluoroethylene mesh after ventral hernia repair. *Ostomy Wound Management* 2002:**48**:40–2,44–5.
35. Bleichrodt RP, Simmermacher RK, van der Lei B, Schakenraad JM. Expanded polytetrafluoroethylene patch versus polypropylene mesh for the repair of contaminated defects of the abdominal wall. *Surg Gynecol Obstet* 1993;**176**:18–24.
36. Brown GL, Richardson JD, Malangoni MA, *et al.* Comparison of prosthetic materials for abdominal wall reconstruction in the presence of contamination and infection. *Ann Surg* 1985;**201**(6):705–11.
37. McNeeley SG Jr. Hendrix SL, Bennett SM, *et al.* Synthetic graft placement in the treatment of fascial dehiscence with necrosis and infection. *Am J Obstet Gynecol* 1998;**179**:1430–5.
38. Shulman AG, Amid PK, Lichtenstein IL. The safety of mesh repair for primary inguinal hernias: results of 3019 operations from five diverse sources. *Am Surg* 1992;**58**:255–7.
39. Berliner SD. Clinical experience with an inlay expanded polytetrafluoroethylene soft tissue patch as an adjunct in

inguinal hernia repair. *Surg Gynecol Obstet* 1993;**176**: 323–6.

40. Gilbert AI, Felton LL. Infection in inguinal hernia repair considering biomaterials and antibiotics. *Surg Gynecol Obstet* 1993;**177**:126–30.
41. Thill RH, Hopkins WM. The use of mersilene mesh in adult inguinal and femoral hernia repairs: a comparison with classic techniques. *Am Surg* 1994;**60**:553–7.
42. Arnaud JP, Eloy R, Adloff M, Grenier JF. Critical evaluation of prosthetic materials in repair of abdominal wall hernias. *Am J Surg* 1977;**133**:339–45.
43. Mann DV, Pout J, Havranek E, Gould S, Darzi A. Late-onset deep prosthetic infection following mesh repair of inguinal hernia. *Am J Surg* 1998;**176**:12–14.
44. Stone HH, Fabian TC, Turkleson ML, Jurkiewicz MJ. Management of acute full-thickness losses of abdominal wall. *Ann Surg* 1981;**193**:612–18.
45. Boyd WC. Use of marlex mesh in acute loss of the abdominal wall due to infection. *Surg Gynecol Obstet* 1977;**144**:251–2.
46. Kaufman Z, Engelberg M, Zager M. Fecal fistula a late complication of Marlex mesh repair. *Dis Colon Rectum* 1981;**24**:543–4.
47. Leber GE, Garb JL, Alexander AI, Reed W. Long-term complications associated with prosthetic repair of incisional hernias. *Arch Surg* 1998:**133**:378–82.
48. Amid PK. Classification of biomaterials and their related complications in abdominal wall hernia surgery. *Hernia* 1997;**1**:15–21.
49. Phillips EH, Arregui M, Carroll BJ, *et al.* Incidence of complications following laparoscopic hernioplasty. *Surg Endosc* 1995;**9**:16–21.
50. Avtan L, Avci C, Bulut T, Fourtanier G. Mesh infections after laparoscopic inguinal hernia repair. *Surg Laparosc Endosc* 1997;**7**:192–5.
51. Ferzoco LB, Paptopoulos V, Silen W. Acute diverticulitis. *N Engl J Med* 1998;**338**:1521–6.
52. Minardi AJ Jr, Johnson LW, Sehon JK, Zibari GB, McDonald J. Diverticulitis in the young patient. *Am Surg* 2001;**67**:458–61.
53. Acosta JA, Grebenc ML, Doberneck RC, *et al.* Colonic diverticular disease in patients 40 years old or younger. *Am Surgeon* 1992;**58**:605–7.
54. Konvolinka CW. Acute diverticulitis under age forty. *Am J Surg* 1994;**167**:562–5.
55. Madiba TE, Mokoena T. Pattern of diverticular disease among Africans. *East Afr Med J* 1994;**71**:644–6.
56. Miura S, Kodiara S, Shatari T, *et al.* Recent trends in diverticulosis of the right colon in Japan: retrospective review in a regional hospital. *Dis Colon Rectum* 2000;**43**:1383–9.
57. Stollman NH, Rakin JB. Diverticular disease of the colon. *J Clin Gastroenterol* 1999;**29**:241–52.
58. Whiteway J, Morson BC. Pathology of the ageing – diverticular diseas. *Clin Gastroenterol* 1985;**14**:829–46.
59. Burkitt DP, Walker ARP, Painter NS. Dietary fiber and disease. *JAMA* 1974;**229**:1068–74.
60. Hinchey EJ, Schaal PH, Richards GK. Treatment of perforated diverticular disease of the colon. *Adv Surg* 1978;**12**:85–109.
61. Boulos PB. Complicated diverticulosis. Best *Prac Res Clin Gastroenterol* 2002;**16**:649–62.
62. Labs JD, Sarr MG, Fishman EK, Siegelman SS, Cameron JL. Complications of acute diverticulitis of the colon: improved early diagnosis with computerized tomography. *Am J Surg* 1988;**155**:331–6.
63. Rao PM, Rhea JT, Novellin RA, *et al.* Helical CT with only colonic contrast material for diagnosing diverticulitis: prospective evaluation of 150 patients. *Am J Roentgenol* **170**:1445–9.
64. McKee RF, Deignan RW, Krukowski ZH. Radiological investigation in acute diverticulitis. *Br J Surg* 1993;**80**:560–6.
65. Ferzoco LB, Raptopoulos V, Silen W. Acute diverticulitis. *N Engl J Med* 1998; 338;**21**:1521–6.
66. Neff CC, van Sonnenberg E. CT of diverticulitis: diagnosis and treatment. *Radiol Clin N Am* 1989;**27**:743–52.
67. Tsai SC, Chao TH, Lin WY, Wang SJ. Abdominal abscesses in patients having surgery: an application of Ga-67 scintigraphic and computed tomographic scanning. *Clin Nucl Med* 2001;**26**:761–4.
68. Halligan S, Saunders B. Imaging diverticular disease. *Best Prac Res Clin Gastroenterol* 2002;**16**:595–610.
69. Ambrosetti P, Becker C, Terrier F. Colonic diverticulitis: impact of imaging on surgical management – a prospective study of 542 patients. *Eur Radiol* 2002;**12**:1145–9.
70. Buchanan GN, Kenefick NJ, Cohen CR. Diverticulitis. *Best Prac Res Clin Gastroenterol* 2002;**16**:**4**:635–47.
71. Solokin JS, Reinhart HH, Dellinger EP, *et al.* Results of a randomized trial comparing sequential intravenous/oral

treatment with ciprofloxacin plus metronidazole to imipenem/cilastatin for intra-abdominal infections. The Intra-Abdominal Infection Study Group. *Ann Surg* 1996;**223**:303–15.

72. Maltezou HC, Nikolaidis P, Lebesii E, *et al.* Piperacillin/tazobactam versus cefotaxime plus metronidazole for treatment of children with intra-abdominal infections requiring surgery. *Eur J Clin Microbiol Infect Dis* 2001; **20**:643–6.
73. Yellin AE, Hassett JM, Fernandez A, *et al.* The 004 intra-abdominal infection study group. Ertapenem monotherapy versus combination therapy with ceftriaxone plus metronidazole for treatment of complicated intra-abdominal infections in adults. *Int J Antimicrob Agents* 2002;**20**:165–73.
74. Shyr YM, Lui WY, Su CH, Wang LS, Liu CY. Piperacillin/tazobactam in comparison with clindamycin plus gentamicin in the treatment of intra-abdominal infections. *Zhonghua Yi Xue Za Zhi (Taipei)* 1995;**56**:102–8.
75. Kellum JM, Sugerman HJ, Coppa GF, *et al.* Randomized, prospective comparison of cefoxitin and gentamicin-clindamycin in the treatment of acute colonic diverticulitis. *Clin Ther* 1992;**14**:376–84.
76. Ambrosetti P, Robert J, Witzig JA, *et al.* Acute left colonic diverticulitis: a prospective analysis of 226 consecutive cases. *Surgery* 1994;**115**:546–50.
77. Ambrosetti P, Robert JH, Witzig JA, *et al.* Incidence, outcome, and proposed management of isolated abscesses complicating acute left-sided colonic diverticulitis. A prospective study of 140 patients. *Dis Colon Rectum* 1992;**35**:1072–6.
78. Stabile BE, Paccio E, Van Sonnenberg E, Neff CC. Prospective percutaneous drainage of diverticular abscesses. *Am J Surg* 1990;**159**:99–105.
78. Kurkowski ZH, Matheson NA. Emergency surgery for diverticular disease complicated by generalized and faecal peritonitis: a review. *Br J Surg* 1984;**71**:921–7.
80. Zeitoun G, Laurent A, Rouffet F, *et al.* Multicenter randomized clinical trial of primary versus secondary sigmoid resection in generalized peritonitis complicating sigmoid diverticulitis. *Br J Surg* 2000;**87**:1366–74.

15
Infections in the thermally injured patient

Edward E Tredget, Robert Rennie, Robert E Burrell, Sarvesh Logsetty

Case presentation

A 37-year-old male pipe fitter was tightening pipes in a petrochemical refining facility when a pipe burst, spewing him with a hot water/liquid ethylene glycol solvent mixture over 40% of his total body surface area (TBSA) including his upper extremities, chest, abdomen, and back. On the burns unit, routine admission wound, nose, rectum, and throat cultures were performed. He was resuscitated with fluids and nutritional support was provided by enteral feeding commenced at 24 hours post burn according to a routine protocol. His wounds were treated with topical silver sulfadiazine cream and his dressing was changed daily in a Hubbard tank hydrotherapy facility. After 5 days in hospital he underwent debridement and split-thickness skin grafting to his upper extremities; 3 days later he became acutely confused, tachypneic, hypotensive (80/60 mmHg), and oliguric. The patient was treated empirically with piperacillin 4 g intravenously every 8 hours and gentamicin 350 mg daily. His blood cultures grew *Pseudomonas aeruginosa* in both vials and methicillin-susceptible *Staphylococcus aureus* and *Enterococcus faecium* in one of two vials. The antibiotics were switched to amikacin 1 g daily, ceftazidime 2 g every 8 hours and vancomycin 1 g every 12 hours. He required massive fluid resuscitation with crystalloids, fresh frozen plasma, and albumin totaling 35 liters over 30 hours as well as intravenous vasopressors, initially dopamine and dobutamine, but ultimately noradrenalin before he was stabilized and his urine output recovered.

Serious infections remain a common complication in thermally injured patients contributing substantially to burn morbidity and mortality. Despite advancements in medical and surgical care of burns patients, no significant improvement in mortality has been documented over a 25-year period in one major institution caring for burns patients once bacteremic with *Pseudomonas aeruginosa*.[1] Much of the evidence guiding management of infections in thermally injured patients is based on case series where bacteriological results have been reported. Therefore a review of the bacteriology of burns is essential to understanding the evidence-base for current practice.

Bacteriology of burns patients

The types of bacteria that colonize and infect burns patients, as well as their susceptibilities to antimicrobials, is highly variable between burns units. It is influenced by both the topical antimicrobial and wound care policies of the burns center as well as the approach to usage of systemic antibiotics. In India, Revathi *et al.* reviewed their experience with 600 infections in burns patients[2] and, similar to many burns centers, found that the most frequent and severe infections were caused by *Pseudomonas* spp followed by *Staphylococcus aureus* and then by other gram-negative organisms including *Klebsiella* spp., *Acinetobacter* spp., *Escherichia coli*, *Enterococcus faecalis*, and *Proteus* sp. In a survey of 176 burn care centers in North America, *P. aeruginosa* was considered the most serious cause of life-threatening infections in thermally injured patients.[3] Similarly, in a 25-year review of *Pseudomonas* bacteremia in burns patients by McManus *et al.*, an overall burn mortality of 77% with *P. aeruginosa* bacteremia was documented, 28% above predicted rates.[1] A comparison of two 10-year periods of gram-negative isolates in pediatric burns patients demonstrated that in the 1990s, *P. aeruginosa* accounted for 35% of the gram-negative organisms from all sites of infections, as compared with 34% in the 1980s. Most recently, however, *Acinetobacter* spp. have replaced *Klebsiella* spp. as the second most common gram-negative bacteria causing infections in children with burns.[4] Similarly, in an overview of wound isolates in burns centers in the United Kingdom, an increasing prevalence of *Acinetobacter* spp. has been described.[5] It is important to note that *Aeromonas* sp. is an uncommon, but rapidly aggressive gram-negative burn wound pathogen that can lead to early burn wound sepsis (within the first burn week) commonly after patients have been exposed to lake or slough water post injury.[6]

In a large case series of established infections in the US army burns center, Pruitt *et al.* reported that 25% of infections were due to pneumonia, 22% to urinary tract, 26% to primary blood stream infections, and 5% to invasion of the burn wound.[7] Of the 57 documented cases of invasive wound infection that occurred in burns patients treated during the 1986–1995 period, there were 26 cases of secondary bacteremia due to *P. aeruginosa*. In this major academic American military burns center where early burn wound excision, avoidance of immersion hydrotherapy, dependence on quantitative and histologic evidence for burn wound infection, and topical sulfamyalon are routine practices, a high rate of yeast and fungal infections occurred in burns of 50% or more of the total body surface area. Most of these fungal infections were in massive burn injuries and were due to *Candida* spp., which on average, colonized the burn wound on post-burn day 30, infected the urinary tract on day 48, and other sites at day 41.[7] Filamentous fungi such as *Aspergillus* spp. and *Fusarium* spp. have also been reported to cause invasive infection.[8] Predisposition of burns patients to fungal infections has been identified when strong dependence on topical mafenide acetate solutions is used to control gram-negative bacteria in the burn wound.[9]

Diagnosis

Clinical presentation

Approximately 400 000 cases of sepsis occur in the USA each year with 30–45% mortality.[10] The clinical spectrum of burns patients resembles that of other septic patients.[11] Fever and inflammation following a burn injury is a very common response to localized microbial invasion to the burn wound. However, when the size of the burn increases beyond 15–20% of the total body surface area, release of cytokines and eicosanoid mediators leads to a systemic inflammatory response syndrome (SIRS), in the presence or the absence of a definable bacteriologic infection.[11] With progressive bacterial or fungal colonization of the burn wound, sepsis progressing to multiple organ dysfunction syndrome (MODS) and septic shock may occur. There are, to date, no clinical features that have been found distinguishing a burns patient with SIRS from a septic burns patient without hypotension. A thorough physical examination and septic workup (blood, wound, and urine cultures; chest radiograph, and urinalysis) is necessary for the initial investigation of the burns patient with symptoms and signs of infection.[12]

Evaluation of infected thermally injured patients is a challenge for clinicians. The clinical presentation of infection can range from an acute (such as the patient presented) to a chronic onset. This may range from low grade cellulitis or minor skin graft infection to fulminant septic shock and widespread infection of skin graft donor site wounds and complete non-take of split-thickness skin grafts in the postoperative period.[7] Classically, bacterial colonization of the burn wound and eschar leads to progressive increases in the numbers of bacteria and penetration of the eschar from superficial to deep into the eschar before invasion into healthy uninjured tissue leads to bacteremia and sepsis.[7] Altered mental status, tachypnea, paralytic ileus, hyper- or hypothermia (> 38·5°C or < 36·5°C), hypotension and oliguria, associated with leukocytosis $> 15{\cdot}0 \times 10^3$ cells/mm^3 or leukopenia $< 3{\cdot}5 \times 10^3$ cells/mm^3, thrombocytopenia < 50 000 platelets/mm^3, hyperglycemia, and unexplained acidosis are cardinal signs of burn wound sepsis.[7] Local evidence of invasive wound infection includes black or brown patches of wound discoloration, rapid eschar separation, conversion of partial thickness wounds to full thickness injuries, spreading peri-wound erythema, punctate hemorrhagic, subeschar lesions, and, with *P. aeruginosa*, violaceous or black lesions in unburned tissue termed 'ecthyma gangrenosum'.[13]

Microbiology cultures

Commonly, wound infection is diagnosed clinically and wound swabs of potentially contaminated tissues are obtained. Surface wound cultures are considered only partially representative of the bacterial flora contained within the wound.[14] For this reason, burn wound biopsies have been employed by many burn care centers to allow quantitation of the numbers of bacteria present within the wound where > 10^5 organisms/g of wet tissue is considered evidence of wound infection, which will prevent successful wound closure surgically.[14] Recently, Steer *et al.* used parallel cultures from 141 samples in 74 burns patients to demonstrate that recovery of the same set of species of bacteria from a burn wound biopsy versus a surface swab was 54%, and the predictive value of the counts obtained by one method to predict the counts obtained by the other was poor, owing, in part, to wide variation in bacterial densities from simultaneous cultures taken from the same burn wound.[14] Further, in burns > 15% TBSA, quantitative bacteriology by burn wound biopsy or surface swab did not aid in the prediction of sepsis or graft loss.[14] By definition, burn wound invasion leading to bacteremia, is a histologic diagnosis where microscopic evidence of invasion of non-burned tissue with bacteria occurs, a finding which McManus found was present in only 36% of biopsies with positive cultures (> 10^5 organisms/g).[15] Unfortunately, burn wound biopsies are expensive, invasive because a section of unburned tissue needs to be included with the biopsy, and associated with considerable variability between adjacent sites of the burn wound.[16] These facts together with more aggressive wound debridement, newer topical antimicrobials, and improved nutritional support and intensive care have limited the use of burn wound biopsy in many burns centers.[17]

Laboratory diagnosis of infection in the burns patient also includes blood cultures, urine and respiratory cultures, depending on clinical clues such as sepsis, pyuria, and evidence of pulmonary infiltrates.

To date, there is little evidence to support the routine use of blood culture testing in burns patients. Keen *et al.* in a small retrospective analysis of 47 burns patients found that positive blood cultures were more common in patients who were in shock, had larger burn wounds, were receiving more antibiotics, and who had indwelling catheters.[18] Reduced frequency of blood cultures was not associated with increased length of stay, ventilator days, or mortality.[18] The small size of this study, however, probably precludes the ability to detect differences. Henke *et al.* conducted a retrospective analysis of 1040 routine blood cultures in 121 surgical patients (including 31 burns patients):[19] 48 positive blood cultures led to a change in management or therapy in 19 (40%). Of interest is the fact that the mortality rate was highest in burns patients who had positive blood cultures (39%) as compared with those with negative blood cultures (7%).[19]

It is routine practice for many burns units to perform cultures of the burn wounds, throat, nose, and rectum upon admission to identify any unusual or high-risk pathogens. However, there are no data to support this practice. Although many burns centers perform routine weekly cultures on patients with open wounds, there is little evidence to support routine wound cultures and the practice is expensive and time-consuming.[20] In addition, considerable data suggest that surface swabs of burns and other wounds are often not representative of the major bacteria present in the wound[14–19] and therefore quantitative burn wound biopsy and histology, with their inherent limitations as discussed earlier, is employed in many but not all burns centers.

Prevention of infection

Topical antimicrobials

The burn eschar is a relatively avascular mass of necrotic material in which therapeutic levels of systemically administered antibiotics are difficult to achieve.[21] Topically applied antimicrobials provide high concentrations of drug at the wound surface acting as a barrier to infection and penetrate the eschar to varying extents, significantly delaying the onset of invasive infection.[22] Much of the evidence on the use of topical antimicrobials in thermally injured patients is based on small clinical trials that used bacteriological primary outcomes or bacteriological considerations alone. Choice of topical agents often also depends on ease of use and other treatment modalities being offered to burns patients.

Silver sulfadiazine is synthesized from silver nitrate and sodium sulfadiazine and is easily applied to burn wounds and does not stain the environment. Although this used to be a common prophylactic topical agent in burns patients, its white, water-soluble cream base interacts with the wound to produce a yellow mucopurulent exudate that needs to be washed off the wound before reapplication every 12 hours as recommended by the supplier.[23] Clinical experience suggests that silver sulfadiazine reduces wound bacterial density and delays colonization with gram-negative organisms but that treatment failures occur frequently in large burns > 50% TBSA.[24] Because this agent is of limited spectrum in the large burn and requires hydrotherapy, which is an established risk factor for nosocomial infections, its usefulness in established *Pseudomonas* infections appears to be low, and its use combined with hydrotherapy predisposes major burns patients to early *Pseudomonas* colonization of the burn wound. Systemic absorption and multi-organ toxicity of silver is high in major burns, often unrecognized, and severe in patients with compromised renal function, the kidney being the principal route of excretion of absorbed silver.[25]

Historically, **silver nitrate** was the first topical agent employed to delay burn eschar colonization based on it's effectiveness against most strains of *Pseudomonas* and *Staphylococcus*. New topical agents were then developed to improve on the limitations of silver nitrate, including limited penetration of the burn eschar and environmental staining.[26] However, there has been a resurgence in the use of silver nitrate based on the recognition that, as a solution, it avoids the mucopurulent exudate common with cream-based topicals, and therefore does not require hydrotherapy. In addition, with the use of new skin and dermal substitutes, topical therapy without hydrotherapy is imperative and effective. Finally, eliminating the use of hydrotherapy not only reduces the risk of nosocomial infection (as discussed below),[27] it reduces the frequency of dressing change to once per day, significantly decreasing the dressing-related pain and cold stress endured by patients during hydrotherapy sessions, and also substantially lowers the overall cost of care of both the topical agents required but primarily of the staffing required for twice daily wound care and hydrotherapy sessions.[3,27]

Mafenide acetate is a topical burns agent with activity primarily against gram-negative organisms including *Pseudomonas*,[24] where its efficacy has been established *in vivo* based on the Walker burns model in rats, where both topical 5% mafenide acetate solution and 10% cream significantly reduced *Pseudomonas* colonization to < 10% organisms/g over 48 hours in standardized full-thickness burns.[28] Using ^{14}C-labelled mafenide acetate, Harrison demonstrated rapid penetration of this topical antimicrobial through burned skin.[29] It has minimal antifungal activity and limited activity against *Staphylococcus aureus*, particularly methicillin-resistant strains. It is formulated as an 11·1% cream or more recently as a 5% solution.[28] Mafenide is a potent carbonic anhydrase inhibitor; hyperchloremic metabolic acidosis limits its application to < 20% TBSA; otherwise, severe hyperventilation can develop as respiratory compensation for the metabolic acidosis. For established *Pseudomonas* infections, mafenide acetate solutions can be combined with nystatin for improved antifungal activity and effectiveness in serious infections; it is often alternated every 12 hours with 0·5% $AgNO_3$ or other topical agents.[30]

Acticoat is a new topical agent that is a novel nanocrystalline silver complex that has been widely tested and effective *in vitro* against a broad range of gram-negative and positive organisms including multiply resistant strains,[31–33] and it possesses strong antifungal properties.[30] It releases silver in aqueous solutions and therefore must be moistened with sterile water for activity, but thereafter can be left in place for up to 72 hours; it also does not normally require hydrotherapy for wound cleansing before reapplication.[17] *In vivo* studies have been completed on the antimicrobial barrier properties of the Acticoat dressing[34] as well as on the healing rates of skin graft donor sites[35] and contaminated full-thickness burn wounds.[36] One small randomized controlled trial in patients with major burns suggests that Acticoat treatment may be associated with lower rates of burn wound sepsis and fewer secondary bacteremias.[27] Using a matched pairs design of patients with symmetric wounds, one wound in each of 15 pairs was randomized to receive Acticoat, the other standard therapy (0·5% silver nitrate solution). Five cases of burn wound sepsis-based on quantitative wound biopsy cultures (> 10^5 organisms per gram of tissue), associated with one secondary bacteremia were noted in the Acticoat group compared with 16 positive wound biopsies and five secondary bacteremias with silver nitrate standard therapy. Other small uncontrolled clinical trials have been supportive of its use in burn wounds.[37,38]

Other topical agents for wound care include nitrofurazone, chlorhexidine, providone–iodine, nystatin, cerium nitrate and combinations of agents, but are of limited proven efficacy and safety in *Pseudomonas* infections as yet.[24] Similarly, infusion of antibiotics under the burn eschar, termed "subeschar lysis" has been performed but has not yet been tested in randomized controlled trials.[39]

Surgery

Prompt surgical excision of the burn wound and timely closure have significantly reduced the occurrence of invasive burn wound infection and its related mortality; however, as wound closure is delayed in patients with massive burns, the potential of invasive wound infection remains.[40] Two randomized controlled trials have reported no survival advantage with early total excision as compared with conservative treatment commencing at the day 10–14 post burn.[41,42] However, Tompkins *et al.* reviewed mortality in adult burns patients from Massachusetts General Hospital during a period prior to early excision and after prompt eschar excision and immediate wound closure. Using logistical regression of 1103 patients over a 10-year period encompassing both surgical approaches, the data showed a reduction in mortality from 24% to 7% ($P < 0{\cdot}001$) associated with a significant reduction in length of stay in hospital from 32 to 22 days.[42] Staged surgical wound closure beginning within 10 days of injury and continuing at 7-day intervals remains the most common surgical approach to the burn wound at present.[41] The supporting evidence for this approach is limited to observational studies. In one study, this approach was associated with a 6-fold reduction in mortality in patients with burns > 50% TBSA, with delayed surgical excision commencing after 7–10 days post injury.[43] In a single center retrospective analysis of 3561 burns patients over a 14-year period, Munster *et al.* reported significant reductions in mortality, length of stay, and cost of care with more aggressive staged surgical excision of the burn wound in the later 7-year period compared with the early era.[41] However, comparison with historical cohorts is a substantial limitation of the study.[1] Large, adequately powered randomized controlled trials are needed to establish optimal timing of surgery. In patients who already have established *Pseudomonas* infection including ecthyma gangrenosum, surgical debridement of infected tissues and temporary wound closure with allograft skin or autograft once the patient has stabilized is considered crucial to survival.[13,44,45]

Empiric antibiotic treatment

Unstable septic patients often require empiric therapy usually guided by initial cultures taken on admission. Initial antibiotic therapy is based on these swabs and tailored once further cultures and susceptibilities become available. Leibovici *et al.* surveyed 296 episodes of gram-negative bacteremia in 286 patients aged 13–99 years and found that thermal trauma, hospital acquisition of the infection, antibiotic treatment before the bacteremic episode, and endotracheal intubation were variables that independently predicted subsequent isolation of a multiresistant strain.[46] In a second group of 144 episodes of gram-negative bacteremia, the predictive index derived from these variables for optimizing empiric treatment maintained good discriminative power and improved empiric antibiotic treatment in 24% of patients.[46]

Pseudomonal sepsis is a significant cause of burn-associated mortality and morbidity requiring systemic antimicrobial therapy. McManus found that 10% of all burns patients developed pseudomonal bacteremia.[1] Unfortunately, with the development of multidrug-resistant *Pseudomonas*, the choice of antibiotics for empiric therapy becomes more difficult.

Case presentation (continued)

Septic workup cultures in the unstable burns patient were positive for *P. aeruginosa*, which was quantified in burn wound biopsies $> 10^8$ organisms per gram of tissue, and skin graft donor sites from multiple regions of the body including his chest, back, both lower extremities, face and scalp, as well as his blood cultures. The organism was resistant to gentamicin, tobramycin, carboxy- and ureidopenicillins. The patient's topical antimicrobial therapy for all infected wounds was switched to mafenide acetate twice daily. Once hemodynamically stable, the patient underwent a series of seven surgical debridements under general anesthetic for infected burn wounds and donor sites, but also for other infected wounds, which were not in the original burn areas but were hematogenously disseminated wounds in the scalp and other areas in which *Pseudomonas* was recovered on culture of the debrided tissue. Early surgical procedures were directed at debridement of *Pseudomonas*-infected tissues and avoidance of creation of any new skin graft donor wounds until reduction of bacterial load had been achieved, evidenced by adherence of fresh allograft skin to the debrided wounds. Despite secondary urine and wound infection with *Candida albicans*, the patient recovered after 77 days of intensive care in the burns unit. He spent 2 months in a rehabilitation hospital before being able to return home; he recommenced his work approximately 1 year after his original injury.

Infection control

Pseudomonas aeruginosa is the most important cause of nosocomial infection in the burns patient. However, only 6–8% of burns patients have rectal colonization.[27] Nosocomial acquisition of *P. aeruginosa* and other gram-negative bacteria arises from contamined water and aqueous solutions used in Hubbard tanks, ventilators, nebulizers, intravenous solutions, and hemodialysis systems.[47] During wound care, hand-to-hand transmission is considered to be the major preventable mode of transmission.

Both the experimental and observational evidence to support infection control interventions in burns units are extremely limited. Strict handwashing is considered the cornerstone in preventing transmission of antibiotic-resistant organisms. Ongoing surveillance of infections in the burns unit is important to defect new resistant organisms so that infection control precautions can be quickly instituted.[48] Isolation and performing admission swabs for culture of new patients can potentially identify new pathogens, especially those from patients who have received care in another institution.[49] However, there are no comparative studies at present that have validated this. Strict barrier precautions are used in many burns units. On entry into the burns patient's room, all personnel and visitors are required to wear a disposable gown and mask and wash their hands.[50] For all direct contact with patients sterile gloves are worn. Hands are washed with an antibacterial soap or alcohol-based hand disinfectants, and all protective garments are changed after each patient encounter. Individualized rooms and beds are cleansed and walls washed with a quarternary ammonium disinfectant between patient admissions. Again, however, comparative evidence for various levels of barrier precautions in burns units and terminal cleaning are lacking.

Improperly designed sinks that have short trap drains and deficient splash guards in themselves can be a source of hand and subsequently wound contamination.[51,52] This is very difficult to detect and establish as a mechanism of transmission of nosocomial infection but has been reported[53–55] and corrected by redesign and implementation of appropriate facilities for safe hand washing. Each individual piece of equipment is soaked with full strength (12%) sodium hypochlorite solution if positive surveillance cultures are obtained.[1]

Selective decontamination of the gastrointestinal flora of the burns patient has been tried without success to reduce burn wound infection by either direct contact or by bacterial translocation of organisms from the gut.[56] Small numbers of burns patients treated with selective gut decontamination compared with historical controls found lower but not significantly reduced rates of wound colonization and respiratory infection, but a subsequent prospective randomized double-blind study of 23 pediatric burns patients demonstrated comparable rates of colonization and infection as compared with the blinded placebo controls.[57]

The role of hydrotherapy in burn wound management

There are no randomized controlled trials that have compared hydrotherapy to no hydrotherapy for burn wound management and its use appears to have developed from a practical desire to wash burn wounds and the need to remove topical antimicrobial creams prior to reapplication of fresh agents. However, observational data of harm related to this therapy exists. Following an outbreak of *P. aeruginosa* linked to hydrotherapy in one burns unit, the incidence of *P. aeruginosa* infections in equal periods of time before and after discontinuation of hydrotherapy was compared.[27] Demographic data showed no difference in burn size, age of patient, or duration of hospitalization or sample size. However, a significant reduction in overall mortality (14 *v* 6, $P < 0{\cdot}05$), septic mortality (8 *v* 1, $P < 0{\cdot}05$) and *Pseudomonas*-associated septic deaths (6 *v* 0, $P < 0{\cdot}05$) was found in the non-hydrotherapy group. There was a significant reduction in the nosocomially-acquired organisms (29 *v* 18, $P < 0{\cdot}05$), and in the number of aminoglycoside resistant strains of Pseudomonas sp. (20 *v* 4, $P < 0{\cdot}05$) in the non-hydrotherapy group. Avoidance of hydrotherapy was also associated with a delay in appearance of *Pseudomonas* sp. in the burn wound (10·1 *v* 16·5 days) and a delay in the onset of aminoglycoside resistance (10·3 *v* 19·5 days), such that the appearance of an aminoglycoside-resistant organism in the burns patient was delayed approximately 16 days longer in the non-hydrotherapy group (20·4 *v* 36·0 days).[27] During the post-hydrotherapy period, an elimination of *Pseudomonas* sp. infection from traditionally clean wounds of the skin graft donor site was achieved (5 or 2·3% *v* 0, $P < 0{\cdot}05$). During the period prior to and after discontinuing hydrotherapy, the cost of care for patients in this burns unit was also analyzed where, from 1987–1991, silver sulfadiazine cream and hydrotherapy was routine before hydrotherapy was discontinued and topical 0·5% silver nitrate solution was substituted.[58] By using mathematical modelling to control for the number of burns patients and severity of injury during each period, substantial reduction in overall costs were predicted and savings in excess of the predicted were actually achieved. The majority of reduction in cost of care (shown in Canadian dollars) was not in the expense of the topical antimicrobials employed for wound care ($29 623 *v* $10 145 per month), but in the reduced labor/nursing costs ($112 046 *v* $91 256 per month) associated with elimination of hydrotherapy and once daily dressings within the patient's isolation room. An important limitation of this study, however, is the use of an historical cohort for comparison.

Similarly, many burns centers are experiencing an increase in *Acinetobacter* infections that are nosocomial in origin. Wisplinghoff *et al.* demonstrated that, in 367 patients hospitalized with severe burn injury where *Acinetobacter baumannii* was endemic (attack rate of 7·9%), 29 patients developed bloodstream infections.[59] When compared with 58 non-infected matched controls, the mortality rates were 31% and 14% respectively, and two deaths were directly attributable to *Acinetobacter* infections. Pulsed-field gel electrophoresis demonstrated three common strains, which were multidrug resistant. Multivariate analysis showed that bloodstream infection was independently associated with the severity of burn injury, prior nosocomial colonization at a distant site, and the use of hydrotherapy, again emphasizing the importance of effective infection control in other types of gram-negative infections.

In summary, there are no trials that establish the efficacy or benefit of hydrotherapy for burn wounds. However, for substantial risk of cross-contamination of multiresistant bacteria owing to hydrotherapy is well documented. This has lead many burns centers to avoid using immersion hydrotherapy.[4]

Prognosis

Based on retrospective, multifactorial logistical regression and probit analysis of 1705 burns patients, the mortality and morbidity of burns patients is related to the age of the patient, the total area of the burn wound (TBSA), and the presence or absence of concomitant inhalation injury,[43] which resemble the findings of other burns centers.[60] Measures of the severity of injury after burns injury such as burn surface areas are often only broad insensitive predictors of outcome. This is because of the failure to recognize the importance of inhalation injury and the depth of burn as a reflection of the volume or magnitude of necrotic tissue.[61] For example, superficial sun burns over 90% of the TBSA without inhalation injury can be considered in the same category of severity as full thickness flame burns after a house fire, where the same TBSA is recorded but the patient also sustained a significant inhalation injury. Despite these limitations, predictive equations derived from one burns center would suggest that the illustrated index case would have a 75% probability of survival, where the total burn surface area, age of the patient, and presence or absence of inhalation injury are independent variables.[43]

Inhalation injury and or adult respiratory distress syndrome (ARDS) and sepsis, ranging from SIRS to frank septic shock are the major causes of mortality in burns patients.[62] Surveys from burns centers identify gram-positive organisms including MRSA as the most frequent cause of burn wound and skin graft infection.[63] However, the evidence suggests that gram-negative bacteria including *K. pneumoniae*, *E. coli* and *Acinetobacter* spp. as well as *P. aeruginosa* are the major causes of mortality in burns centers. McManus *et al.* reported that 10% of all burns patients develop *Pseudomonas* bacteremia, carrying a mortality rate of 80%.[1,64] The risk of *Pseudomonas* infection increases substantially in burns > 30% of the TBSA.

Emerging data for major burns involving more than 30–35% of the TBSA suggests that they do not necessarily all become infected with *P. aeruginosa.*[65] However, *Pseudomonas* morbidity and mortality may be reduced by measures taken to avoid nosocomial infection or to delay the onset of infection as long as possible.[27] One study of burns patients, using historical controls, suggested that the delay in the onset of resistant infections led to a 9-day or more infection free period, enough time for surgical procedures to remove potentially infected burns tissue and close wounds with skin grafts.[27] McManus *et al.* reported similar findings after moving into a new burns center and avoiding transmission of an endemic strain of *Pseudomonas* in the old center by cohort nursing and avoidance of moving patients in the old burns center into the new center.[64]

Avoidance of nosocomial *Pseudomonas* infections is most important for patients with larger or deeper wounds, or in those who are older, have inhalation or other risk factors that put them at high risk of death from burn injury.[1] Recently, a review of mortality in burns > 50% TBSA demonstrated a 6-fold lower risk of death when a setting with better control of nosocomial infection[51] was compared with historic controls in the same setting at a time when nosocomial infections were more common, and shared practices, facilities, or equipment for wound care (such as hydrotherapy) occurred. Recent improvements in outcomes may be due to additional factors such as earlier surgical care, newer skin substitutes, or better intensive care. However, reports exist where these factors did not significantly improve outcomes over a similar time period.[60] To date, a number of other reports of nosocomial *Pseudomonas* outbreaks in other burns centers have emerged resembling that described herein, where mortality was very high in the infected patients.[47,66–69]

In burns centers that use silver nitrate as a topical agent for the burn wounds, thus avoiding hydrotherapy and maintaining high levels of reverse isolation in laminar flow units, the cross-contamination rate with multidrug-resistant organisms is extremely low, 3·2 cases per 1000 patient days.[70] Other centers where similar isolation is not possible have demonstrated that 74% of burns patients wounds become colonized with *P. aeruginosa*, > 95% of which are resistant to multiple antibiotics including gentamicin, when only 4·75% of patients are contaminated at the time of admission.[71] Such dramatic differences in infection rates between burns centers illustrate the broad range of treatment approaches practiced and the difficulty and deficiency of clinical trails addressing isolation procedures and antimicrobial therapy in burns centers.

New preventive strategies: vaccines

The serious nature of infections caused by *P. aeruginosa* has led to concerted efforts by many investigators to develop candidate vaccines for prevention of *Pseudomonas* infections in the burned patient and in persons with cystic fibrosis. Lipolysaccharide (LPS) vaccines conjugated to carriers have been produced. While they showed good immunogenicity in human trials, toxicity from the lipid A portion of the LPS has prevented their use.[72,73] Whilst there have been some studies with flagellar vaccines, their efficacy in humans has not been clearly identified.[74,75] Recently, outer membrane proteins (OMPs) have also been used as targets for *P. aeruginosa* vaccines. In human volunteers, recombinant OMPs expressed in *E. coli* showed good immunogenicity.[76,77] In one recent study in burns patients, a composite OMP vaccine showed promise in reduction of sepsis caused by *P. aeruginosa*.[78] Peptide vaccines are also being investigated. They have been derived from OMPs[79,80] or are being produced synthetically as consensus sequences from pilin proteins.[81,82] These compounds may be conjugated to other proteins (for example, tetanus toxoid) as haptens, to improve their immunogenicity. These consensus sequence peptides are strongly immunogenic in animal models, and are now undergoing phase I human clinical trials. It is still unknown if any of these candidate vaccine molecules will come into routine clinical use. It has been observed that the immune response following thermal injury may not be optimal[83] and therefore immunogenicity of these vaccines in animals or in healthy persons may not translate into efficacy in the burned patient.

Acknowledgments

The authors acknowledge the research support of the Alberta Heritage Foundation for Medical Research and the Canadian Institute for Health Research, as well as the Firefighters' Burn Trust Fund of the University of Alberta Hospital.

References

1. McManus AT, Mason AD, Jr., McManus WF, Pruitt BA, Jr. Twenty-five year review of *Pseudomonas aeruginosa* bacteremia in a burn center. *Eur J Clin Microbiol* 1985;**4**: 219–23.
2. Revathi G, Puri J, Jain BK. Bacteriology of burns. *Burns* 1998;**24**:347–9.
3. Shankowsky HA, Callioux LS, Tredget EE. North American survey of hydrotherapy in modern burn care. *J Burn Care Rehabil* 1994;**15**:143–6.
4. Heggers JP, McCauley R, Herndon DN. Antimicrobial Therapy in Burns patients. *Surg Rounds* 1992:613–17.

5. Frame JD, Kangesu L, Malik WM. Changing flora in burn and trauma units: experience in the United Kingdom. *J Burn Care Rehabil* 1992;**13**:281–6.
6. Barillo DJ, McManus AT, Cioffi WG *et al.* Aeromonas bacteremia in burns patients. *Burns* 1996;**22**:48–52.
7. Pruitt BA, Jr., McManus AT, Kim SH, Goodwin CW. Burn wound infections: current status. *World J Surg* 1998; **22**:135–45.
8. Pruitt BA, Jr. Phycomycotic infections. In: Alexaner JW, ed. *Problems in General Surgery*. Philadelphia: Lippincott, 1984.
9. Kucan JO, Smoot EC. Five percent mafenide acetate solution in the treatment of thermal injuries. *J Burn Care Rehabil* 1993;**14**:158–63.
10. Wendt C, Messer SA, Hollis RJ *et al.* Molecular epidemiology of gram-negative bacteremia. *Clin Infect Dis* 1999;**28**:605–10.
11. Definitions for sepsis and organ failure and guidelines for the use of innovative therapies in sepsis. In: American College of Chest Physicians/Society of Critical Care Medicine Consensus Conference; 1992: *Critical Care Medicine*, 1992.
12. Vindenes HA, Ulvestad E, Bjerknes R. Concentrations of cytokines in plasma of patients with large burns: their relation to time after injury, burn size, inflammatory variables, infection, and outcome. *Eur J Surg* 1998;**164**: 647–56.
13. Bisno AL. Cutaneous infections: microbiologic and epidemiologic considerations. *Am J Med* 1984;**76**:172–9.
14. Steer JA, Papini RP, Wilson AP, McGrouther DA, Parkhouse N. Quantitative microbiology in the management of burns patients. I. Correlation between quantitative and qualitative burn wound biopsy culture and surface alginate swab culture. *Burns* 1996;**22**:173–6.
15. McManus AT, Kim SH, McManus WF, Mason AD, Jr., Pruitt BA, Jr. Comparison of quantitative microbiology and histopathology in divided burn-wound biopsy specimens. *Arch Surg* 1987;**122**:74–6.
16. Williams HB, Breidenbach WC, Callaghan WB, Richards GK, Prentis JJ. Are burn wound biopsies obsolete? A comparative study of bacterial quantitation in burns patients using the absorbent disc and biopsy techniques. *Ann Plast Surg* 1984;**13**:388–95.
17. Tredget EE, Shankowsky HA, Groeneveld A, Burrell R. A matched-pair, randomized study evaluating the efficacy and safety of Acticoat silver-coated dressing for the treatment of burn wounds. *J Burn Care Rehabil* 1998;**19**: 531–7.
18. Keen A, Knoblock L, Edelman L, Saffle J. Effective limitation of blood culture use in the burn unit. *J Burn Care Rehabil* 2002;**23**:183–9.
19. Henke PK, Polk HC, Jr. Efficacy of blood cultures in the critically ill surgical patient. *Surgery* 1996;**120**:752–9.
20. Miller PL, Matthey FC. A cost-benefit analysis of initial burn cultures in the management of acute burns. *J Burn Care Rehabil* 2000;**21**:300–3.
21. Nagesha CN, Shenoy KJ, Chandrashekar MR. Study of burn sepsis with special reference to *Pseudomonas aeruginosa*. *J Indian Med Assoc* 1996;**94**:230–3.
22. Moncrief JA, Lindberg RB, Switzer WE, Pruitt BA, Jr. The use of a topical sulfonamide in the control of burn wound sepsis. *J Trauma* 1966;**6**:407–19.
23. George N, Faoagali J, Muller M. Silvazine (silver sulfadiazine and chlorhexidine) activity against 200 clinical isolates. *Burns* 1997;**23**:493–5.
24. Monafo WW, West MA. Current treatment recommendations for topical burn therapy. *Drugs* 1990;**40**:364–73.
25. Sano S, Fujimori R, Takashima M, Itokawa Y. Absorption, excretion and tissue distribution of silver sulphadiazine. *Burns Incl Therm Inj* 1982;**8**:278–85.
26. Klasen HJ. A historical review of the use of silver in the treatment of burns. II. Renewed interest for silver. *Burns* 2000;**26**:131–8.
27. Tredget EE, Shankowsky HA, Joffe AM *et al.* Epidemiology of infections with *Pseudomonas aeruginosa* in burns patients: the role of hydrotherapy. *Clin Infect Dis* 1992;**15**:941–9.
28. Murphy RC, Kucan JO, Robson MC, Heggers JP. The effect of 5% mafenide acetate solution on bacterial control in infected rat burns. *J Trauma* 1983;**23**:878–81.
29. Harrison HN, Blackmore WP, Bales HW, Reeder W. The absorption of C 14-labeled Sulfamylon acetate through burned skin. I. Experimental methods and initial observations. *J Trauma* 1972;**12**:986–93.
30. Wright JB, Lam K, Hansen D, Burrell RE. Efficacy of topical silver against fungal burn wound pathogens. *Am J Infect Control* 1999;**27**:344–50.
31. Yin HQ, Langford R, Burrell RE. Comparative evaluation of the antimicrobial activity of ACTICOAT antimicrobial barrier dressing. *J Burn Care Rehabil* 1999;**20**:195–200.

32. Wright DG, Hansen DL, Burrell R. The comparative efficacy of two antimicrobial barrier dressings: In vitro examination of two controlled release of silver dressing. *Wounds* 1998;**10**:179–88.
33. Wright JB, Lam K, Burrell RE. Wound management in an era of increasing bacterial antibiotic resistance: a role for topical silver treatment. *Am J Infect Control* 1998;**26**:572–7.
34. Burrell RE, Heggers JP, Davis GJ, Wright JB. Effect of Silver Coated dressings on Animal Survival in a Rodent Burn Sepsis Model. *Wounds* 1999;**11**(4):64–71.
35. Olson ME, Wright JB, Lam K, Burrell RE. Healing of porcine donor sites covered with silver-coated dressings. *Eur J Surg* 2000;**166**:486–9.
36. Wright JB, Lam K, Buret AG, Olson ME, Burrell RE. Early healing events in a porcine model of contamined wounds: effects of nanocrystalline silver on matrix metalloproteinases, cell apoptosis and healing. *Wound Repair Regen* 2002;**10**:141–51.
37. Voigt DW, Paul CN. The use of Acticoat silver impregnated telfa dressing in a regional burn and wound care center: The clinician's view. *Wounds* 2001;**13**:5–12.
38. Kirsner RS, Orsted H, Wright JB. Matrix metalloproteinases in normal and impaired wound healing: A potential role for nanocrystalline silver. *Wounds* 2001;**13**: 5–12.
39. Baxter CR, Curreri PW, Marvin JA. The control of burn wound sepsis by the use of quantitative bacteriologic studies and subeschar clysis with antibiotics. *Surg Clin North Am* 1973;**53**:1509–18.
40. Herndon DN, Spies M. Modern burn care. *Semin Pediatr Surg* 2001;**10**:28–31.
41. Munster AM, Smith-Meek M, Sharkey P. The effect of early surgical intervention on mortality and cost-effectiveness in burn care, 1978–91. *Burns* 1994;**20**:61–4.
42. Tompkins RG, Burke JF, Schoenfeld DA *et al.* Prompt eschar excision: a treatment system contributing to reduced burn mortality. A statistical evaluation of burn care at the Massachusetts General Hospital (1974–1984). *Ann Surg* 1986;**204**:272–81.
43. Tredget EE, Shankowsky HA, Taerum TV, Moysa GL, Alton JD. The role of inhalation injury in burn trauma. A Canadian experience. *Ann Surg* 1990;**212**:720–7.
44. Ng W, Tan CL, Yeow V, Yeo M, Teo SH. Ecthyma gangrenosum in a patient with hypogammaglobulinemia. *J Infect* 1998;**36**:331–5.
45. Eldridge JP, Baldridge ED, MacMillan BG. Ecthyma gangrenosum in a burned child. *Burns Incl Therm Inj* 1986;**12**:578–85.
46. Leibovici L, Konisberger H, Pitlik SD, Samra Z, Drucker M. Predictive index for optimizing empiric treatment of gram-negative bacteremia. *J Infect* Dis 1991;**163**:193–6.
47. Kolmos HJ, Thuesen B, Nielsen SV *et al.* Outbreak of infection in a burns unit due to *Pseudomonas aeruginosa* originating from contaminated tubing used for irrigation of patients. *J Hosp Infect* 1993;**24**:11–21.
48. Roberts SA, Findlay R, Lang SD. Investigation of an outbreak of multi-drug resistant Acinetobacter baumannii in an intensive care burns unit. *J Hosp Infect* 2001;**48**:228–32.
49. Cook N. Methicillin-resistant *Staphylococcus aureus* versus the burns patient. *Burns* 1998;**24**:91–8.
50. Marvin J. Burn care protocols-infection control in burn unit. Review of infection control procedure at Jackson Memorial Hospital Burn Center, From Harborview Hospital, Seattle. *J Burn Care Rehabil* 1987;**8**:71.
51. Tredget EE, Anzarut A, Shankowsky H, Logsetty S. Outcome and quality of life of massive burn injury: The impact of modern burn care. In: American Burn Association Annual Meeting; 2002; Chicago, Illinois; 2002.
52. Berrouane YF, McNutt LA, Buschelman BJ *et al.* Outbreak of severe *Pseudomonas aeruginosa* infections caused by a contaminated drain in a whirlpool bathtub. *Clin Infect Dis* 2000;**31**:1331–7.
53. Doring G, Ulrich M, Muller W *et al.* Generation of *Pseudomonas aeruginosa* aerosols during handwashing from contaminated sink drains, transmission to hands of hospital personnel, and its prevention by use of a new heating device. *Zentralbl Hyg Umweltmed* 1991;**191**: 494–505.
54. Doring G, Jansen S, Noll H *et al.* Distribution and transmission of *Pseudomonas aeruginosa* and *Burkholderia cepacia* in a hospital ward. *Pediatr Pulmonol* 1996;**21**:90–100.
55. Doring G, Horz M, Ortelt J, Grupp H, Wolz C. Molecular epidemiology of *Pseudomonas aeruginosa* in an intensive care unit. *Epidemiol Infect* 1993;**110**:427–36.
56. Manson WL, Westerveld AW, Klasen HJ, Sauer EW. Selective intestinal decontamination of the digestive tract for infection prophylaxis in severely burned patients. *Scand J Plast Reconstr Surg Hand Surg* 1987;**21**:269–72.

57. Barret JP, Jeschke MG, Herndon DN. Selective decontamination of the digestive tract in severely burned pediatric patients. *Burns* 2001;**27**:439–45.
58. Inkson TI, Shankowsky HA, Brown K *et al.* Cost comparison of silver sulfadiazine and silver nitrate for burn wound care. In: American Burn Association meeting, Chicago, Illinois, 1993.
59. Wisplinghoff H, Perbix W, Seifert H. Risk factors for nosocomial bloodstream infections due to *Acinetobacter baumannii*: a case-control study of adult burns patients. *Clin Infect Dis* 1999;**28**:59–66.
60. Ryan CM, Schoenfeld DA, Thorpe WP *et al.* Objective estimates of the probability of death from burn injuries. *N Engl J Med* 1998;**338**:362–6.
61. O'Keefe GE, Hunt JL, Purdue GF. An evaluation of risk factors for mortality after burn trauma and the identification of gender-dependent differences in outcomes. *J Am Coll Surg* 2001;**192**:153–60.
62. Gullo A. Sepsis and organ dysfunction/failure. An overview. *Minerva Anesthesiol* 1999;**65**:529–40.
63. Taylor GD, Kibsey P, Kirkland T, Burroughs E, Tredget E. Predominance of staphylococcal organisms in infections occurring in a burns intensive care unit. *Burns* 1992;**18**: 332–5.
64. McManus AT, McManus WF, Mason AD, Jr., Aitcheson AR, Pruitt BA, Jr. Microbial colonization in a new intensive care burn unit. A prospective cohort study. *Arch Surg* 1985; **120**:217–23.
65. Tredget E, Shankowsky H, Lee J, Swanson T. The impact of nosocomial resistant pseudomonas infections in a burn unit. In: American Burn Association Annual Meeting, Miami, Florida, 2003.
66. Perinpanayagam RM, Grundy HC. Outbreak of gentamicin-resistant *Pseudomonas aeruginosa* infection in a burns unit. *J Hosp Infect* 1983;**4**:71–3.
67. Douglas MW, Mulholland K, Denyer V, Gottlieb T. Multi-drug resistant *Pseudomonas aeruginosa* outbreak in a burns unit - an infection control study. *Burns* 2001;**27**:131–5.
68. Hsueh PR, Teng LJ, Yang PC *et al.* Persistence of a multidrug-resistant *Pseudomonas aeruginosa* clone in an intensive care burn unit. *J Clin Microbiol* 1998;**36**: 1347–51.
69. Fujita K, Lilly HA, Ayliffe GA. Spread of resistant gram-negative bacilli in a burns unit. *J Hosp Infect* 1982;**3**: 29–37.
70. Weber JM, Sheridan RL, Schulz JT, Tompkins RG, Ryan CM. Effectiveness of bacteria-controlled nursing units in preventing cross-colonization with resistant bacteria in severely burned children. *Infect Control Hosp Epidemiol* 2002;**23**:549–51.
71. Rastegar Lari A, Bahrami Honar H, Alaghehbandan R. Pseudomonas infections in Tohid Burn Center, Iran. *Burns* 1998;**24**:637–41.
72. Cryz SJ, Jr., Sadoff JC, Cross AS, Furer E. Safety and immunogenicity of a polyvalent *Pseudomonas aeruginosa* O-polysaccharide-toxin A vaccine in humans. *Antibiot Chemother* 1989;**42**:177–83.
73. Jones RJ, Roe EA, Gupta JL. Controlled trials of a polyvalent pseudomonas vaccine in burns. *Lancet* 1979;**2**:977–82.
74. Doring G, Dorner F. A multicenter vaccine trial using the *Pseudomonas aeruginosa* flagella vaccine IMMUNO in patients with cystic fibrosis. *Behring Inst Mitt*, 1997.
75. Holder IA, Wheeler R, Montie TC. Flagellar preparations from *Pseudomonas aeruginosa*: animal protection studies. *Infect Immun* 1982;**35**:276–80.
76. von Specht BU, Lucking HC, Blum B *et al.* Safety and immunogenicity of a *Pseudomonas aeruginosa* outer membrane protein I vaccine in human volunteers. *Vaccine* 1996;**14**:1111–17.
77. Mansouri E, Gabelsberger J, Knapp B *et al.* Safety and immunogenicity of a *Pseudomonas aeruginosa* hybrid outer membrane protein F-I vaccine in human volunteers. *Infect Immun* 1999;**67**:1461–70.
78. Kim DK, Kim JJ, Kim JH *et al.* Comparison of two immunization schedules for a *Pseudomonas aeruginosa* outer membrane proteins vaccine in burns patients. *Vaccine* 2000;**19**:1274–83.
79. Hughes EE, Gilleland LB, Gilleland HE, Jr. Synthetic peptides representing epitopes of outer membrane protein F of *Pseudomonas aeruginosa* that elicit antibodies reactive with whole cells of heterologous immunotype strains of *P. aeruginosa*. *Infect Immun* 1992;**60**:3497–503.
80. Hughes EE, Gilleland HE, Jr. Ability of synthetic peptides representing epitopes of outer membrane protein F of *Pseudomonas aeruginosa* to afford protection against *P. aeruginosa* infection in a murine acute pneumonia model. *Vaccine* 1995;**13**:1750–3.
81. Sheth HB, Glasier LM, Ellert NW *et al.* Development of an anti-adhesive vaccine for *Pseudomonas aeruginosa*

targeting the C-terminal region of the pilin structural protein. *Biomed Pept Proteins Nucleic Acids* 1995; **1**:141–8.

82. Cachia PJ, Glasier LM, Hodgins RR *et al.* The use of synthetic peptides in the design of a consensus sequence vaccine for *Pseudomonas aeruginosa*. *J Pept Res* 1998;**52**:289–99.

83. Lawrence MH, de Riesthal HF, Calvano SE. Changes in memory and naive CD4+ lymphocytes in lymph nodes and spleen after thermal injury. *J Burn Care Rehabil* 1996;**17**:1–6.

16
Infections in healthcare workers

Brian J Angus, Fiona Smaill

Case presentation 1

A phlebotomist presents to you with a needlestick injury from a patient known to have advanced HIV infection and hepatitis C infection. She had used the needle to draw blood and had injected a small amount of blood into her finger accidentally while re-sheathing the needle before disposal. She had been fully vaccinated against hepatitis B and had her antibody levels checked within the last 6 months. You counsel her about the risk of transmission of HIV and hepatitis C and consider her to be in the high-risk group.

Burden of illness/relevance to clinical practice

It is estimated that American healthcare workers suffer between 400 000 and 800 000 needlestick and other sharps injuries every year.[1] The American Hospital Association estimates that one case of serious infection by a blood-borne pathogen can result in expenditures of $1 million or more for testing, follow up, time lost from work, and disability payments. The cost of follow up for a high-risk exposure is almost $3000 per needlestick injury, even when no infection occurs.[2]

HIV: risk assessment of needlestick injuries

A summary of 25 case control studies (22 seroconversions in 6955 exposed people) found that the risk of HIV transmission after percutaneous exposure was 0·32% (95% CI 0·18–0·45) and the risk after mucocutaneous exposure was 0·03% (95% CI 0·006–0·19%).[3] Certain factors predict the likelihood of transmission of HIV to healthcare workers after percutaneous exposure (see Table 16.1).[4] The average hollow-bore needlestick transmission risk is 0·3% but is predicted to be higher if the source is seroconverting to HIV or has late stage disease with a high HIV viral load.[5]

The case control study from the USA and France evaluated outcomes in 31 healthcare workers who acquired HIV infection after occupational exposure and outcomes in 679 controls who did not acquire HIV infection despite occupational exposure.[4] This study included people followed up for at least 6 months after exposure. HIV infection was less likely in people who received post-exposure prophylaxis compared with those who did not (reduction in OR by 81%, 95% CI 43–94%). There is some indirect evidence for[6] and against[7] post-exposure prophylaxis from studies in primates. It is also extrapolated from the placebo controlled, randomized controlled trials of zidovudine[8] and nevirapine[9] in pregnant women, which found reduced frequency of mother-to-child HIV transmission and this is thought to be caused in part by a post-exposure prophylaxis effect.

There are no studies of post-exposure prophylaxis using combinations of antiretroviral drugs. Randomized controlled trials have found that combinations of two, three, or more antiretroviral drugs are more effective than single

Table 16.1 Factors predicting transmission of HIV to HCWs after percutaneous exposure[4]

	Adjusted odds ratio	95% CI
Deep (intramuscular) injury	16·1	6·1–44·6
Visible blood on device	5·2	1·8–17·7
Needle used to enter blood vessel	5·1	1·9–14·8
Source patient with terminal AIDS	6·4	2·2–18·9
Zidovudine prophylaxis used	0·2	0·1–0·6

drug regimens in suppressing viral replication for the treatment of HIV infection. Combination therapy may also become increasingly necessary because of transmission of and primary infection with drug-resistant virus. Primary infection with resistant virus was 4% in St Louis from 1996 to 1998, but increased to 17 % during 1999 to 2001.[10] In the Swiss cohort, the prevalence of resistance in primary infections for successive years was 8·6% in 1996, 14·6% in 1997, 8·8% in 1998, and 5·0% in 1999.[11] A survey from the USA showed an increase in resistance among patients recently infected with HIV from 3·4% in 1998 to 12·4% in 2000.[12] Zidovudine alone may not prevent transmission of zidovudine resistant strains of HIV.

The Centers for Disease Control and Prevention (CDC) guidelines recommend a basic 4-week regimen of two drugs (zidovudine [ZDV] and lamivudine [3TC]; 3TC and stavudine [d4T]; or didanosine [ddI] and d4T) for most HIV exposures and an expanded regimen that includes the addition of a third drug (usually a protease inhibitor) for HIV exposures that pose an increased risk for transmission.[13] Where possible, viral genotyping of the source patient to detect drug-resistant virus may be useful to determine which regimen to use but treatment should not be delayed awaiting results.

Short-term toxicity (including fatigue, nausea, and vomiting) and gastrointestinal discomfort have been reported by 50–75% of people taking zidovudine and caused 30% to discontinue post-exposure prophylaxis.[14] Treatment studies suggest that the frequency of adverse effects is higher in people taking a combination of antiretroviral drugs (reported in 50–90%), which may reduce adherence to post-exposure prophylaxis (24–36% discontinued overall). The risk of drug interactions is also increased. The increased risk of side effects with protease inhibitors did not lead to more discontinuation in one study.[15] Drug-induced hepatitis in persons taking combination post-exposure prophylaxis was 0·5 and 25 per 100 person months in protease- and nevirapine-including regimens respectively.[16] Because of reports of severe toxicity with nevirapine its use as a prophylactic agent is not recommended.

There is good evidence from clinical trials that determining the HIV antibody status of the source patient using a rapid screening test is associated with significant reduction in psychological stress in the healthcare worker, antiretroviral drug use, and cost.[17,18]

A Cochrane Library systematic review has shown that condoms were effective in reducing transmission of HIV.[19] Although HIV infection following an occupational exposure is infrequent, healthcare workers should be counselled to use condoms or exercise sexual abstinence to prevent sexual transmission for at least 6–12 weeks after exposure.

Hepatitis B virus (HBV) infection

Healthcare workers have been historically recognized as being at increased risk of HBV infection. Effective vaccines are available to prevent HBV infection and universal immunization programs are now advocated. Following a needlestick injury, the risk of developing HBV infection ranges from 1–6% when HBeAg is absent, to 19–40% when it is present.[20] While needlestick injuries are one of the most efficient modes of HBV transmission, most transmission in the healthcare setting probably occurs in the absence of a documented percutaneous injury.

There is evidence from a Cochrane Library systematic review to support occupational health guidelines that all healthcare workers should be offered HBV vaccination and that the vaccine is safe.[21] Studies reported in the early 1980s showed an overall benefit of plasma derived HBV vaccine for preventing HBV infection in healthcare workers [OR 0·33; 95% CI 0·21, 0·53], although the differences were not significant for the low-risk healthcare workers [OR 0·33, 95% CI 0·05, 1·30]. Recombinant DNA HBV vaccines have been shown to be as safe and immunogenic as the original plasma-derived vaccine[22] and any differences in immunogenicity between the licensed preparations of recombinant HBV vaccine are of little clinical or public health importance.[23]

Approximately 10% of healthcare workers may fail to respond to HBV immunisation. Factors that were significantly associated with failure to develop protective levels of antibodies in an HBV vaccine study of healthcare workers included increasing age, obesity, smoking, and male gender.[23] An open prospective study administering intradermal HBV vaccine to healthcare workers who had failed to respond to an initial course reported response rates of 88% but comparative studies are needed.[24]

There is no evidence that booster doses are necessary to maintain positive HBs titers.[25] Although not prospectively evaluated, most guidelines recommend serological testing for hepatitis antibody after a primary immunization course has been completed, and for non-responders, screening for markers of present or past infection, administering a second vaccine series and consideration of hepatitis B immune globulin (HBIG) after significant exposure.[13]

For those healthcare workers who have not been immunized, HBIG and HBV vaccine are recommended after a significant exposure. Although the effectiveness of HBIG and HBV vaccine has not been evaluated in the occupational health setting, the increased efficacy of this combination compared with HBIG alone in preventing perinatal transmission is presumed to apply to the occupational health setting.[26] When compared with immune serum globulin, HBIG alone was shown to be 75% effective in preventing HBV infection in the occupational setting,[27] although a further analysis of this study questioned whether some of the immunoglobulin preparations contained HBsAg and active immunity to HBV was induced.[28]

Hepatitis C infection

Cohort studies have shown that healthcare workers are at a small but increased risk for acquiring hepatitis C virus (HCV) infection as a result of occupational exposure.[29] The average risk of hepatitis C seroconversion following parenteral exposure from an HCV positive source as determined from longitudinal and prospective studies is 1·9% [95% CI 1·4, 2·5; range 0–22%] (44 infections out of 2357 exposures) but the actual risk is probably lower. There have been no clinical trials to characterize the factors associated with occupational transmission of hepatitis C. In one descriptive study, transmission only occurred with a hollow-bore needlestick compared with injury from other sharps.[30] No transmission has been documented from intact or non-intact skin exposures, and epidemiological data do not support environmental contamination nor exposure to fluids or tissues other than blood as a significant risk for transmission.

There is no evidence of a benefit of immunoglobulin prophylaxis for hepatitis C and its use is not recommended.[13] There have been no clinical trials evaluating the efficacy of antiviral agents to prevent or treat HCV infection following occupational exposure. In an open-label study of treatment of acute hepatitis C, which included 14 healthcare workers, single-agent therapy with interferon-alfa 2b was effective in 98% of patients, strikingly different from the treatment outcomes for chronic hepatitis C infection.[31] Treatment was well tolerated. While the current CDC guidelines recommend measuring HCV antibody at 4–6 months to detect infection,[13] there has been no prospective evaluation comparing this approach with PCR testing for HCV viremia and pre-emptive treatment with interferon with or without ribavirin if infection is documented. Currently there are no data to establish an optimal approach for healthcare workers exposed to or occupationally infected with hepatitis C.

Prevention

There have been few randomized controlled trials evaluating the effectiveness of interventions to reduce needlestick injuries in healthcare occupations. In one systematic review that included 11 randomized trials, mostly evaluating interventions during surgical procedures, a 'no-touch' technique compared with the traditional 'hand-in' method of wound closure was associated with a statistically significant reduction in the number of glove perforations favouring the 'no-touch' technique.[32] The use of specialized needles during surgical wound closure also decreased the number of glove or skin perforations. Needleless intravenous devices have been shown to decrease sharps injuries[32] but other studies have shown variable results[33] explained in part by problems with product acceptance and worker behavior.

Summary

One case–control study found limited evidence suggesting that post-exposure prophylaxis with zidovudine may reduce the risk of HIV infection over 6 months. Evidence from other settings suggests that a combination of antiretroviral drugs is likely to be more effective than zidovudine alone. There is good evidence to support occupational health guidelines that all healthcare workers should be offered HBV vaccination and that the vaccine is safe but that there is weak evidence supporting the use of HBV immunoglobulin for post-exposure. There are no data on how best to manage occupational exposures to hepatitis C.

Case presentation 2

At the end of his 24 hours on-call shift, the resident asks his attending staff to look at his rash. It is obviously chickenpox. The Infection Control and Occupational Health Services are promptly called for advice regarding management of the resident and his contacts. As part of their investigation, the Occupational Health Services identify that the resident thought he must have had chickenpox as a child, but had not been tested further. They have no records for the attending staff physician who could not recall whether he had previously had chickenpox but did know he had neither been tested for immunity nor received any vaccinations. As a result of this exposure, 15 healthcare workers spent 14 days of paid leave off work and eight exposed patients needed to be kept in respiratory isolation during the period that they were potentially infectious. At the next meeting of the Infection Control Committee a recommendation is made for a thorough review of the screening protocols for healthcare workers and policies for vaccine preventable infections.

Varicella zoster infections

Varicella (i.e. chickenpox) is usually an uncomplicated infection in children, with rash, mild fever, and systemic symptoms. While most skin infections following chickenpox are mild and other complications are rare, chickenpox has been shown to dramatically increase the likelihood of invasive group A streptococcal infections in children (relative risk 58; 95% CI 40–85%).[34] Disease in adults and immunocompromised persons is more severe, with higher rates of pneumonia, encephalitis, and death reported.[35] The risk of congenital varicella syndrome following maternal infection during the first trimester of pregnancy has been estimated to be 2·2% (95% CI 0–4·6%).[36] Nosocomial transmission of varicella infection is recognized frequently enough that control measures in healthcare facilities are strongly recommended.[37]

The long-term effectiveness of the varicella vaccine in children, based on results from randomized trials, has been estimated at 95%.[38] Prospective cohort studies of the effectiveness of the vaccine estimate that the vaccine will provide 70–90% protection against infection and 95% protection against severe disease.[35] Although there have been no controlled trials of the effectiveness of the vaccine in adults or healthcare workers, a prospective evaluation of healthcare workers who received the vaccine showed that the attack rate following household and hospital exposure was reduced from an estimated 90% to 18% and 8% respectively, that all illness was mild to moderate (mean 40 vesicles), and that 96% of healthcare workers developed antibodies to varicella.[39] Based on these data, current guidelines recommend that all susceptible healthcare workers be immunized with two doses of varicella vaccine.[40]

No clinical trials have examined the cost effectiveness of varicella vaccination in the healthcare setting. Using a simulation model, however, Gray *et al.* found that serotesting all staff with an uncertain history or no report of previous varicella and vaccinating those negative for antibodies was a cost-effective strategy.[41] This approach is supported by other studies and reviews.[42–44] The sensitivity of a history of chickenpox for predicting serologic immunity in healthcare workers ranges from 79 to 100%[45–48] but, although the positive predictive value is high (98–100%), the negative predictive value is as low as 10%.

Varicella vaccine has been shown to be effective in preventing or reducing the severity of varicella if given to a susceptible individual within 3 days after exposure, although this approach has not been evaluated in the healthcare setting. In one study, none of 26 vaccinated contacts developed chickenpox compared with all 19 in the control group.[49] A prospective observational study in a homeless shelter estimated the post-exposure effectiveness of varicella vaccine at 95·2% (95% CI 81·6–98·8) for prevention of any disease and 100% for moderate or severe disease.[50]

Although there are no data to support acyclovir prophylaxis after exposure in the healthcare setting, this strategy has been studied in household contacts. In two small studies, 7·4% and 16% of contacts given acyclovir developed disease compared with 77% and 100% of contacts in the control groups who were not given acyclovir.[51,52] Although both the use of post-exposure vaccination and acyclovir may modify illness in the individual healthcare worker, based on the available evidence they cannot be advocated as an acceptable alternative to current management guidelines for the exposed healthcare worker.[37]

Given that 99% of adults after immunization will develop antibodies, routine serologic testing after vaccination is not recommended but can be considered after exposure to varicella.[35]

Healthcare workers who do not have detectable antibody may need to be removed from the patient care setting, but there are no data from controlled trials on how best to manage vaccinated healthcare workers exposed to varicella.

Varicella-zoster immune globulin (VZIG) has been shown in observational studies to be effective in preventing or modifying varicella in immunocompromised patients exposed to chickenpox.[53,54] Although varicella is a more severe illness in adults, there is no evidence to support the routine use of VZIG in healthcare workers exposed to chickenpox. Because pregnant women are considered to be at higher risk of complications from varicella, VZIG is recommended for susceptible pregnant women,[35] although there is no evidence from controlled trials to support this approach nor that this treatment prevents infection of the fetus.

Influenza

Influenza is an important cause of acute respiratory illness. Typical symptoms are fever, myalgias, sore throat, headache, and non-productive cough. Those groups at increased risk for pneumonia, hospitalization, and death related to influenza are the elderly and persons with chronic underlying illnesses. Nosocomial transmission of influenza occurs during community outbreaks. Guidelines from the Advisory Committee on Immunisation Practices supported by other national bodies strongly recommend annual influenza vaccine for all healthcare workers.[40,55]

A Cochrane Library systematic review to assess the effectiveness of the influenza vaccine in healthy adults showed a benefit in reducing serologically confirmed cases of influenza by 48% (95% CI 24–64) for the live aerosol vaccine and by 68% (95% CI 49–79) for the inactivated vaccine, but only a modest effect on clinical disease of 13% and 24% respectively.[56] Use of the vaccine, however, was associated with a significant reduction in time spent off work. One study included in the review that enrolled healthcare workers, however, showed no difference between subjects compared with the placebo group for influenza-like illness and absenteeism, which was explained by a drift of the prevalent influenza strain away from the vaccine type.[57] In another randomized, placebo-controlled trial from two pediatric hospitals in Finland, where the vaccine strain more closely matched the circulating strain, immunization was significantly associated with fewer days lost work because of respiratory infections (1·0 *v* 1·4 days, $P = 0·02$).[58]

Immunization of healthcare workers has been shown to reduce the morbidity and mortality of their patients. In a study of 12 Scottish long-term care facilities, where healthcare workers were offered vaccination, vaccination of healthcare workers was associated with reduction in total patient mortality from 17–10% (OR 0·56; 95% CI 0·40–0·80) while vaccination of patients was not associated with significant effects on mortality.[59] Similar results were obtained in a study of 20 long-term care facilities in the UK, randomized to be offered or not offered influenza vaccine. Influenza vaccine uptake was 50·9% in hospitals where vaccine was offered, compared with 4·9% where it was not. There was a significant reduction in uncorrected mortality in patients from 22·4% to 13·6% (OR 0·58; 95% CI 0·40–0·84) between no vaccine and vaccine hospitals.[60]

Although there are no data from controlled trials, guidelines for the management of non-immunized healthcare workers during an outbreak of influenza recommend antiviral prophylaxis. A Cochrane Library systematic review of neuraminidase inhibitors for prophylaxis in adults showed that neuraminidase inhibitors were 74% effective in preventing clinical influenza, although none of the studies was performed in healthcare workers.[61] Another Cochrane Library systematic review of amantadine and rimantadine showed that amantadine prevented 23% of clinical influenza cases (95% CI 11–34) and 63% of serologically confirmed influenza, but was associated with significant gastrointestinal side effects.[62] Rimantidine was associated with fewer side effects. Some of these studies enrolled healthcare workers.

The uptake of influenza vaccine amongst staff is reported to be as low as 2 to 5% despite intensive promotional programs.[63] In a cross-sectional survey, addressing employee concerns about vaccine safety, removal of barriers to vaccination, such as inconvenience and cost, and an explanation of the reasons for targeting healthcare workers, were identified as strategies to improve immunization levels in healthcare workers.[64] However, in a randomized controlled trial, an intensive promotional campaign could not be shown to increase the uptake of vaccination against influenza among healthcare workers.[65] In healthcare workers in whom concern about side effects is an impediment to vaccination, there is good evidence from a placebo-controlled trial that acetaminophen will significantly reduce any symptoms of sore arm and nausea associated with the vaccine.[66]

Prevention of other infections in healthcare workers

Nosocomial transmission of measles and rubella is well documented.[67] A number of observational studies have shown that serological screening of healthcare workers before immunization is cost-effective for measles.[68–71] A history of disease or vaccination can be unreliable.[68] Immunization of healthcare workers who do not have evidence of immunity against measles, mumps, and rubella is strongly recommended[40,55] with recent evidence from case control and cohort studies supporting a vaccine efficacy of greater than 95%.[72–74]

Invasive meningococcal disease is associated with a high case fatality rate of up to 10%. There are no controlled trials on the effects on prophylactic antibiotics on the incidence of meningococcal disease nor good evidence to identify which contacts should be treated.[75] Although there are reports of transmission of infection to healthcare workers, nosocomial transmission is extremely rare. In a retrospective survey from England and Wales the risk of invasive meningococcal disease in healthcare workers exposed to meningococcal disease was 0.8 per 100 000 HCWs at risk and, although this was 25 times that in the general population, the authors of the study concluded that the excess risk was small.[76] However, based on case reports of meningococcal infection in healthcare workers with unprotected airway exposure to respiratory droplets from patients with meningococcal infection, occupational health guidelines recommend prophylaxis in these settings.[55] There is evidence from randomized trials, using eradication of *Neisseria meningitidis* as the endpoint, to support the use of rifampin, single dose ceftriaxone, or single dose ciprofloxacin for post-exposure prophylaxis.[77,78]

The Centers for Disease Control and Prevention retrospectively collected data on cases of laboratory-acquired invasive meningococcal disease and estimated an increased attack rate of 13 per 100 000 population (95% CI 5–29) and based on this observation recommended that vaccination be considered for laboratory workers working with isolates of *Neisseria meningitidis*.[79] The vaccine, however, will only protect against meningococcal disease caused by serogroups contained in the vaccine.

Summary

There is good evidence, in many instances from controlled trials, to support current guidelines as advocated by the Advisory Committee on

Immunization Practices[40] and other national organisations for the screening and immunization of healthcare workers against vaccine preventable infections.

References

1. Henry K, Campbell S. Needlestick/sharps injuries and HIV exposure among health care workers. National estimates based on a survey of U.S. hospitals. *Minn Med* 1995; **78**:41–4.
2. Occupational Safety and Health Administration. *Record Summary of the Request for Information on Occupational Exposure to Bloodborne Pathogens Due to Percutaneous Injury* (Washington, D.C.: Occupational Safety and Health Administration, May 1999), http://www.osha-slc.gov/html/ndlreport052099.html.
3. Public Health Laboratory Service. *Occupational transmission of HIV. Summary of published reports.* London: PHLS, 1997.
4. Cardo DM, Culver DH, Ciesielski CA, *et al.* A case-control study of HIV seroconversion in health care workers after percutaneous exposure. Centers for Disease Control and Prevention Needlestick Surveillance Group. *N Engl J Med* 1997;**337**:1485–90.
5. Gerberding JL. Management of occupational exposures to blood-borne viruses. *N Engl J Med* 1995;**332**:444–51.
6. Tsai CC, Emau P, Sun JC, *et al.* Post-exposure chemoprophylaxis (PECP) against SIV infection of macaques as a model for protection from HIV infection. *J Med Primatol* 2000;**29**:248–58.
7. Le Grand R, Vaslin B, Larghero, J *et al.* Post-exposure prophylaxis with highly active antiretroviral therapy could not protect macaques from infection with SIV/HIV chimera. *AIDS* 2000;**14**:1864–6.
8. Connor EM, Sperling RS, Gelber R, *et al.* Reduction of maternal-infant transmission of human immunodeficiency virus type 1 with zidovudine treatment. Pediatric AIDS Clinical Trials Group Protocol 076 Study Group. *N Engl J Med* 1994;**331**:1173–80.
9. Guay LA, Musoke P, Fleming, T *et al.* Intrapartum and neonatal single-dose nevirapine compared with zidovudine for prevention of mother-to-child transmission of HIV-1 in Kampala, Uganda: HIVNET 012 randomised trial. *Lancet* 1999;**354**:795–802.
10. Ristig MB, Arens MQ, Kennedy M, Powderly W, Tebas P. Increasing prevalence of resistance mutations in antiretroviral-naive individuals with established HIV-1 infection from 1996–2001 in St. Louis. *HIV Clin Trials* 2002;**3**:155–60.
11. Yerly S, Vora S, Rizzardi P, *et al.* Acute HIV infection: impact on the spread of HIV and transmission of drug resistance. *AIDS* 2001;**15**:2287–92.
12. Little SJ, Holte S, Routy J-P, *et al.* Antiretroviral-Drug Resistance among Patients Recently Infected with HIV. *New Engl J Med* 2002;**347**:385–94.
13. Centers for Disease Control and Prevention. Updated U.S. Public Health Service Guidelines for the Management of Occupational Exposures to HBV, HCV, and HIV and Recommendations for Postexposure Prophylaxis. *MMWR* 2001;**50**(RR-11):1–52.
14. Puro V, De Carli G, Orchi N, *et al.* Short-term adverse effects from and discontinuation of antiretroviral post-exposure prophylaxis. *J Biol Regul Homeost Agents* 2001;**15**:238–42.
15. Braitstein P, Chan K, Beardsell, A *et al.* Safety and tolerability of combination antiretroviral post-exposure prophylaxis in a population-based setting. *J Acquir Immune Defic Syndr* 2002;**29**:547–8.
16. Puro V, Soldani F, De Carli G, *et al.* Italian Registry of Antiretroviral HIV post-exposture prophylaxis. *AIDS* 2003;**17**:1988–90.
17. King AM, Osterwalder JJ, Vernazza PL. A randomized prospective study to evaluate a rapid HIV-antibody assay in the management of cases of percutaneous exposure amongst health care workers. *Swiss Med Wkly* 2001; **12**:10–3.
18. Kallenborn JC. Price TG, Carrico R, Davidson AB. Emergency department management of occupational exposures: cost analysis of rapid HIV test. *Infect Control Hosp Epidemiol* 2001;**22**:289–93.
19. Weller S, Davis K. Condom effectiveness in reducing heterosexual HIV transmission. (Cochrane Review) In: *The Cochrane Library*, Issue 1, 2003. Oxford: Update Software.
20. Werner BG, Grady GF. Accidental hepatitis B surface antigen positive inoculations: use of e antigen to estimate infectivity. *Ann Intern Med* 1982;**97**:367–9.
21. Jefferson T, Demicheli V, Deeks J, *et al.* Vaccines for preventing hepatitis B in health care workers (Cochrane

Review) In: Oxford: Update Software. *The Cochrane Library*, Issue 1, 2003.

22. Andre FE. Summary of safety and efficacy data on a yeast-derived hepatitis B vaccine. *Am J Med* 1989;**87**:14S–20S.
23. Averhoff F, Mahoney F, Colemen P, *et al.* Immunogenicity of hepatitis B vaccines. Implications for persons at occupational risk of hepatitis B infection. *Am J Prev Med* 1998;**15**:1–8.
24. Levitz RE, Cooper BW, Regan HC. Immunization with high-dose intradermal recombinant hepatitis B vaccine in healthcare workers who failed to respond to intramuscular immunization. *Infect Control Hosp Epidemiol* 1995;**16**:88–91.
25. European Consensus Group on Hepatitis B Immunity. Are booster immunisations needed for lifelong hepatitis B immunity? *Lancet* 2000;**355**:561–5.
26. Beasley RP, Hwang L-Y, Steven CE, *et al.* Efficacy of hepatitis B immune globulin for prevention of perinatal transmission of the hepatitis B virus carrier state: final report of a randomized double-blind, placebo controlled trial. *Hepatology* 1983;**3**:135–41.
27. Veterans Administration Cooperative Study. Type B hepatitis after needlestick exposure: prevention with hepatitis B immune globulin. Final report of the Veterans Administration Cooperative Study. *Ann Intern Med* 1978:**88**:285–93.
28. Hoofnagle JH, Seeff LB, Bales ZB, Wright EC, Zimmerman HJ. Passive-active immunity from hepatitis B immune globulin. Reanalysis of a Veteran Administration cooperative study of needle-stick hepatitis. *Ann Intern Med* 1979;**91**:813–18.
29. Henderson DK. Managing Occupational Risks for Hepatitis C transmission in the Health Care setting. *Clin Micro Reviews* 2003;**16**:546–68.
30. Puro V, Petrosillo N, Ippolito G, Italian Study Group on Occupational Risk of HIV and other bloodborne infections. Risk of hepatitis C seroconversion after occupational exposure in health care workers. *Am J Infect Control* 1995;**23**:273–7.
31. Jaeckel E, Cornberg M, Wedemeyer H, *et al.* Treatment of acute hepatitis C infection with interferon alfa-2b. *N Engl J Med* 2001;**345**:1452–7.
32. Rogers B, Goodno L Evaluation of interventions to prevent needlestick injuries in health care occupations. *Am J Prev Med* 200;**18**:90–8.
33. L'Ecuyer PB, Schwab EO, Iademarco E, *et al.* Randomized prospective study of the impact of three needleless intravenous systems on needlestick injury rates. *Infect Control Hosp Epidemiol* 1996;**17**:803–8.
34. Laupland KB, Davies HD, Low DE, *et al.* Invasive group A streptococcal disease in children and association with varicella-zoster virus infection. Ontario Group A Streptococcal Study Group. *Pediatrics* 2000;**105**:E60.
35. Centers for Disease Control and Prevention. Prevention of varicella: recommendations of the Advisory Committee on Immunization Practices (ACIP). *MMWR* 1996;**45** (RR11):1–36.
36. Pastuszak AL, Levy M, Schick B, *et al.* Outcome after maternal varicella infection in the first 20 weeks of pregnancy. *N Engl J Med* 1994;**330**:901–5.
37. Weber DJ, Rutala WA, Hamilton H. Prevention and control of varicella-zoster infections in healthcare facilities. *Infect Control Hosp Epidemiol* 1996;**17**:694–705.
38. Kuter BJ, Weibel RE, Guess HA. Oka/Merck varicella vaccine in healthy children: final report of a 2–year efficacy study and 7–year follow up studies. *Vaccine* 1991;**9**:643–7.
39. Saiman L, LaRussa P, Steinberg SP, *et al.* Persistence of immunity to varicella-zoster virus after vaccination of healthcare workers. *Infect Control Hosp Epidemiol* 2001;**22**:279–83.
40. Centers for Disease Control and Prevention. Immunization of Healthcare Workers: Recommendations of the Advisory Practices and the Hospital Infection Control Practices Advisory Committee. *MMWR* 1997;**46**(RR-18):1–43.
41. Gray AM, Fenn P, Weinberg J, Miller E, McGuire A. An economic analysis of varicella vaccination for health care workers. *Epidemiol Infect* 1997;**119**:209–20.
42. Weinstock DM, Rogers M, Lim S, Eagan J, Sepkowitz KA. Seroconversion rates in healthcare workers using a latex agglutination assay after varicella virus vaccination. *Infect Control Hosp Epidemiol* 1999;**20**:504–7.
43. Gayman J. A cost-effectiveness model for analysing two varicella vaccination strategies. *Am J Health Syst Pharm* 1998;**15**:S4–8.
44. Thiry N, Beutels P, Van Damme P, Van Doorslaer E. Economic evaluations of varicella vaccination programmes: a review of the literature. *Pharmacoeconomics* 2003;**21**: 13–38.
45. Ferson MJ, Bell SM, Robertson PW. Determination and importance of varicella immune status of nursing staff in a children's hospital. *J Hosp Infect* 1990;**15**:347–51.

46. Vandersmissen G, Moens G, Vranckx R, de Schryver A, Jacques P. Occupational risk of infection by varicella zoster virus in Belgian healthcare workers: a seroprevalance study. *Occup Environ Med* 2000;**57**: 621–6.
47. Waclawski ER, Stewart M. Susceptibility to varicella-zoster virus in applicants for nurse training in Scotland. *Commun Dis Public Health* 2002;**5**:240–2.
48. Gallagher J, Quaid B, Cryan B. Susceptibility to varicella zoster virus infection in health care workers. *Occup Med* 1996;**46**:289–92.
49. Asano Y, Nakayama H, Yazaki T, Kato R, Hirose S. Protection against varicella in family contact by immediate inoculation with live varicella vaccine. *Pediatrics* 1977;**59**:3–7.
50. Watson B, Seward J, Yang A, *et al.* Postexposure effectiveness of varicella vaccine. *Pediatrics* 2000;**105**:84–8.
51. Asano Y, Yoshikawa T, Suga S, *et al.* Post-exposure prophylaxis of varicella in family contact by oral acyclovir. *Pediatrics* 1993;**92**:219–22.
52. Lin TY, Huang YC, Ning HC, Hsueh C. Oral acyclovir prophylaxis of varicella after intimate contact. *Pediatr Infect Dis J* 1997;**16**:1162–5.
53. Balfour HH Jr, Groth KE, McCullough J, *et al.* Prevention or modification of varicella using zoster immune plasma. *Am J Dis Child* 1977;**131**:693–6.
54. Orenstein WA, Heymann DL, Ellis RJ, *et al.* Prophylaxis of varicella in high risk children: dose response effect of zoster immune globulin. *J Pediatr* 1981;**98**:368–73.
55. Health Canada. Prevention and control of occupational infection in health care. an infection control guideline. *CCDR* 2002;**28S1**:1–264.
56. Demichell V, Rivetti D, Deeks JJ, Jefferson TO. Vaccines for preventing influenza in healthy adults. (Cochrane Review) In: *The Cochrane Library*, Issue 3, 2003. Oxford: Update Software.
57. Weingarten S, Staniloff H, Ault M, *et al.* Do hospital employees benefit from the influenza vaccine? A placebo-controlled clinical trial. *J Gen Intern Med* 1988;**3**:32–7.
58. Saxen H, Virtanen M. Randomized, placebo-controlled double-blind study on the efficacy of influenza immunization on absenteeism of health care workers. *Pediatr Infect Dis J* 1999;**18**:779–83.
59. Potter J, Stott DJ, Roberts MA, *et al.* Influenza vaccination of health care workers in long-term care hospitals reduces the mortality of elderly patients. *J Infect Dis* 1997;**175**:1–6.
60. Carman WF, Elder AG, Wallace LA, *et al.* Effects of influenza vaccination of healthcare workers on mortality of elderly people in long-term care: a randomized controlled trial. *Lancet* 2000;**355**:93–7.
61. Jefferson T, Demisheli V, Deeks J, Rivetti D. Neuraminidase inhibitors for preventing and treating influenza in healthy adults (Cochrane Review). In: *The Cochrane Library*, Issue 3, 2003. Oxford: Update Software.
62. Jefferson TO, Demicheli V, Deeks JJ, Rivetti D. Amantadine and rimantadine for preventing and treating influenza in adults (Cochrane Review). In: *The Cochrane Library*, Issue 3, 2003. Oxford: Update Software.
63. Smedley J, Palmer C, Baird J, Barker M. A survey of the delivery and uptake of influenza vaccine among healthcare workers. *Occup Med* 2002;**52**:271–6.
64. Nichol KL, Hauge M. Influenza vaccination of healthcare workers. *Infect Control Hosp Epidemiol* 1997;**18**:189–94.
65. Dey P, Halder S, Collins S, Benons L, Woodman C. Promoting uptake of influenza vaccination among health care workers: a randomized controlled trial. *J Public Health Med* 2001;**23**:346–8.
66. Aoki FY, Yassi A, Cheang M, *et al.* Effects of acetaminophen on adverse effects of influenza vaccination in health care workers. *CMAJ* 1993;**149**: 1425–30.
67. Atkinson WL, Markowitz LE, Adams NC, Seastrom GR. Transmission of measles in medical settings – United States, 1985-89. *Am J Med* 1991;**91**:320S–324S.
68. Ziegler E, Roth C, Wreghitt T. Prevalence of measles susceptibility among health care workers in a UK hospital. Does the UK need to introduce a measles policy for its healthcare workers? *Occup Med* 2003;**53**:398–402.
69. Ferson MJ, Roberston PW, Whybin LR. Cost-effectiveness of prevaccination screening of healthcare workers for immunity to measles, rubella and mumps. *Med J Aust* 1994;**18**:478–82.
70. Sellick JA Jr, Longbine D, Schideling R, Mylotte JM. Screening hospital employees for measles immunity is more cost-effective than blind immunization. *Ann Intern Med* 1992;**116**:982–4.

71. Stover BH, Adams G, Keubler CA, Cost KM, Rabalais GP. Measles-mumps-rubella immunization of susceptible hospital employees during a community measles outbreak: cost-effectiveness and protective efficacy. *Infect Control Hosp Epidemiol* 1994;**15**:18–21.
72. Hennessey KA, Ion-Nedeleu N, Craciun MD, *et al.* Measles epidemic in Romania, 1996–1998: assessment of vaccine effectiveness by case-control and cohort studies. *Am J Epidemiol* 1999;**150**:1250–7.
73. Rivest P, Bedard L, Arruda H, Trudeau G, Remis RS. Risk factors for measles and vaccine efficacy during an epidemic in Montreal. *Can J Publ Health* 1995;**86**:86–90.
74. Janaszek W, Gay NJ, Gut W. Measles vaccine efficacy during an epidemic in 1998 in the highly vaccinated population of Poland. *Vaccine* 2003;**21**:473–8.
75. Correia J, Hart C. Meningococcal disease. *Clinical Evidence.* London: BMJ Publishing Group, 2003.
76. Gilmore A, Stuart J, Andrews N. Risk of secondary meningococcal disease in healthcare workers. *Lancet* 200;**356**:1654–5.
77. Schwartz B, Al-Tobaiqi Al-Ruwais A, *et al.* Comparative efficacy of ceftriaxone and rifampicin in eradicating pharyngeal carriage of group A Neisseria meningitidis. *Lancet* 1988;**1**:1239–42.
78. Dwarozack DL, Sanders CC, Horowitz EA, *et al.* Evaluation of single-dose ciprofloxacin in the eradication of Neisseria meningitidis from nasopharyngeal carriers. *Antimicrob Agents Chemother* 1988;**32**:1740–1.
79. Laboratory-acquired meningococcal disease – United States, 2000. *MMWR* 2002;**51**:141–4.

Index

Abbreviations: STIs, sexually-transmitted infections